The Foundations of Bioethics

The Foundations of Bioethics

H. Tristram Engelhardt, Jr.

New York   Oxford
OXFORD UNIVERSITY PRESS
1986

Oxford University Press

Oxford   New York   Toronto
Delhi   Bombay   Calcutta   Madras   Karachi
Petaling Jaya   Singapore   Hong Kong   Tokyo
Nairobi   Dar es Salaam   Cape Town
Melbourne   Auckland

and associated companies in
Beirut   Berlin   Ibadan   Nicosia

Published by Oxford University Press, Inc.,
200 Madison Avenue,
New York, New York 10016.

Oxford is a registered trademark of Oxford University Press

Library of Congress Cataloging in Publication Data

Engelhardt, H. Tristram (Hugo Tristram)
The foundations of bioethics.

Includes bibliographies and index.
1. Medical ethics.   2. Bioethics.   I. Title.
[DNLM: 1. Bioethics.   2. Delivery of Health Care.
3. Ethics, Medical.   W 50 E57f]
R724.E54   1985   174′.2   84–29572
ISBN 0–19–503608–5

Printing (last digit):   9 8 7 6 5 4

Printed in the United States of America

To the memory of
Josef Karl Tristram
and
Elsie Tristram Engelhardt,
who introduced me to philosophy—
the first in the spirit and the second in the flesh

Preface

Bioethics has become a household word because the moral issues raised by health care touch everyone. Questions about contraception, abortion, consent to treatment, and the allocation of funds to health care are of concern to nearly every individual at some time in his or her life. Many of these issues occasion bitter disputes: abortion clinics are bombed, patients sue their physicians claiming they were not adequately informed, some theologians argue that genetic engineering of the human germline offends against the Deity, and major controversies exist in every industrialized democracy about how to allocate funds for health care and how to contain health care costs. These controversies captivate our attention and engage our imagination. They involve the very ways in which we understand ourselves as humans, the ways in which we understand the proper ways to live, to control disease and illness, and to care for the dying. Because of the emotions they evoke, these controversies are the stuff of newspaper headlines. There is hardly a literate individual who has not heard or discussed one of the major controversies in bioethics.

The problem is how to find one's way through such controversies. How ought an individual or a society decide on a correct abortion policy or a just way to distribute resources for health care? How should the concern not to alarm a patient uselessly with remote and farfetched risks be balanced with a patient's right to information about treatment? The widespread interest in answering such questions in a sensible fashion has given a new public life to philosophy, which has of late often been characterized by an interest in esoteric puzzles that plague philosophers much more than they interest ordinary men and women. The moral and conceptual problems associated with health care and the biomedical sciences have called philosophy back to questions that are part of everyday life, even if it is the life of a society characterized by new and expensive medical technology. In medical schools from Germany to the United States and from Sweden to Argentina and Beijing, philosophers have been invited to participate in forming public policy bearing on health care, to serve on ethics committees, or to participate in teaching medical students. Bioethics has taken shape as a philosophical discipline recognized across the globe.

A philosophical analysis of the character of bioethical debates reveals deep divisions of opinion. Numerous ideological and religious viewpoints bring special answers to the moral questions raised by bioethical disputes. Insofar as these special answers cannot be justified in terms of general rational analysis and argument, a gulf yawns between the bioethics of general secular philosophy and the bioethical analyses undertaken within the embrace of particular religious and ideological viewpoints. Secular pluralism has become a watchword for moral crisis. This book sustains that concern. Much that one would like to prove regarding the nature of the good life and/or the authority to enforce it appears unavailable. The life of reason, unlike the life of belief or special grace, appears impoverished.

Some may wish to see this volume as a defense of a secular pluralist ethic. That would be a mistake. My intent has not been to defend that ethic but rather the very opposite. I have endeavoured to find grounds for establishing by reason a particular view of the good life and securing by general rational arguments the authority for its establishment. To my dismay and sorrow, such have not been available. Rather than as a manifesto on behalf of secular pluralist ethics, this volume is offered as an acknowledgment of its inevitability. Insofar as people live together without the benefit of a common grace of belief and a concrete understanding of the good life and of proper health care, there will be a tension between what they know through special grace and intuition and what they can prove and enforce with rational authority. Even the person of belief will feel the tension between what can be established and enforced with rational authority and that which may be believed. In addition to this profound tension there will also be tensions within ethics itself that will have wide-reaching consequences for bioethics. Autonomy and beneficence, for instance, which lie at the very foundations of bioethics, are principles at tension.

If such conflicts and tensions are as irremediable as this volume suggests, we will need to rethink many of the ways in which we approach public policy in general and health care policy in particular. That such a task awaits us should not be unexpected. Our philosophical and public policy acknowledgment of the fact that we live in secular societies with a wide plurality of beliefs is a relatively recent one. We have only begun to look at the consequences of living in peaceable secular pluralist societies. Taking these circumstances seriously has implications for law and public policy. Though the volume offers no legal advice, it does offer points of departure for reassessing both law and public policy. It offers an examination of moral and philosophical roots. To meet the challenges of the future within the constraints of human finitude, we will need to learn to deliver health care in a context of a plurality of moral viewpoints, where there is limited moral authority to impose one understanding on all without their consent. In understanding the limits of reason and the moral authority to use force, we will come to learn much about the human condition.

Houston   H. T. E.
November 1985

Acknowledgments

I am in deep debt to many who gave generously to the development of this book. They have provided criticism, support, and help in fleshing out its ideas. They are responsible for its virtues but for none of its shortcomings and vices. In particular, I wish to acknowledge my colleagues at the Institute for the Medical Humanities in Galveston, the Kennedy Institute of Ethics of Georgetown University, and the Center for Ethics, Medicine, and Public Issues, who discussed many elements of this work as it took shape. I am especially grateful to Thomas J. Bole III, James F. Childress, Xavier de Callataÿ, S. G. M. Engelhardt, Lee Friedman, Mary Ann Gardell, Stanley Hauerwas, Ross Kessel, Michael Rie, Hans-Martin Sass, Earl E. Shelp, Stuart F. Spicker, and Lawrence T. Ulrich, who read through the final manuscript and some of its antecedent versions. To them and many more whom I cannot name here, I give thanks for their collegial support, their vigorous criticism, and their friendship.

Contents

The Foundations of Bioethics

. . . . hvars þú böl kannt,
kveð þú þér bölvi at
ok gef-at þínum fjándum frið.

. . . . illu feginn
ver þú aldregi,
en lát þér at góðu getit.

Hávamál, 127, 128

1

The Emergence of a Secular Bioethics

Bioethics and the crisis in values

Bioethical questions arise against the backdrop of a moral crisis that is closely tied to a series of losses of both ethical and ontological conviction in the West. When Martin Luther nailed his ninety-five theses to All Saints' Church in Wittenberg on Halloween in 1517, he marked a new era for the West, and the crumbling of the presumed possibility of a uniformity of moral viewpoint. One could no longer hope to live in a society that could aspire to a single moral viewpoint governed by a single supreme moral authority. In little over a century this would lead to the Thirty Years' War. The Pax Westphalica that followed in 1648 signaled the unlikelihood of ever cementing Europe in one Christian vision. And while the religious roots of ethical and metaphysical consensus were fragmenting, progress in the sciences undermined established understandings of man's place in the cosmos. When the first copy of Nicolaus Copernicus's *De revolutionibus orbium coelestium* was placed on his deathbed on May 24, 1543, a bequest was made to a shift in ideas that was to become the metaphor for dramatic and extensive changes in world views. This Copernican revolution was one of the many changes in ideas that would leave us devoid of a sense of absolute or final perspective: man was to cease to be the center of the cosmos, and the established Christian view of the cosmos was to be overturned.

As the religious synthesis weakened, the Enlightenment hope arose that reason alone (through philosophy) could disclose the character of the good life and the general canons of moral probity. As Alasdair MacIntyre and others have shown, this hope has proven vain.[1] Rather than philosophy being able to fill the void left by the collapse of the hegemony of Christian thought in the West, competing philosophies and philosophical ethics have become ever more academic and therefore ever more removed from practical cultural needs. This volume is thus set against a background of considerable skepticism. One must wonder to what extent a moral viewpoint can be elaborated and justified outside a nest of supporting premises fashioned by a particular religious or other cultural tradition.

The discussion of issues in bioethics now transpires within the compass of secular pluralist societies. That such societies are secular is in part the result of recent historical forces that have led to the major institutions of most democracies no longer being associated in a significant fashion with an established church, even where vestiges may remain. Such societies are pluralistic in encompassing a wide divergence of moral sentiments and beliefs. Such divergence has likely always been present, however hidden. Europe of the Middle Ages, though nominally Catholic, included significant populations of Jews, in addition to heretics and some agnostics. In order to fashion a society that is not pluralist, one quite likely must settle for a society on a very small scale, probably not exceeding the compass of a Greek city-state. Whenever one considers a society of greater scope, or for that matter a society that has not voluntarily assembled around a full, willing, and complete submission to a particular moral or ideological perspective, one will have a pluralism of moral beliefs. It is this ever-present inclination to diversity of opinions that makes the single heretic so to be feared. In this volume I will talk of peaceable secular pluralist societies so as to indicate societies including a diversity of moral viewpoints, and enjoying in addition a freedom of moral opinion without the fear of repression. "Peaceable secular" is best interpreted broadly to indicate the absence of any particular religious or moral orthodoxy imposed by force. I place among the religions of the world, at least by metaphor, such Christian heresies as Marxism. The problem is how to fashion an ethic for biomedical problems that can speak with rational authority across the great diversity of moral viewpoints. This problem is especially acute given the collapse of many of the traditional certainties.

Philosophical reflections have been directed to health care because of (1) major and rapid technological changes that have created pressures to reexamine the underlying assumptions of established practices (e.g., the advent of transplantation contributed to interests in a brain-oriented definition of death);[2] (2) rising health care costs, which have occasioned questions about the allocation of resources; (3) the frankly pluralistic context in which health care is now delivered (e.g., physicians and nurses can no longer presuppose that they share a view in common with their patients, or with each other, or that the conduct of their practice will be framed within acknowledged Judeo-Christian assumptions); and (4) the expansion of publicly recognized rights of self-determination (e.g., the 1965 Supreme Court ruling *Griswold* v. *Connecticut,* holding unconstitutional laws forbidding the distribution of contraceptives to married couples).[3] If these changes render the answers of the past suspect, and if there is no accepted or imposed orthodoxy to provide answers, both answers and a conceptual framework must be fashioned anew.

The history of bioethics over the last two decades has been the story of the development of a secular ethic. Initially, individuals working from within particular religious traditions held the center of bioethical discussions. However, this focus was replaced by analyses that span traditions, including particular secular traditions. As a result, a special secular tradition that attempts to frame answers in terms of no particular tradition, but rather in ways open to rational individuals as such, has emerged. Bioethics is an element of a secular culture and the great-grandchild of the Enlightenment. Because the 1980s have been marked in Iran, the United States, and elsewhere by attempts to return to traditional values and the certainties of religious beliefs, one must wonder what this augurs for bioethics in this special secular sense. However, because the world does not appear on the brink of embracing a particular orthodoxy, and if an orthodoxy is not imposed, as say in Iran or the Soviet Union, bioethics will inevitably develop as a secular fabric of rationality in an era of uncertainty. That is, the existence of open peaceable discussion among divergent groups, such as atheists, Catholics, Jews, Protestants, Marxists, heterosexuals and homosexuals, about public policy issues bearing on health care, will press unavoidably for a neutral common language. Bioethics is developing as the lingua franca of a world concerned with health care, but not possessing a common ethical viewpoint.

It is not hyperbolic to claim that health care and the biomedical sciences are playing a central role in a major cultural change. For instance, in the last hundred years, the United States has gone from a paternalistic view of patients' rights, a free enterprise system of health care delivery, and the legal proscription of abortion and contraception on request, to enforcing rights to free and informed consent, providing health care as a part of a federal welfare system, and legalizing abortion and contraception. These changes constitute a major cultural development, which is the outcome of an interplay between technology and culture.

Changes in technology and the acquisition of new knowledge have contributed ideas that have shaped our appreciation of the human condition. For example, the development of an evolutionary understanding of human origins has made neo-Aristotelian notions of natural and unnatural acts

difficult to credit, at least in secular terms. How, for example, could one hold
on nonreligious grounds that homosexuality is unnatural if human nature is
the product of evolutionary processes that may even have developed genes
for homosexuality, given the advantages of the trait in certain circumstances?[4] In any event, the outcomes of evolution would be without intrinsic
normative force. Evolution is, after all, a morally blind process that has at
best adapted us to environments in which we no longer live. A better
knowledge of human origins has implications for arguments in bioethics, if in
no other way, through undercutting the rhetorical force of certain kinds of
arguments in ethics. Further, the technological developments of the biomedical sciences have themselves influenced the understanding of moral issues.
The wide availability of effective contraception has suggested the feasibility
of lifestyles that were more difficult in the past (e.g., women being fully
sexually active and controlling reproduction, while participating fully in
demanding occupations), and offered new areas of possible responsibility
(e.g., the obligation to avoid the birth of seriously defective children, as
suggested in *Curlender* v. *Bio-Science Laboratories*).[5]

Bioethics, unlike many codes of ethics, tends not to be national or
parochial, because these developments in health care and in the biomedical
sciences are tied generally to the development of industrial societies. Though
bioethics is a major focus of Western society, that society itself is ever less
parochial, and embraces not only North America and Europe, but societies
such as Japan and Taiwan as well. Western health care and its problems are
no longer solely Western problems. As it addresses this wide range of
societies and their difficulties with "Western" biomedicine, bioethics draws
on a tradition of the West that in fact attempts to step outside the constraints
of particular cultures, including Western culture itself, by giving reasons and
arguments anyone should accept. In this sense, bioethics is a general attempt
in secular ethics. Although specific problems surely are tied to the particular
health care systems of particular cultures, throughout the world the number
of areas of common concern is growing. In every country, for example, a
contraceptive ethos is in place, and amniocentesis and abortion are available
nearly everywhere. The result has been a need to reconsider sexual and
reproductive mores. The general availability of expensive life-sustaining
technology has made the use of extraordinary care an issue for at least a few
in every country. And every nation faces choices regarding the allocation of
its resources to health care endeavors. In short, elements of Western culture
are international, bound to the character of industrial or industrializing
society. These give a common cast to health care and its problems, and evoke
international interest in bioethics. In the latter part of the twentieth century,
one finds bioethics spanning national boundaries as well as religious and
political groups.

Bioethics: taking ideas seriously and reexamining cultural assumptions

As an undertaking in philosophy, bioethics is an attempt to clarify concepts and to search for conceptual presuppositions. It is an intellectual endeavor. But one must recognize that intellectual undertakings have concrete roots that touch us in our everyday lives. For example, the widespread use of IUDs (intrauterine devices) for contraception, with few of the users feeling any guilt in the matter, presumes that: (1) people do not find such a practice unnatural, or if they do, they judge that state of affairs to be of little or no moral consequence, and (2) people do not find the wastage of zygotes that do not implant as a result of the use of IUDs to involve the taking of the lives of persons, or if they do, they judge the circumstances to have no serious moral significance in that context. When one then wishes to know whether one ought to use an IUD, one will likely be pressed to clarify such views. One will need to examine concepts of unnatural actions and their moral implications, if any. One will need to draw distinctions between human biological and human personal life. Such are intellectual undertakings, philosophical endeavors. However, they spring from practical interests, in this case choosing an acceptable means to avoid an unwanted pregnancy.

One has no intellectual problems, no philosophical problems, if one does not worry about giving reasons. However, not attending to reasons and the implications of choices would mean eschewing conversations about moral matters with oneself as well as with others. It would involve acting without concern for consequences. As soon as one wonders whether certain choices are better and how one can tell, the intellectual endeavor is joined. As one attempts to justify actions to others, or to persuade others that their actions are wrong, the intellectual undertaking assumes social dimensions. Such social dimensions exist as soon as one tries to justify one's choices as a patient, physician, or nurse, to another patient, physician, or nurse, or to society in general. The endeavors of health care are public concerns that lead to philosophical questions. This work is written on this premise: bioethics springs naturally from the concerns of patients, physicians, and nurses.

The questions addressed by bioethics are not restricted to the province of physicians, but concern nurses, other health care professionals, patients, and laymen. The term *bioethics* in fact encompasses issues that fall outside health care ethics in the strict sense of an exploration of the *moral* issues raised by health care and the biomedical sciences. Issues concerning *nonmoral* values regarding what ought to be treated (e.g., signaling a state of affairs as pathological, as physiologically or psychologically abnormal), and ontological issues concerning when persons begin and cease (e.g., questions about the point at which fetuses should be acknowledged as persons), are also customarily gathered within the compass of bioethics (bioethics in a broad sense).

These issues have a breadth that transcends particular professional boundaries because the differences among the various health care professions primarily represent differences in economic advantages, status, and power within health care institutions and practices.[6] As a result, I will not use the term *health care* in the narrow sense (i.e., as the preservation or promotion of health) that contrasts with the narrow sense of *medical care* (the treatment of disease). Instead I will favor the broad sense of health care that includes a collection of somewhat competing professions (e.g., doctors of medicine, doctors of osteopathy, nurses, dentists, occupational therapists, physician assistants, clinical psychologists) with differing but overlapping interests, who face a common set of puzzles regarding the rights and obligations of professionals, patients, and societies concerning health care. In this volume I will not attempt to draw a systematic distinction or set of distinctions between medical care and health care; both are so intimately intertwined, and both terms possess strategic ambiguities. These professions are involved in a set of general cultural unclarities. They share in a set of uncertainties that transcend their particular professional boundaries.

Bioethics, in addressing these uncertainties, is philosophy engaged in one of its central tasks: aiding a culture to clarify its views of reality and of values. Philosophy done well is a culture examining its own conceptual and value presumptions. It is through applying the language of bioethics that health care understands its place in a culture, and the culture comprehends the significance of health care practices and the biomedical sciences it sustains. Bioethics plays a central role in the mutual intellectual adaptation of culture and biomedical technology. This is not simply an isolated, academic endeavor. However, to be much use it must be an academic endeavor in the sense of providing disciplined analyses. Insofar as one asks an intellectual question, one seeks more than consciousness raising, emotional refreshment, or a chance to exchange ideas over a drink. One strives to get ideas clearer because it is important to decide how one ought to resolve the disputes occasioned by the health care arts and sciences. Because they bear on life, death, and the quality of life, one must with care and discipline attend to drawing conceptual distinctions. For example, deciding when human life ends signals the difference between describing the removal of a heart from a body as murder or as harvesting an organ. Such conceptual niceties (i.e., what is the difference between human biological and human personal life) carry practical weight. Finally, such tasks of intellectual clarification have merit, even when they do not lead to the definitive resolution of a problem. Greater clarity about a problem is better than more confusion, even when final answers are elusive. Philosophical progress is usually incremental:

cautious steps forward, not final steps into the light. On this point, it is worth noting that it is frequently difficult to know in advance where such reflection will lead. One often discovers, with chagrin, that one's most heartfelt convictions are indefensible prejudices.

This is apparent on a large scale when one observes changes in public policy due to conceptual refinements. Though at the beginning of this century, for example, it was easy to hold a whole-body-oriented definition of death, that is no longer the case. In fact, now the very contrary holds: a living body with a completely dead brain is most easily seen as no longer a person. This shift occurred over time, following major advances in our understanding of our bodies. One might think of the initial lay reflections concerning cardiac transplants and the possible influence of the donor's heart on the recipient's personality.[7] There was over time a change in the understanding of what it meant to be alive, embodied in this world.[8] One was moving from a whole-body-oriented definition of life and death to a brain-oriented definition. One was as well drawing distinctions between principles of organic life and principles of personhood, of existing as a person in this world.[9] These changes in ontological view influenced bioethical reflections, which in turn have shaped our general understandings of ourselves. Bioethics is a philosophical undertaking that springs naturally from the delivery of health care and the development of the biomedical sciences in social contexts marked by pluralism and rapid technological change, but without an imposed orthodoxy. Bioethics is the disciplined puzzling of people attempting to understand the significance of birth, copulation, illness, and death, especially as these are touched on by health care and the biomedical sciences. Such reflections lead to changes in established cultural views and practices. Bioethics is a central element of a culture's self-understanding and self-transformation.

The place of philosophy

Since any particular culture is likely to contain a cluster of somewhat contrary, if not actually contradictory, presumptions, one is brought to sketch a rational, consistent account insofar as one is looking for rational, consistent answers. This will require one to be a geographer of concepts and values, analyzing and criticizing the advantages and disadvantages of alternative projections and mappings of concepts and values. Such an undertaking is philosophical; it is not one of empirical anthropology or sociology. It is an attempt to resolve an intellectual quandary: "How can I consistently understand what is right conduct in the health care professions and in the biomedical sciences, and justify it to others?" It is not the attempt to decide what people usually hold about right conduct in a particular society, nor is it an attempt to determine what viewpoint would be most credible to most people. Rather, it is an endeavor to look at reasons and to determine what reasons should be credited by impartial, unprejudiced, nonculturally biased reasoners, whose only interests are in the consistency and force of rational argument. Though no such culturally unprejudiced viewpoint can be fully achieved, the goal of its achievement can serve as a guiding ideal, suggesting a direction to proceed in attempting to clarify one's ideas on a subject. This approach, even when it cannot produce final answers (and, though, as we will see, it cannot ground a concrete ethic), can at least make progress by providing some tentative answers, and by suggesting why some resolutions of moral questions are better than others in terms of consistency, scope, and strength of possible rational justifications.

This intellectual approach to a set of very important questions (e.g., Do we declare this patient dead now? May we morally expend these funds on good Scotch whiskey, rather than on treating the hypertension of indigent populations?) is ultimately unavoidable. One can decide to choose to one's best advantage, using whatever means are available, and think no further. Or one can appeal to intuitions, to one's conscience, to what feels right, and let that suffice. In either case, one rejects morality as a peaceable bond among persons. In the first case, one is not concerned with others as either moral objects or subjects. In the second case, the matrix for possible moral action with others is irrational, surd, and inexplicable for those who do not share the same moral intuitions. One simply affirms one's feelings and holds those who disagree to be wrong, in that they fail to have the grace of one's own true insights. In either case, there is no bond through which to fashion the moral community, if one means by that a community founded on mutual respect, not force. However, insofar as one is concerned to have a justification that can appeal to other reasonable individuals, one enters into a fabric of ideas and justifications. As soon as one makes a choice, as a decision one would seek to justify, that choice and the actions it supports fit into a geography of ideas that requires philosophical or ethical analysis to provide orientation and justification. (E.g., "I am going to declare that patient dead, because his entire brain is dead." Why is that sufficient ground? "Because being a person requires at least a minimal level of sentience, and the capacities for sentience are supported by the brain.")

In justifying biomedical decisions, one is embedded in a matrix of conceptual and value presuppositions. Making a biomedical decision involves bioethics. The health professions are practiced within a terrain of concepts and values that presupposes particular relations between concepts and values for which philosophers function as the geographers. This is both a forward, as well as a humble, claim. On the one hand, philosophy cannot pull conceptual rabbits out of hats. Philosophers cannot disclose something on the terrain of ideas and values that was not already there, at least implicitly as an element of human reality. Philosophers can call attention to neglected features, forgotten relationships, and unforeseen contradications. Philosophers can aid in better mapping and in critically evaluating the conceptual and value commitments involved in particular actions and choices.

This should signal certain obvious points about the role of bioethics and of books on bioethics. First, bioethics is not to be understood as a surrogate religion that will convert the evil from the errors of their ways. It will not likely render the uncaring humane, though in some cases it might (some portrayals of ideas capture the imagination and motivate action). Nor is bioethics a basis for a genre of moral counseling that would provide unique answers to particular questions. Such directive counseling is usually beyond its scope, though in some restricted areas bioethics may indeed serve this function. Its role usually will be to provide moral guidance in the sense of giving instruction regarding the likely character of the moral world and the moral significance of choices in biomedicine. This last function, the primary function of bioethics, is a central goal of the humanities generally: to provide an understanding of the human condition through a disciplined examination of the ideas, values, and images that frame the significance of the human world and guide human practices, here those of health care. As an undertaking of men and women, not a deliverance of the gods, its conclusions are likely to be, and probably in most cases will be, tentative.

Secular versus religious bioethics

There are numerous competing secular views of the good life and of the canons of moral probity. These are grounded in particular traditions and in particular moral senses. Unless I indicate otherwise, when I speak of secular bioethics, I mean bioethics in the first sense, as the attempt to find those understandings that can be justified across particular moral communities, traditions, and ideologies, including not only particular religious communities, but particular secular communities of thought as well. If one attempts to chart the conceptual and value commitments of individuals in approaching and resolving biomedical problems—simply as rational individuals without the special illumination of some divine grace—one will find a world view that is secular, though not antireligious. Indeed, as this work will argue, the peaceable context of a neutral secular understanding provides the circumstances within which religious views and special secular traditions can be embraced and pursued in security. A general secular bioethics must function as the logic of a pluralism, as the means for the peaceable negotiation of moral intuitions.

Secular bioethics as the provision of a neutral framework to address moral problems in biomedicine is a peaceable solution to the problems of delivering health care, when physicians, nurses, patients, and individuals generally hold a diversity of moral views. If one is not to embark on an inquisitorial quest of imposing by force or coercion a religiously or metaphysically grounded view of moral probity, or even a *particular* secular tradition, then one will need to content oneself with a general moral framework that lacks such moorings. Without such moorings, there may be a consequent loss of societal certainties. The deliverances of bioethics will often be weaker than a religious thinker, or a partisan of a particular secular moral viewpoint, might wish. Secular bioethics reflections may not support all the moral restraints that religious individuals or partisans of a particular ideology may want. As this volume will show, there will be few serious general secular moral objections to abortion on request. A secular bioethics is unlikely to develop convincing arguments for forbidding many actions that our Western Christian societies have taken to be morally wrong, such as "unnatural sexual activities," suicide, or the active euthanasia of severely defective newborns. In addition, secular bioethics will usually qualify its answers, leaving vexing areas of uncertainty. This will not be out of a pursuit of a minimalist ethics, such as Daniel Callahan has criticized,[10] but rather out of a recognition of the limitations of secular reasoning. These conclusions about the capacities of bioethics will require changes in public policy. If a secular society does not possess general rational arguments to show that certain actions are wrong, the moral authority to enforce such prohibitions weakens. Though this volume is not a volume in law and medicine and does not pretend to give legal advice, it will offer moral and philosophical reassessments of much of law and public policy in medicine.

Threats to traditional certainties may make an imposed orthodoxy appear attractive. There may seem to be greater security for one's beliefs (if one has the good luck of having the same beliefs as the moral oppressors) through suppressing discussion of the fundamental intellectual foundations of the good life and of the canons of moral probity. In the absence of such an imposed orthodoxy, one sees unveiled the faltering attempts of men and women to come to terms with the task of fashioning an account of the moral life. If one is accustomed to the sure answers of a religiously grounded ethics, a general secular bioethics may occasion frustration when one is forced into lengthy chains of reasoning, and disappointment when final answers are not forthcoming.

With all its defects, however, a secular bioethics has numerous virtues. It promises the possibility of providing a context for health care that can encompass in toleration health care givers and receivers with diverse moral perspectives. Believers should also recognize that a secular bioethics can provide the peaceable neutral framework through which they can reach out to others beyond their own particular religious tradition and convert through witness and example, even if not through force. A secular bioethics is also a check against the temptation to flee to false prophets of private intuition for answers that are best achieved through careful analyses sustained by communities of inquiring individuals. It recalls one to the reality of modern medical practice in a pluralist context. Its failings must be seen in the light of the human condition: secular bioethics is framed by men and women, not gods and goddesses. Those with religious persuasions should know that grace makes plain what reason cannot discern. The grace of conversion is not the force of coercion, but rather a divine gift.

The distinctions drawn in this volume between a general secular morality and the moralities of particular moral communities are related to the traditional distinction between what unaided reason can establish and what revelation can teach.[11] Unsupplemented by some special source of knowledge, our understandings of morality and of the ultimate purpose of our lives must remain impoverished.[12] Most of the traditional questions of Western metaphysics concerning the significance of human existence will go at least partially unanswered.[13] The differences between the conclusions in this volume and those offered by traditional natural law theory, such as that of St. Thomas Aquinas, will lie in the limitations of reason that this volume will acknowledge.[14] If one cannot establish through reason alone the great body of Judeo-Christian precepts, there will be, as we shall see, a sharp contrast between secular ethics and the ethics of particular moral communities that rely on special traditions or special revelations. The gulf between church and state will widen, and one will find oneself living a moral life within two complementary but distinct moral perspectives.

Apart from any arguments in principle on behalf of this view of toleration (which arguments will indeed be given in this volume), one might ask under what circumstances there could ever be a peaceable union of the peoples of the earth, save through acquiescing in the policy that persons may do with themselves and consenting others whatever they wish, despite what others might think and feel in the matter. The risk to humanity from war and brutal repression in the name of religious and ideological rectitude far outweighs the harms likely to come from tolerating such evils as self-determination, abortion, and infanticide. Perpetual peace in the absence of repression will likely come, if ever, when we are willing to endure the choices persons make with themselves, consenting others, and their private resources. This volume will explore a number of these themes. Here it is enough to underscore that the purchase price of such peace is toleration of personal tragedy—the toleration of deviant lifestyles, if they are peaceable, and the acceptance of the tragedies that persons experience as the result of their own free choices. To hope to be discharged from such payments is to aspire to the life of the gods, which aspiration is surely to be punished by the plagues that follow hubris.

This gulf and the tensions it engenders characterize the contemporary moral predicament. As we shall see, they are the result of the respect owed to persons, the limits of reason, and the limits on the authority to use force. The purchase price of freedom is tragedy and diversity. It is tragedy because individuals in their freedom will choose in ways that others find to be ill-considered and harmful. Such choices will lead to an untidy diversity of competing moral viewpoints, often making common actions in many areas impossible. Because one is obliged to tolerate such tragedy and diversity, the moral life becomes an ambiguous undertaking. One must often tolerate on moral grounds that which one must condemn on moral grounds. For example, as the reader shall see, there are limits on the public authority to use force in order to compel charity.[15] However, the reader should understand that the author holds just as strongly that charity is central to the good moral life and is one of the proper responses to a universe blind to human sufferings, where persons are often deaf to the needs of others. Such tolerance has not been traditional in many societies of the West. St. Thomas Aquinas recommends that the stubborn or relapsing heretic be exterminated from the world by death.[16] We will need to learn to be tolerant, even about issues less important than the salvation of immortal souls. We will need to eschew contemporary versions of the *writ de haeretico comburendo* (i.e., the writ for the burning of a heretic).

The conclusions in this volume are at times perturbing and upsetting. The reader should be advised that the author also was often disturbed by many of the conclusions. The unbiased analysis of settled moral viewpoints has the danger of undermining cherished moral sentiments—or at least of showing that they must be recognized as a part of a community's special moral commitments and not amenable to general rational justification. Then, of course, it would be too much to hope that all of one's culture's mores could find general rational justification. Philosophical analysis is a form of intellectual adventure. One may perhaps arrive at viewpoints one would not have anticipated.

Notes

1. Alasdair MacIntyre, *After Virtue* (Notre Dame, Ind.: University of Notre Dame Press, 1981).
2. Ad Hoc Committee of the Harvard Medical School to Examine the Definition of Brain Death, "A Definition of Irreversible Coma," *Journal of the American Medical Association* 205 (Aug. 1968): 336–40.
3. Griswold v. Connecticut, 381 U.S. 479, 85 S.Ct. 1678. 14 L.Ed.2d 510 (1965). Similar constitutional protection was extended to the right of unmarried indi-

viduals to have access to contraception in Eisenstadt v. Baird, 405 U.S. 438, 92 S.Ct. 1029, 31 L.Ed.2d 349 (1972).

4. It is interesting to note that some individuals have provided arguments to support the notion that homosexuality evolved because it maximized inclusive fitness. For such an argument, see Robert Trivers, "Parent-Offspring Conflict," *American Zoologist* 14 (1974): 249–64.

5. Curlender v. Bio-Science Laboratories and Automated Laboratory Sciences, 165 Cal. Rptr. 477 (Ct. App. 2nd Dist. Div. 1, 1980). I cite this case to illustrate a moral point, even though the decision has since been overturned by a California law (Cal. Cir. Code, sec. 43.6 [1982]), as well as there being a contrary ruling in Turpin v. Sortini, 119 Cal. App. 3rd 690 (1981).

6. H. T. Engelhardt, Jr., "Physicians, Patients, Health Care Institutions—and the People in Between: Nurses," in A. H. Bishop and J. R. Scudder (eds.), *Caring, Curing, Coping: Nurse, Physician, Patient Relationships* (University, Ala.: University of Alabama Press, 1985) pp. 62–79.

7. See, for example, Kenneth Vaux, "A Year of Heart Transplants: An Ethical Valuation," *Postgraduate Medicine* 45 (Jan. 1969): 201–5. Irving S. Wright, "A New Challenge to Ethical Codes: Heart Transplants," *Journal of Religion and Health* 8 (1969): 226–41. Patricia MacMillian, "But My Heart Belongs to Me...," *Nursing Times* 76 (April 1980): 677.

8. For a study of the development of concepts of the cerebral localization of mental capacities, see Robert Young, *Mind, Brain, and Adaptation in the Nineteenth Century* (Oxford: Clarendon Press, 1970); S. F. Spicker and H. T. Engelhardt, Jr. (eds.), *Philosophical Dimensions of the Neuro-Medical Sciences* (Dordrecht: Reidel, 1976).

9. H. Tristram Engelhardt, Jr., "Defining Death: A Philosophical Problem for Medicine and Law," *American Review of Respiratory Diseases* 112 (Nov. 1975): 587–90. Though, as I shall argue in this volume, the brain-oriented definition of death is best understood as the recognition of the brain as the sponsor of consciousness, there have been attempts to avoid this recognition. See, for example, the President's Commission for the Study of Ethical Problems in Medicine and Biomedical and Behavioral Research, *Defining Death* (Washington, D.C.: U.S. Government Printing Office, 1981), esp. pp. 31–43.

10. Daniel Callahan, "Minimalist Ethics," *Hastings Center Report* 11 (Oct. 1981): 19–25.

11. Classically, there was a distinction made between what can be concluded by natural reason, by reason unaided by grace and revelation, and what can be known through revelation. As St. Thomas stated, "It was therefore necessary that, besides the philosophical disciplines investigated by reason, there should be a sacred doctrine by way of revelation." *Summa Theologica* I, art. 1. *The Basic Writings of Saint Thomas Aquinas*, Anton C. Pegis (ed.), vol. 1 (New York: Random House, 1945), p. 6.

12. Here one must include not only grace and revelation but also special moral traditions and moral senses.

13. Metaphysics in the West has classically included natural theology and discussions on the immortality of the soul. One might think here of the three questions of Kant: "1. What can I know? 2. What ought I to do? 3. What may I hope?" *Critique of Pure Reason* A805 = B833. Norman Kemp Smith (trans.), *Immanuel Kant's Critique of Pure Reason* (London: Macmillan, 1964), p. 635. I, following Kant, consider the limits of our ability to answer such questions.

14. The Roman Catholic Church contends that on the basis of natural reason one can demonstrate the existence of God and the immorality of contraception.

15. One should note that Jesus is reported to have said, "If thou wilt be perfect, go and sell that thou hast, and give to the poor, and thou shalt have treasure in heaven . . ." (Matthew 19:21). There is no evidence that he said, "If you would be perfect, establish a progressive redistributive tax system." Being committed to aiding the poor is not equivalent to being committed to using state force to compel others to be beneficent.

16. St. Thomas Aquinas, *Summa Theologica* II, Q. IX, art. iii–iv. In this regard, St. Thomas was reflecting the general ethos of the time. The Fourth Lateran Council, for instance, granted the same indulgences to those who exterminated heretics at home as to those who went to the Holy Land. "Catholici vero qui, crucis assumpto charactere, ad haereticorum exterminium se accinxerint, illa gaudeant indulgentia, illoque sancto privilegio sint muniti, quod accedentibus in Terrae sanctae subsidium conceditur." "Concilium Lateranese IV" [1215], *Conciliorum Oecumenicorum Decreta* (Basil: Herder, 1962), *Constitutiones* 3, p. 210.

2

The Intellectual Bases of Bioethics

The problem of objectivity in morals

A serious controversy in ethics leads to the roots of human values. Bioethical controversies are no exception. What might appear an isolated biomedical choice will in the end be found to be embedded in a matrix of public policies, rooted in concepts of the good life, the nature of rights and duties, and the standing of moral objects and subjects. Consider a thirty-six-year-old woman seeking amniocentesis to determine whether her fetus has Down's syndrome, with a view under those circumstances to having an abortion. The example involves a person at an increased risk (around 1 in 250) due to age of giving birth to a child with Down's syndrome.[1] Such a child has a higher than usual chance of being a drain on limited societal resources.[2] Moreover, if the child is born with Down's syndrome, it would not meet this woman's view of an acceptable child. How should a physician, or for that matter society, respond? If the woman is indigent, should there be public support for the cost of the amniocentesis and the abortion? What if one of the nurses who assisted the physician during the amniocentesis objected to abortion? What is the moral standing of the fetus? Does it have a right to life, and if so, how strong a right and in what circumstances? Does the woman have a right to avoid giving birth to a defective child? For that matter, what rights and obligations do parents have to avoid the birth of defective children? What rights do parents have to control the quality of the children they will have? What do such terms as *rights* and *obligations* mean in these contexts? What are the bases for holding certain children to be "defective" and therefore less valuable than others? Does society have a legitimate interest in minimizing the costs it would incur in the care of defective children by preventing their births? Is amniocentesis a truly medical procedure? What are the goods to be found in having children and being a parent? What are the virtues at stake in the use of amniocentesis and abortion?

Such ethical questions (e.g., would it be good to aid this woman in securing amniocentesis and abortion, should she want them?) and ontological questions (are fetuses persons?) are found in a nexus of controversies. These involve matters of dispute both within and across cultures. To look for answers one will need to ask how such disputes could in principle be resolved. The procedures for fashioning an answer to a question disclose both the meaning of the question and the significance of the answer. If, for example, one wants to know a patient's serum glucose level, one needs to know how it will be determined in order to know the significance of the results. The meaning of the answer will depend on how one understands the question, which itself will depend on the ways in which one performs the determination, in this case, of the serum glucose level. Similar constraints apply to ethical questions. To decide which choice is better requires deciding better *for whom* and *with respect to what criteria*. To have meaning, actual determinations of facts and ethical issues require specification of the criteria employed. Each such specification is, however, likely to have both its strengths and weaknesses; these will be determined in part by the capacities of the knowers or the evaluators. Also, certain forms of acquiring knowledge will be too costly or in fact impossible. And, as in the case of the pregnant woman, all actual tests for Down's syndrome will have some risk of false positive or false negative findings, no matter how remote.[3] Moreover, it will always be very difficult if not impossible to predict all the relevant moral consequences of a decision to seek an abortion. The predicament of the finite knower and evaluator will be conditioned by incomplete knowledge and partial understanding of the circumstances.

One may have a notion of an ideal determination, so that one can rank some answers in terms of that ideal as being clearly better than others. Put most generally, the search for a flawless answer can be understood as an attempt to achieve the position of the perfect knower, ideally and traditionally the viewpoint of the Creator, God. The Deity (a perfectly advantaged, totally unbiased Knower) would be able to provide the best of answers. The Deity's answers are taken to be impeccable, because there is no better-placed knower. No one could rebut the answers of the Deity by claiming a more advantaged position. Furthermore, if the Deity created things, there is the presumption that He (She? or It?) knows them from the inside out. After all, the Deity created them, even their hidden essences. One could attempt to imagine, therefore, a reality as known by the Deity, in comparison with which all other portrayals of reality, all other understandings of things, would be deficient cases. What the Deity holds to be the nature of reality is the nature of reality, for it is the Deity's will, informed by Its understanding of reality, that forms the source of the structure of reality. Thus, the Deity cannot be wrong. Moreover, it is not simply that the Deity's view of reality cannot fail to accord with things in themselves; in addition, the Deity's account is the paradigm of an all-encompassing coherent account of reality. In short, in the Deity's case, criteria for truth based on the agreement between the knowledge claim and the object to be known and criteria for truth based on ideal conditions for intersubjective agreement coincide. The Deity satisfies both correspondence and coherence conditions for truth.

This privilege of the Deity is usually held to obtain for issues of both fact and value. The Deity knows the structure of reality because It can best examine reality and because reality is Its own creation. Similarly, in the case of values, the Deity can best judge the consequences of various possible choices, and can therefore offer the most exhaustive evaluation of their comparative merits in this regard. Even if values, like rules of logic, are beyond the Deity's control, still the Deity should be uniquely placed to judge and compare them. In this sense, the Deity offers the existential realization of the philosophical device of the ideal disinterested observer who judges moral choices, uninfluenced by prejudice and supported by an exhaustive knowledge of the relevant facts. The Deity can provide the perfect answers to the perfect questions.

However, the Deity does not appear to speak to all directly. As a consequence, there is general disagreement about the perfect questions and their perfect answers. Nonetheless, some have attempted to employ the notion of the Deity's viewpoint as a guiding intellectual construct, a regulative ideal against which to measure particular attempts to assess reality and to judge conduct. One might think here of the importance of the divine perspective for the philosophical accounts offered by René Descartes (1596–1650), Benedict Spinoza (1632–1677), and Gottfried Wilhelm Leibniz (1646–1716), where the Deity possesses the paradigm case of clear and distinct ideas, of clear and distinct perceptions. Such viewpoints presume that the world of facts, and often the world of values, has a unique pattern of rational coherence.

This I will term the *monotheistic presumption*: there is one unique vantage point in terms of which a concrete account of knowledge and ethics can be given. If, however, there is no satisfactory access to that one viewpoint, then it will not be clear whether such a viewpoint exists. There might in fact be many gods and goddesses and, as a consequence, many competing viewpoints. Put poetically, insofar as one abandons the presumption of the possibility of a single, authoritative, concrete account of knowledge and ethics, one embraces what could be termed the *polytheistic presumption*. I will thus distinguish between the monotheistic presumption (that there is a unique moral perspective) and the polytheistic presumption (that there are a number of equally defensible, but quite different, moral perspectives). The more one can hope for access to a unique authoritative viewpoint, the more one can hope to give a generally satisfactory answer regarding the treatment of the woman seeking amniocentesis with a view to possible abortion. Insofar as a unique, authoritative viewpoint appears unobtainable, answers will turn more on matters of particular inclination and of common decision, rather than on points open to general resolution through the discovery of correct answers. As this book will argue, the polytheistic presumption, at least in matters of values, appears better founded—especially if the gods and goddesses are seen within a cosmos of general rational restraints.

The very significance of bioethical disputes hinges on fundamental philosophical issues about the possibility of answering ethical and ontological questions. The significance of such disputes must be established through an examination in controversy theory by which one would hope to determine the conditions for the possibility of the resolution of ethical and ontological controversies in general, and those in biomedicine in particular. One will need to determine which ethical and ontological controversies are open to resolution by discovering a correct answer, and which are to be resolved through fair procedures for fashioning an answer. One will need to distinguish among various senses of "fair" or "correct" answers. Insofar as the justification of these answers does not require achieving a divine (absolute) viewpoint, such answers will disclose the deliverances of particular finite reasoners with varying finite (relative) viewpoints and goals. Senses of fairness and of correctness will then vary, at least in part, from community to community, or more precisely, from moral sense to moral sense.

Since the criteria for such views of correctness and fairness will often not be explicitly stated by the members of such communities, it will be necessary for philosophers to give an account of them. Philosophy contributes in part by providing rational reconstructions, maps of the canons of probity and of fairness presupposed by particular communities of knowers and evaluators. Such charting and analysis are enterprises in comparative epistemology and comparative value theory. This is also a project that can be enlightened by studies in the sociology and history of knowledge and evaluation. Different communities of knowers and evaluators, with different rules for recognizing evidence and reasoning on its basis, are likely to perceive and understand facts and values quite differently.

One will hope to find a sense of the enterprise of knowing and valuing that will allow one to hold that some criteria for knowing or valuing correctly are better, that is, more defensible, than others. Even if a final, absolute, or divine perspective is not accessible, one can still ask what answers should rationally resolve controversies regarding facts and values. In conflicts among rival empirical accounts, one will have the advantage of being able to compare their predictive power, given a sufficiently common understanding of what is at stake. One can determine how one could decide what the etiologic infectious agent for yellow fever is. Disputants can test the competing accounts with reality and thus falsify some competitors and strengthen the claims of others. Some accounts will stand out as preferable in being simpler accounts of the facts with fewer anomalies and with fewer ad hoc assumptions. The "facts" can cause difficulties for many conjectures concerning reality.

In the case of conflicts of morals, such appeals to "facts" do not appear to be as forceful, since what is at stake are not simply the "facts," but evaluations of the "facts." Consider how different the question regarding the morally proper balance between investment in preventive medicine and in individual health care is from the question regarding the cause of yellow fever. Unless one is going to make morality depend on the views of particular individuals and their particular interests, in order to resolve ethical disputes one will need to find a set of criteria, somewhat on the model of those canons one might hope to derive from the Deity's standpoint, were that standpoint accessible. One will need an objective viewpoint, such as that one might seek from testing empirical theories against facts. Secular surrogates for the objectivity of the Deity's viewpoint are likely to be convincing only if they disclose the very conditions for the possibility of particular kinds of knowledge or of values. If ethics does not have material facts by which to resolve arguments, it will need to appeal to formal constraints. That is, the resolution of ethical controversies will need to depend on an inescapable and important understanding, so that in asking the question one discovers the answer. In other words, the inescapable question must itself predestine the answer. Such circularity will be tolerable only if the circle is sufficiently encompassing so that following it around is in fact illuminating.

Arguments of this sort have a kinship with the transcendental arguments of Immanuel Kant (1724–1804). Kant despaired of being able to settle arguments concerning the nature of reality by appeals to reality as it is in itself (i.e., reality untouched by the conditions of human experience, reality as it is known by the Deity). Instead, he appealed to the conditions of human experience. Knowledge of a spatiotemporal, sensible world has conceptually expressible preconditions. For there to be experience, there must be points of permanence in that experience. Changes must occur with some regularity, and the points of permanence with their changes must be in correlation with each other. These are necessary conditions for the possibility of coherent experience, for there being a commonly shared phenomenal world.[4] Kant thus attempted to sketch the general conceptual framework within which particular empirical claims can be framed and tested. In giving his account, Kant abandoned the search for reality as the Deity knows it and sought instead to account for reality as humans have empirical experience of it.[5] This involved a singular shift of philosophical attention. Kant's point of departure for justifying his account of the nature of reality is not that of the divine perspective, but that of the possible community of finite knowers who know spatiotemporally and sensibly.[6]

I will not be quite as confident as Kant that there is only one such finite perspective for humans.[7] In fact, I will proceed with the presumptions that (1) there may be many special human realities (e.g., the reality of macro- versus microphysics), and (2) that the portrayal of the conditions of reality in any detail is itself conditioned by the perspective of a particular historical period.[8] I will agree in part with Kant that we can at least gesture in the direction of truth, even if the truth we actually know is only a truth of finite knowers and valuers. We can discern what should count as better answers in terms of becoming clearer about what the best ways of putting questions should be. Like Hegel (1770–1831), I will hold that one should not see an unbridgeable cleft between subject and object, between thought and being.[9] As one more clearly sees how one can think about reality, one at the same time discerns more clearly reality's rational structures.[10] I will attempt here to outline the nature of ethics by indicating what is involved in the general enterprise of asking ethical questions and ontological questions that bear on ethical issues in health care.

These philosophical considerations are important in deciding the significance of an answer concerning the morality of amniocentesis and abortion in the case of the thirty-six-year-old pregnant woman. One would hope, for example, to be able to decide whether the standing of pregnant women and of fetuses is equal. Are both persons? Are both persons in the same sense? If not, what are their moral rights given the circumstances of this case? What obligations to society do persons have when reproducing? What is the standing of societal claims? One would want to know the extent to which such distinctions and determinations are open to objective discovery and the extent to which they are deliverances of a historically formed consensus, or of a formal agreement. Answering moral questions regarding the circumstances under which it would be allowable to perform amniocentesis and abortion, and the extent to which the costs of such procedures for the indigent should be borne by society, depends on judgments about the nature of ethics and of ontological views regarding the nature of persons. In the next section of this chapter, I will explore problems involved in developing a general, secular ethics and suggest the extent to which such an ethics can be justified intellectually.

The nature of ethics

Some meanings of ethics

The term *ethics* is ambiguous. First, as its etymology suggests, ethics can mean that which is customary. As that which is habitual to a people, ethics is similar in meaning to the root of the word morals, *mos* (pl. *mores*), the customs of a people, a sense that is close to the meaning of the English word mores. In medical ethics, these senses are found in many of the Hippocratic works portraying the Greek physician.[11] In such cases, one is dealing with taken-for-granted webs of moral values that constitute the character of the everyday lifeworlds of medical practice. It is in terms of ethics, in this sense, that most of us live most of our lives, and in terms of which most health care is provided. From within an assumed matrix of values, we derive many of our moral intuitions and have our consciences formed for us before we become self-conscious moral reasoners. When physicians speak of having learned about the character of good medicine from the example of an excellent teacher, they often are referring to the initiation into a lifeworld of virtue and purpose that such distinguished "role models" provide. If the community within which one lives is small and not subject to technological developments and other forces that abet social change, this taken-for-granted sense is likely not only to be unquestioned, but also to appear to be unquestionable. It provides, in any event, a point of departure for most ethical reflections.

Ethics is also used to identify the rules of conduct of special professional groups, as in the ethics of lawyers, of accountants, or of physicians and nurses. When these are articulated as specific canons of probity for the conduct of such professions, and when the focus is primarily on issues of professional decorum, ethics in this sense is best understood as etiquette. In fact, this is how some of the codes of medical ethics were styled[12] prior to the American Medical Association's adoption of its first code of medical ethics in May 1847.[13] A major portion of the issues addressed in such codes of etiquette were not moral issues in an immediate and strict sense, but rather questions of fees, advertisement, and the relation of physicians with non-orthodox practitioners. Such rules are not trivial. Codes of etiquette formally describe an important dimension of the mores of a group or profession. They are like laws. They are explicit enactments or precedents that reflect moral principles and political agreements. But unlike laws, they usually possess only the sanctions of professional disapproval or ostracism. Professional etiquette possesses a more restricted scope and source of authority than the law.

The canons of proper conduct as determined by law are often taken to be equivalent to canons of ethics. However, one speaks not only of good laws and bad laws, but also of laws that ought or ought not to be obeyed. Thus, laws restricting basic personal freedoms are held by many, if not most, not only to be improper, but also to merit disobedience. As a creature born of political forces and of compromise, the law is likely at best to reflect only in part the mores of a society. This is more clearly the case the more a legal framework binds together a number of communities with somewhat divergent views of the good life. The more such communities differ in their accepted canons of moral probity, the more explicit laws and bureaucratic rules will need to be.[14] In such cases, laws and rules will be relied on as the social cement to hold together communities that do not share such a matrix of values. Different communities with different mores will have framed common rules for common action.[15] The price of life in a heterogeneous society spanning numerous distinct and contrasting moral communities is a body of bureaucratic rules and regulations. Where communities do not share a common sense of moral propriety, detailed formal regulations are often needed. Also, laws as formal deliverances may develop more slowly than changes in societal mores. As a result, the ethical views embodied in laws will at times reflect largely abandoned moral viewpoints. For example, in a number of states of the United States, oral intercourse is a felony, even between married individuals,[16] though surveys conducted indicated in 1972 that about 90 per cent of married couples under age twenty-five had engaged in oral intercourse at least once in that year.[17]

Religions constitute another major source of ethical viewpoints. Depending on the character of a society, the contributions of religions may in various degrees be separated from a society's mores and its laws. A secular society is likely to have customs, taken-for-granted understandings of proper conduct, that have little religious coloring and are not substantially rooted in religious understandings. One might think here of the rules for free and informed consent in health care. In other societies, these may be inseparably bound. One might think here of laws against elective abortions in many Catholic countries. In particular, religious ethics have the distinction of being founded on claims of transcendent moral truths. As a consequence, they are often difficult to defend or understand in general rational terms. The Jehovah's Witnesses' opposition to blood transfusions provides a good example.[18] A rational argument regarding the virtues of such transfusions is unlikely to be accepted as defeating a religious claim. Ethics, in the sense of secular customs, may be arbitrary, but the sources are usually acknowledged to be explicable in the history and traditions of a people. Codes of etiquette and the laws of a community as secular institutions can similarly be traced to formal or informal attempts to establish rules of conduct. Considered as secular phenomena, they can be justified in terms of their fairness, usefulness, the service they perform for the interests of particular individuals, special groups, or the community in general, or their justifiability by appeal to rationally supported or supportable moral principles. However, religious ethics, especially those of revealed religions, claim a grounding in a transcendent reality. Insofar as the nature of that ultimate reality is disclosed via some special revelation, it purports to fall beyond the power of a secular society to examine adequately its claims to correctness.

It is because of such attempts at justification that revealed religions have both their strengths and weaknesses. On the one hand, they speak with an authority and certainty that are often reassuring. They account for the state of the world, its purposes, and the goods of human life from the purported vantage point of the Deity's understanding or from some ultimate account of the meaning of things. They can state without qualification that sterilization is morally improper, or that one must surgically repair duodenal atresia in an infant born with Down's syndrome. On the other hand, even a revelation of the Deity, if it is not to be a mystic encounter of each person face-to-face with his or her own god or goddess, will need to be mediated by men and women. The word of God must be put in human language and will then inextricably be subject to the weaknesses and limitations of those languages. Languages and their speakers are mired in history.

Individuals within a tradition can attempt to refashion doctrines by reinterpreting language. Such hermeneutical endeavors have produced attempts by liberal Roman Catholic theologians to alter Catholic opposition to all forms of artificial birth control.[19] As a consequence, much of the certainty claimed on the basis of the Deity's authority is lost in the uncertainties of human history and human messengers. Further and more important, it is difficult to test the authority claimed for a revelation as a revelation, in that special revelations require privileged access to the Truth by grace of the Deity. Since such privilege has transcendent origins, the only circumstances under which one could test for the truth of such claims, beyond a critique based on logical contradictions or violations of the general canons of secular morality, would be with the receipt of the grace of true belief, or by an appeal to publicly witnessed and inspected miracles that violated the very laws of nature, transcended the possibility of immanent explanation, and whose very character unambiguously supported one particular system of belief.

Because not all are favored by such grace, and because there is no generally acceptable evidence that such miracles do occur, the world is explained by prophets of competing accounts, and the cacophony of their contradictory claims can be heard in any large society. There appears to be no greater

uniformity among religions than among the partisans of secular philosophies. If anything, there may be more divergence among the prophets of
religion. Truly secular philosophers who eschew the transcendent claims of
metaphysics (a special surrogate for revealed religion)[20] are for the most part
siblings descended from the Western Enlightenment and therefore share
more assumptions than do the advocates of the various religious ethics.

Absent either a general conversion to one religion, or the existence of a
generally imposed orthodoxy, one will need to search for common grounds
to bind rational individuals in a peaceable community. Such a search will be
a quest for ethics in the sense of the canons of proper action that could be
peaceably established on the basis of principles commonly discovered, or
chosen by common agreement. This sense of ethics is that of a secular,
philosophical ethics, introduced in chapter 1. It is an ethics that aspires to
provide a logic for a pluralism of beliefs, a common view of the good life that
can transcend particular communities, professions, legal jurisdictions, and
religions, but whose grounds for authority are immanent to the secular
world. One moves to this sense of ethics precisely because particular social
customs, rules of etiquette, codes of laws and religious traditions appear too
parochial or too arbitrary to bind together individuals from varying
traditions and communities. If one is a patient or practices medicine in a
society that includes patients and physicians of radically different communities of moral belief, one will need to appeal to general rational grounds to
justify a moral viewpoint across communities of conviction and belief.

Looking for objectivity in ethics

Here is where the central problem for serious ethical reflection lies: how to
justify *any* set of claims regarding what is right and good. Are moral
cornerstones of medical practice such as free and informed consent and
confidentiality merely arbitrary cultural dispositions? If particular cultural
traditions or religions cannot establish their authority in a general secular
community on the basis of established precedent, divine grace given to
prophets, or the private satisfaction of one's own conscience, how will one be
able to establish authority for any particular set of moral claims? In fact,
moral claims made within a particular moral tradition are liable to appear
strange and exotic to those trying to weigh claims on rational grounds alone.

Consider, for example, the argument by the Protestant theologian Paul
Ramsey against such techniques as artificial insemination from a donor:

We need rather the biblical comprehension that man is as much the body of his soul as
he is the soul of his body. The single word *sarx* in the "one-flesh" unity of marriage
and parentage is sufficient to impel us to think with the Jews and Christians in all ages
who have affirmed a unity between the vocations of soul and body. They therefore

affirmed the biological to be *assumed into* the personal and in some ultimate sense believed there is a linkage between the love-making and the life-giving.[21]

It is difficult to understand fully what is being claimed, much less credit the justification for the claims, outside the particular tradition within which the claims are made. The claims are grounded in certitudes (e.g., a particular inspired literature and tradition), which are taken for granted only within particular communities of religious belief.

In contrast, in science, claims can, up to a point, be tested so that at least the predictive value of some scientific accounts can be assessed. Thus, for example, given the recent exploration of the planets (e.g., Venus and Mars), Ptolemy's account of the solar system is shown simply and irrevocably to be false—Flat Earthers, Cardinal Bellarmine, and Pope Urban VIII to the contrary notwithstanding. Of course, in many cases such crisp choices between competitive scientific accounts are not available. One must then also consider the varying explanatory powers of competing theoretical accounts and their ability to encompass different ranges of data in ways that variously promise to be fruitful for further exploration. One must recognize that attempts to test predictions require interpretations of data that are always made within the theoretical and factual expectations of the investigators. Choices of how one will specify the foci of one's inquiry are guided by antecedent theoretical and value commitments.[22] *Ceteris paribus* clauses (i.e., this will obtain, all else being equal) involve decisions made with the guidance of generally accepted scientific paradigms, historically conditioned by the thought styles of the particular scientific communities of the investigators.[23] In short, even science is not an ahistorical deliverance of the gods. Scientific truth, as all human truth, is historically and culturally shaped. However, the empirical sciences benefit from the discipline imposed by an external reality, even when that reality always appears dressed in the expectations of particular times and persons. As a consequence, external reality makes certain accounts of empirical reality difficult, if not impossible, to hold.

Such restraints rarely intrude into the undertakings of ethics or bioethics. Philosophers can speak of what moral agents ought to do, without presuming that such entities in fact exist. The constraints on ethics would appear to be first and foremost logical. If one asserts contradictions, one need not be taken as attempting to offer a serious answer to a rational question about what one ought to do. After all, ethics is an intellectual endeavor. One appeals to philosophical ethics when one wants a reasoned answer to reasonable questions. If one is seeking edification or religious enthusiasm, an intellectual answer may be beside the point. In contrast, in ethics one would want, as in a scientific explanation, to be able to give as encompassing and systematic an account of the moral life, with the least number of ad hoc explanations and the fewest contradictions, as possible. Yet, without the constraints of empirical reality, ethicists, including bioethicists, will enjoy considerable latitude in the development of their accounts of the moral life. Indeed, the problem is how to give intersubjective moral authority to intrasubjective conviction or dispositions of conscience. To speak of truth as a "private truth" is at best a bastard usage. Making a serious rational claim involves asserting intersubjective force for that claim and holding that evidence shows the intellectual costs of disagreeing and that the intellectual benefits of agreeing do in fact favor the claim.

Since science deals with an external reality, this reality imposes different costs and benefits on holders of rival accounts, suggesting which may be more sustainable. However, often even what may appear to be scientific disputes do not always turn on simply empirical matters. Consider the disagreement about the efficacy of laetrile. It is in part a political disagreement regarding the right of individuals to self-medication, independent of the effectiveness of such medication. Or it may reflect deep-seated suspicions regarding the scientific establishment. Yet, insofar as it is a dispute about the nature of the world, it turns on the character of reality and the ways of fashioning generalizations from scientific data. The rational resolution of an empirical scientific controversy in part depends for its correctness on the ability consistently to fashion scientific accounts. Since these reflect the formal character of reasoning itself, if one is interested in rational answers to rational questions about likely outcomes, one will need to conform to such formal constraints. They, however, will not provide content. Such formal considerations, when combined with the constraints of external reality, offer an intersubjective basis for resolving, or at least in principle understanding how one could resolve controversies regarding the efficacy of laetrile. That is, one can in principle understand how one could resolve the question of the efficacy of laetrile by appeal to formal criteria for consistent reasoning and to the nature of external reality.[24]

With regard to moral claims, the question is the extent to which one can secure a similar toehold on intersubjectivity. Are there ways in which one can approach the intersubjectivity available in determinations about matters of fact, when answering questions in bioethics or ethics generally?[25] Here it should be stressed that morality must be a potentially intersubjective endeavor if it is to provide a basis for moral agents being held to have acted wrongly or in a blameworthy fashion. It is surely the case that individuals have various strongly held views about right actions. Patients and physicians disagree regarding the morality of abortion, artificial insemination, and the rights of patients to free health care. The question is whether any of these views is correct such that other moral agents ought rationally to concur with them. Can one provide for morality more than (1) the formal rational constraints of avoiding contradictions and (2) the conditional constraints of embracing the means to the ends one holds to be obligatory insofar as one holds them to be conditionally or overridingly obligatory?

Where then does one turn for criteria to choose among competing versions of the moral life in order to establish foundations for bioethics? For example, how ought one to decide whether it is better morally always to gain the permission of competent patients prior to treatment, or only when it is useful in patient management? One knows that across the world, and within the last fifty years, there have been widely divergent modes of caring for patients. Some have seen patients, or certain classes of patients, as objects (e.g., "teaching material"). Others have been careful to respect the freedom of patients to choose their own destinies. Indeed, a serious inquiry into moral foundations, in order to meet the criteria of intellectual honesty in justifying a general account of moral actions in health care, will need to seek grounds for the most taken-for-granted elements of moral convictions. An ethical investigation focused on health care will need to determine why patients ought to be treated with respect in any circumstance. One will need to establish rational justifications for the moral viewpoints one holds to be proper. Can one establish, for example, that it is morally wrong to let children die who are born with Down's syndrome? Is it wrong actively to kill such children? Such an endeavor in justification will be of intellectual benefit in many circumstances. It will be of special practical importance in the case of bioethics, for bioethics involves the reassessment of practices such as the taking or the preservation of human life (e.g., abortion, decisions regarding who is admitted to intensive care units in hospitals, and the recognition of rights to refuse treatment).

Problems in justifying a particular moral viewpoint

A frank appraisal of the justification of ethics and therefore of bioethics must then begin with the question, What can one in principle establish, and with what certainty, in the area of morals? One will need to know what rational bases exist even for such taken-for-granted rules as "It is immoral to torture and kill the unconsenting innocent for sport." Such an approach does not carry a prejudice against traditional morality, nor is it designed to place the rights of persons or cherished human values in jeopardy. Rather, it involves the honest realization that much of what structures the concrete fabric of the everyday moral life-world has, when explored for its justification, the character of the arbitrary and conventional. This is often most clearly seen in the conflict of cultures.

For example, Captain Cook and his men were shocked by the fact that

Hawaiians thought it quite natural and proper for men and women in certain circumstances to sleep with each other without the benefit of marriage. However, the Hawaiians were disquieted by the fact that the Europeans found it proper for men and women to eat together—this the Hawaiians knew to be taboo:

··· the women never upon any account eat with the men, but always by themselves. What can be the reason of so unusual a custom, it is hard to say; especially as they are a people in every other instance, fond of Society and much so of their Women. They were often asked the reason, but they never gave no other Answer, but that they did it because it was right, and expressed much dislike at the custom of Men and Women eating together of the same Victuals ... more than one-half of the better sort of the inhabitants have entered into a resolution of enjoying free liberty in Love, without being troubled or disturbed by its consequences ... both sexes express the most indecent ideas in conversation without the least emotion, and they delight in such conversation beyond any other. Chastity, indeed, is but little valued ...[26]

Since nearly all would now see no moral difficulty in allowing men and women to eat together, and many would take no exception to unmarried men and women having sex together, this example may not be seen to constitute a serious challenge to the fundamentals of traditional morality. It may lack the heuristic force of more extreme examples.

For such one might consider the Ik, who live in the mountains separating Uganda, the Sudan, and Kenya. They live according to a moral system in which little if any altruism is supported, and where the good is equivalent to a full stomach. Taking food from the starving could thus be termed a good act.

The very word for "good," *marang*, is defined in terms of food. "Goodness," *marangik*, is defined simply as "food," or, if you press, this will be clarified as "the possession of food," and still further clarified as "*individual* possession of food." Then if you try the word as an adjective and attempt to discover what their concept is of a "good man," *iakw anamarang*, hoping that the answer will be that a good man is a man who helps you fill your own stomach, you get the truly Ikien answer: a good man is one who *has* a full stomach. There is goodness in being, but none in doing, at least not in doing to others.[27]

Is the viewpoint of the Iks immoral, and if so, why?

Such anthropological case examples of divergent moral viewpoints bring one home to the central question regarding the justification of moral claims: how can one establish *anything* as morally binding? One possibility might be by showing the consequences of particular actions. One might argue that if one does not seek free and informed consent from patients, the fabric of mutual respect will be weakened. However, such a goal-oriented morality or teleological approach presupposes that one already knows what goals ought to be pursued and when. In order to choose among competing moralities on the basis of the consequences, one will need already to know which

consequences are better or worse than others. Consequentialist ethics presupposes nonconsequentialist ethics. How, for example, does one know which is
preferable for a society—spartan virtues or those of an indulgent latter-day
Athens? Is it better to organize society around the virtues of a St. Francis or a
Samurai warrior? Is it better for a society, and consequently its bioethics, to
be founded on the moral sentiments of the Ik or on those of the Mennonites?
How does one know which choice is better? To answer any of these
questions, one will need to know the answer to two questions in advance:
Better for whom? and Better with respect to which values? To assess
consequences one needs a moral criterion.

One might try to answer these questions by an appeal to the choices a
disinterested, impartial, all-knowing observer would make. However, a
choice on the part of such an observer presupposes a particular moral sense.
A mere description of what disinterested, impartial, all-knowing observers
would choose, devoid of particular moral judgments, will not support any
particular moral choices. Or at the most, the appeal to a disinterested
observer will eliminate those moral viewpoints that involve formal logical
contradictions, or which are grounded on formally fallacious arguments
(appeals to disinterested reasoners can make at least this contribution). The
crucial issue is thus how to decide what moral sense to impute to the
disinterested observer. This last question returns one to the important issue
of how one determines the answer to the questions, Better for whom; and
Better with respect to what? Nor will it do to say that the observer must be
non-partisan. On the one hand, one will need to know why a nonpartisan
observer is to be preferred to a partisan observer who chooses one's own side
(especially if one *believes* one's side is correct or that one's interests are the
morally proper interests). On the other hand, how can a moral judge be truly
impartial and partisan to no side? It will need to decide that some preferences, not others, are to be given precedence. What if, on the basis of one's
moral sense, only a few are tortured and very many enjoy it (imagine a
Roman coliseum on international television)? One is unavoidably brought
back to the central moral issues of embracing a particular ranking of moral
goals (Better with regard to what?) for each particular reference class (Better
with regard to whom?).

To resolve these controversies, one will need to distinguish among three
issues: (a) the genesis of a moral viewpoint, (b) the justification of a moral
viewpoint, and (c) the grounds for being rationally motivated to act morally.
Actual moral viewpoints are fashioned under the force of various sociohistorical influences. This condition is shared by morality with the sciences.
That the Western world has the science and technology it possesses today is
the deliverance of past sociohistorical circumstances. However, this genesis
of Western science does not thereby render it parochial, or nonobjective, or

merely Western. The issue of the scope of its validity turns on its justification. In order to justify a practice such as science or morals, one will need to show why it is intrinsic to the undertakings of rational persons. In part, this is done for science by showing that when one commits oneself to making empirical claims about the character of the external world, one at the same time commits oneself to certain intersubjective ways of resolving disputes regarding the character of that external world. The same is true with regard to morals. It is in terms of such a justification that one could hope to be able to show that concerns with free and informed consent are not simply expressions of Western cultural peculiarities. The justification of the practice of morality must turn on an account of what one could mean by blaming or praising individuals or achieving the common welfare. In both the case of science and morality, in seeking a justification one is asking for the rationality of the activity and is therefore pressed to a rational answer. Justification here must be interpreted as the provision of a rational warrant for holding a particular proposition to be correct.

Morality as a rational endeavor must be taken to refer to a systematically assessed body of claims about the rightness and wrongness of actions and about what it is good or bad to do. Morality or ethics in this sense must then be distinguished from morality as customary rules of taboo and moral probity, just as science as a set of systematic claims about the world must be distinguished from bodies of unexamined opinion. As soon as one attempts to justify particular customs or opinions as those rational individuals ought to acknowledge, one has entered into an attempt to free oneself from merely traditional or accepted viewpoints. One has moved from taking for granted that children with severe spina bifida manifesta must at least be given food and water, to attempting to seek the justification for such practices.

Beyond issues of justification, one must also acknowledge the question of what rational grounds exist to motivate one always to act morally or scientifically. One can clearly imagine circumstances where it might be in one's self-interest to act contrary to the endeavors of science or morality. Instances of fabrications of medical research data provide examples where individuals violate the general canons of both science and morality. To ask for the rational grounds that should motivate individuals not to violate those canons is to ask what sanctions exist apart from the contingent sanctions of the law. I will return to the issue of such sanctions later. Here I turn first to the problem of justifying morality and its claims.

Attempts to justify ethics: why they so often fail

There is a fundamental difficulty in establishing the objectivity of any moral preferences, or of evaluations generally. One is in need of a standard by which to order outcomes. How does one compare the interests of a group of patients who could be treated in a protocol that offers them a considerable amount of noxious side effects and only limited chances of cure, with the interests of future patients who in a decade will very likely be the real beneficiaries of such attempts at treatment through the future advances to which current treatment with its noxious side effects may eventually lead? How does one balance interests in treating a pregnant woman with a drug to control a not immediately fatal but serious disease, with the risk of the drug's damaging the fetus she is carrying? To provide answers one will need to appeal to some standard that would rank one outcome or consideration as more important than another. But where could such a standard be found?

Such standards in ethics can be sought (1) in the very content of ethical claims themselves, in intuitions, in what appears to declare itself to be self-evidently right or wrong; (2) in the consequences of moral choices; (3) in the idea of an unbiased choice or the ideal of an impartial observer or a group of unbiased contractors; (4) in the idea of rational moral choice itself; or (5) in the nature of reality. In summary, a standard can be sought in the content of moral thought (i.e., in intuitions), in the form of moral reasoning (e.g., in the idea of impartiality or rationality), or in some external objective reality (e.g., consequences of actions or the structure of reality). As we shall see, there are problems with all of these endeavors because (1) an appeal to intuition begs the question of a standard, (2) an appeal to a formal structure gives no content, and (3) an appeal to an external reality will show what is, not what ought to be. Somewhat procrusteanly, these alternatives, all of which are unsatisfactory, can be put under five headings for more detailed examination.

First, let us turn to appeals to intuition. One might endeavor to intuit moral standards, constrained by certain disciplines, as was suggested by Henry Sidgwick (1838–1900). To be intuitively grounded a moral precept would need to be clearly and precisely formulated, appear self-evident in careful reflections, be consistent with other intuitively known moral propositions, and be of the kind to be recognized by other moral experts to be correct.[28] Such a procedure may incorporate an endeavor to reach a reflective equilibrium among one's various intuitions and those of others. Indeed, the consequences of holding some intuitions to be true may lead to consequences that one will hold to violate other more deeply established moral intuitions. Thus, if one comes to hold that fetuses are not persons, and if it is clear that newborn infants are not different from late-gestation fetuses, one may be pressed to consider whether infanticide involves any greater intrinsic wrong than abortion. If one holds that abortion is not a very serious moral matter, one may then as a consequence be pressed to embrace a new set of moral and ontological views regarding infants and infanticide. Depending on which intuition one holds to be better established, one will then revise one's intuitions either regarding the propriety of feticide or regarding infanticide. But how could one determine which intuitions ought to be held to be better established? One could appeal to a further intuition, perhaps to the intuition that it is best to go with the preponderance of one's intuitions. But how would one know that this is the tack to take? One will need to appeal to increasingly higher-order intuitions or simply arbitrarily embrace one intuition, or set of intuitions, as final. Intuitionism does not appear able to offer a satisfactory answer, for any one intuition can be countered with a contrary intuition.

Second, given the failure of intuitionist accounts, one could attempt to compare the consequences of different systems of moral choices. But how could one assay the comparative virtues of competing systems without appealing to a background moral theory that would allow one to assess the relative merits of the competing systems? The possibility of establishing such a theory is exactly what is at issue. Imagine a utilitarian attempting to assess the comparative merits of two major methods of distributing health care, one which provides acute and chronic care and some preventive care (one might here imagine something not too distant from the current U.S. health care system) versus a system that concentrates its resources on preventive medicine, but with only a minimal amount of acute care and no chronic health care at all. Each will have different costs, including moral costs. In the first system, since the prime focus is on acute and chronic care, the claims of individuals seeking such treatment will be better met than in the second, where they may be denied with the remark that in the end the greatest good will be achieved through research in, and application of, preventive medicine. Of course, those in the second system will have their interests in preventive medicine addressed more adequately than they would be in the first. If those are held to be very important interests by the proponents of the second system, they too can consistently claim that their system will lead to the greatest good for the greatest number. Who is right, and why? To what extent may one discount the need of those seeking health care now in favor of those who may in the future be secured against the evils of preventable diseases? How does one compare the persons' preferences of those who seek health care now with those seeking better prevention now? One would need to appeal to a particular moral sense in order to decide. One cannot decide on the basis of consequences alone which moral sense to employ, for that would beg the question. One needs to know how to rank the consequences.

To answer such questions, one will need to know which outcomes are indeed more important and which preferences ought to be given priority. However, consequentialist accounts (including utilitarian accounts), which compare outcomes, are no better advantaged than the intuitionists with regard to being able to demonstrate which ranking of benefits and banes is to be preferred, since they all require an authoritative means of ranking benefits and harms.

Third, one might attempt to remedy this circumstance by constructing a hypothetical-choice theory. Such a theory might invoke the notion of a disinterested observer, as have Roderick Firth[29] and Richard B. Brandt,[30] in order to specify what rational individuals would choose, and therefore what one ought to choose if one is seeking a rational choice. But such an observer must be specified in some detail. The observer must be fully informed concerning the consequences of various possible choices and be able to imagine how such consequences will affect those concerned (here the similarities to the Deity are considerable). The observer must also be impartial in weighing everyone's interests and siding with none. However, if the observer meets all of these conditions, how will it be able to perform the task of identifying a morally preferable outcome? The observer cannot be so impartial and dispassionate as not to favor certain consequences over others. If it is not partial to certain choices, the observer could not serve as a guide to moral choices. That is, one must impute to the impartial observer a particular moral sense. But what is at stake, in fact, is how to establish the preferability of a *particular* moral sense, and the ordering of goods it would secure, over alternative moral senses and their orderings of moral goods. Without a solution to this difficulty, one will not be able to appeal to a disinterested observer in order to decide, for example, whether it is preferable painlessly to kill severely affected neonates, which would die anyway, or simply to let them die. Such a decision would require the capacity to weigh alternate benefits and harms. That capacity will in turn depend on making reference to one of many competing hierarchies of benefits and harms, each grounded in an alternative moral sense.

It will not help here to multiply the number of impartial observers as Rawls has done in his hypothetical-contractor theory. John Rawls, in attempting to determine the grounds for identifying just social institutions, appeals to an intellectual device in which one is invited to imagine oneself establishing the basic principles of justice that would govern the constitution and laws of the society into which one will be born.[31] Rawls suggests that one would want to attempt to increase one's share of the primary social goods (rights and liberties, powers and opportunities, income and wealth) as long as this would not be at the expense of one's share in equal liberty.[32] In addition, one would not want to risk losing an acceptable amount of the primary social goods in order to secure the possibility of acquiring an even greater amount of these goods.[33] He therefore invites us to picture a number of rational contractors who are equally ignorant with respect to what their future places in society will be, what their natural assets or abilities will be, what conception of the good they will have, the special features of their psychology, the particular circumstances of the society, or even the generation, into which they will be born.[34] Such strategically ignorant contractors, not knowing what their position will be, should agree, Rawls contends, on an unequal distribution of the primary social goods only if such a distribution were to "the greatest benefit of the least advantaged, consistent with the just savings principle," given that such primary social goods are "attached to offices and positions open to all under conditions of fair equality of opportunity."[35] In addition, Rawls holds that such rational contractors would value liberty more highly than other primary social goods. This approach has been widely applied in discussions of what would count as just distribution of medical resources.

Rawls's view presupposes that such rational contractors also have a particular moral sense. They must (1) rank liberty more highly than other societal goods; (2) be risk aversive; (3) not be moved by envy; and (4) not assign a very high ranking to such goods as living peaceful lives in a state of nature.

On the last point, consider the BaMbuti, the pygmies who inhabit the forests of Zaire. They move about the forest in small bands, living in small villages in relative harmony and free from warfare. They do not invest energies in accumulating goods that could save defective children born into their groups or the elderly in need of special health care.[36] Thus, though they live in near-Rousseauean, idyllic circumstances, they violate the just-savings principle of Rawls. Would they, under the principles of Rawls, be morally compelled to abandon their traditional ways of life? Ought one to hold their society to be unjust, if they could now join the larger society of Zaire and provide health care for such defective children or needy elderly, though such interventions are likely to disturb the cultural integrity of the BaMbuti living in the forests? May the BaMbuti legitimately reject such help because they value their own way of life more highly? The answer will turn on the moral sense of the rational contractors to whom one appeals in order to resolve the issue. It will depend on how they rank particular harms and benefits. In short, Rawls presupposes the legitimacy of a particular moral sense. He is best understood as having engaged in a much more limited, but still important, goal of providing a rational reconstruction of the moral world of a liberal member of the Cambridge, Massachusetts, community.[37]

Fourth, attempts to discover a concrete view of the good life, or of justice through analysis of rationality, neutrality, or impartiality, suffer from the same difficulties as hypothetical-choice theories (e.g., impartial-observer theories and rational-contractor theories). One must know beforehand which sense of rationality, neutrality, or impartiality one ought to choose. Appeals to reason alone will provide only logical constraints, but not moral content. One might think of Bruce Ackerman, who in his *Social Justice in the Liberal*

State imports concepts of entitlement into his neutrality principle in order to impeach privileges due to success in the natural lottery (e.g., being born healthy) and social lottery (e.g., being born rich), even when those privileges do not involve trespasses against others.[38] In short, Ackerman attempts, by embracing a particular liberal interpretation of neutrality, to disallow libertarian arguments such as those of Robert Nozick,[39] who accepts the results of the natural and social lotteries. The importance of rival analyses of rationality can be put into perspective, if such enterprises are understood as rational reconstructions of *particular* liberal theories of justice, not as the establishment of *the* theory of justice. However, when faced with the problem of choosing a just pattern or model of health care distribution, one will need to decide what is *the* just approach.

Finally, one will not be able to resolve moral quandaries simply by an appeal to the structure of reality or to so-called natural law. In order for the character of reality to serve as a criterion for resolving moral disputes, it must be shown to be morally normative. One must be able to show that the general tendencies of nature were established by God, not to test the abilities of humans to redirect them, but to guide humans to their proper goals. To establish such a proposition would require special religious or metaphysical premises not open to a general secular defense. In order to know whether the general tendencies of nature or the structures of reality are to be acknowledged as morally instructive rather than confronted as challenges to human manipulative capacities, one must have standards by which to judge states of affairs or structures of nature or reality to be good or bad, as being that to which one ought to submit or that which one ought to set aside. But the availability of such standards is what is at issue. One must have such standards by which to judge whether what is natural is good or bad. Nature, and the laws of nature, are not by themselves morally normative (a point we will examine further in chapter 5). The traditional sources for moral standards appear unpromising when fashioning a general secular ethic.

On the brink of nihilism

One must appreciate the enormity of this problem. It bears not only against theories of justice, but also against morality generally. If rational arguments are not forthcoming to disclose some lines of conduct as immoral, then the approach to medicine of Albert Schweitzer's hospital and the Nazi death camps will be equally defensible or indefensible. In short, one sits on the brink of a nihilism as one contemplates these difficulties. There appear to be no ways to discover the concrete character of the good life, because one cannot establish an objective method to decide when the morally deviant are also the morally wrong. Even if one attempts a defense of secular ethics on the basis of arguments that are not reducible to intuitionist, consequentialist, or hypothetical-choice arguments, or analyses of the nature of rational choices, such arguments are likely to fail as well and for similar reasons. All concrete moral choices presuppose that a particular moral sense can be identified as authoritative. The difficulty is in establishing any particular concrete moral sense. The force of this point may seem academic to those who live in the embrace of a well-established, commonly accepted moral framework (e.g., Orthodox Jews, Amish, Southern Baptists). However, the general framework for common peaceful actions across communities will be absent, given the failure of the enterprise of philosophical ethics. The action of the oppressor and the saint will be equally justifiable or lacking in justification, at least in general secular terms.

This difficulty is particularly perturbing because Western culture has presumed that there is a fabric of natural law in terms of which one can judge the rightness or wrongness of actions across cultures and times. Such presumptions have guided Western law from the time of the Roman Empire to that of modern times and the Nuremberg trials.[40] Gaius speaks of "the law that natural reason establishes among all mankind [and which] is followed by all people alike, and is called *ius gentium* [law of nations or law of the world] as being the law observed by all mankind."[41] This is a point repeated in the *Institutes of Justinian* [42] and Blackstone's *Commentaries on the Laws of England*.[43] The failure to develop a perspective from which one could rationally choose from among competing views of natural law brings the entire set of moral canons into doubt.

To summarize the difficulty, in order to establish the authority of any particular moral perspective, one will need to establish the authority of a particular moral sense. Establishing the priority of any particular moral sense will require a moral sense to choose the right moral sense. One will have the same difficulty in the case of the selection of that second-order moral sense, and so on *ad indefinitum*. As a consequence, one will not be able to establish, outside of particular, already accepted, moral viewpoints, which concrete moral claims are right or wrong. The prospects for ethics as a serious intellectual undertaking seem, as a result, as bleak as the actual cacophony of competing claims would appear to suggest. It would seem that there cannot be a rational basis for choosing one set of moral views over any others, outside of considerations of one's own personal advantage. So if one were to try to compare the morality or immorality of an Adolf Hitler or a Dietrich Bonhoeffer, one would find no general principles to sustain a conclusion as to which was morally correct. There would be no general basis for distinguishing between the practice of gaining the free and informed consent of research subjects and the practice of pressing subjects into service. Judgments may vary according to inclinations or perceived self-interest.

General grounds for distinguishing morally between such alternatives would not appear to exist. One is left standing on the yawning abyss of nihilism. All bioethics is thus brought into question insofar as it aspires to be anything more than an exegesis and application of the moral presuppositions of a particular culture or world view.

Ethics and the resolutions of controversies: a closer look at the brink

Much can be regained for ethics by remembering what in fact one could hope for from ethics. To ask an ethical question is to seek a rational answer, a ground other than force for resolving a controversy. Ethics is at the very least a means for resolving controversies regarding proper conduct on bases other than direct or indirect appeals to force as the fundamental basis for a resolution. Put in this way, ethics is an enterprise in controversy resolution. Controversies regarding which lines of conduct are proper can be resolved on the basis of (1) force, (2) conversion of one party to the other's viewpoint, (3) sound argument, and (4) agreed-to procedures. The grounds for the resolution of moral controversies are of crucial importance, for they provide the authority for public policy. One must distinguish in this regard between resolutions through what one might term *cloture* (main force) and resolutions that satisfy the intellectual question regarding the correct solution. Using force, even legally authorized force, to close abortion clinics would be by itself simply an act of force. An appeal to force will not answer the ethical question as a *rational* question regarding why the controversy ought to be resolved in a particular fashion. Brute force is simply brute force. A goal of ethics is to determine when force can be justified. Force by itself carries no moral authority.

Justification for the resolution of a moral controversy has often been sought in a commonly held moral viewpoint, a viewpoint to which all in a community have in one sense or another been converted. In great proportion, the appeal to "conversion" involves one of the traditional Western hopes for the resolution of moral controversies. The Christian West, especially prior to the Reformation, envisaged a single authoritative moral viewpoint, available through divine grace, and interpreted by the singular authority of the church, and in particular that of the pope.[44] It completed and fulfilled what reason disclosed regarding the *ius gentium*.[45] The fragmentation of Christendom and the development of a more secular spirit called this ideal into question as a historical possibility.[46] Moreover, the appeal to a transcendent God and His grace cannot resolve controversies in a secular society. Since, by definition, the decisive premises in such a context are available only through divine revelation and grace, they will not be accessible to those not so blessed. Force will need to be employed to coerce those not so favored, and that force will not be justifiable in general rational terms. Religious controversies, which involve other than true believers, will as a result be resolved by force and without the benefit of a generally defensible justification. Such actions will then be against the possibility of a peaceable, generally defensible morality. Indeed, the Christian states of the Middle Ages were without moral authority in much of what they did, as the history of the persecution of Jews and heretics attests.[47] The failure of Christendom's hope is in historical terms a major one.

This failure suggests that it is hopeless to suppose that a general moral consensus will develop regarding any of the major issues in bioethics. There will always be minorities who in a free and open society will take vocal exception to any who claim a consensus. This will be the case from the issue of abortion to that of rights to health care. As a consequence, attempts to forge a general consensus will lack the authority of general endorsement.

The third possibility is that of achieving moral authority through successful rational arguments to establish a particular view of the good moral life. This Enlightenment attempt to provide a rationally justified, concrete view of the good life, and thus a secular surrogate for the moral claims of Christianity, has not succeeded. From the French Revolution to the October Revolution, reason has failed to establish a particular view of the good life as morally authoritative.[48] The problem is as outlined earlier. In order rationally to establish a particular concrete understanding of the nature of the good life as morally authoritative, one will need to appeal to a particular moral sense. However, to justify that moral sense one will need to appeal to a yet higher moral sense, *ad indefinitum*. Nor will Marxist claims regarding the inevitability of the triumph of a communist morality secure the normativeness of that viewpoint. Pessimists have long supposed that the morality of the debased and misguided might in the end universally triumph. In short, force, conversion, and sound argument appear to fail as means for resolving moral controversies in a way the stakeholders should rationally hold to be a proper resolution. The only remaining hope is resolution by agreement.[49]

If one cannot clearly establish by sound rational argument a particular concrete moral viewpoint as properly decisive (and one cannot, because the establishment of such a viewpoint itself presupposes a moral viewpoint, and that is exactly what is at stake), then the only mode of resolution is by agreement. Such agreement can be either free or forced. Free agreement can either be on the basis of sharing moral premises for which general justification cannot be given, or on the basis of nonmoral considerations that lead one to agree to a mechanism or procedure for negotiating disputes. Or to rephrase the point, because it does not appear that there will in fact be decisive arguments to establish one concrete view of the moral life to be better than its rivals (or at least as we shall show, beyond certain general constraints), and since usually all will not convert to a single moral viewpoint, canons of moral probity will often need to be created by commonly accepted procedures. For this to succeed generally, one will need to discover an inescapable procedural basis for ethics. This basis, if it is to be found at all, will need to be disclosable in the very nature of ethics itself. Such a basis appears to be available in the minimum notion of ethics as an alternative to force in resolving moral controversies. If one is interested in resolving moral controversies without recourse to force as the fundamental basis of agreement, then one will have to accept peaceable negotiation among members of the controversy as the process for attaining the resolution of concrete moral controversies.

This condition is the minimum condition, because it commits one to no particular concrete moral view of the good life (e.g., the importance of health care vis-à-vis other human undertakings). Such a concrete view would require either arguments that do not appear to be successful (i.e., establishing a particular view of the good life by general moral arguments) or special premises available only within special communities endorsing particular religious, metaphysical, or ideological presuppositions. It is a minimal condition in simply underscoring what it is to resolve issues peaceably and with moral authority. Such a defining condition (i.e., ethics as a means for commonly and peaceably discerning or creating canons of moral probity— what I shall refer to as the morality of mutual respect and summarize under the rubric of a negative principle of autonomy) offers ethics as an enterprise that can be accepted by all participants. It establishes an equally acknowledgeable authority for its conclusions: the conclusions to the process of ethical reasoning are those that peaceable negotiators have all agreed to accept. If a participant in a negotiation refuses to participate because of an interest in resolving the dispute by an appeal to force, even if supposedly morally justified (e.g. "God tells me that abortions are wrong, so therefore we will forbid them by law"), others can retort: "When you use force against the innocent on the basis of moral claims that are not generally justifiable, or agreed to by all parties concerned, you cannot rationally protest when we employ force to protect ourselves from you and reject your supposed authority. What is asserted without proof can as easily be rejoined with a counterassertion. Moreover, rational beings anywhere in the cosmos who are interested in resolving moral controveries peaceably, and in not using force as the primary basis for the resolution of disputes, should understand you to be an enemy of the moral community, and therefore blameworthy, and hold us to have acted correctly." On the other hand, when an individual refuses to participate in a particular agreement, as long as that refusal does not involve the use of unconsented-to force against the innocent (e.g., breaking a promise), one has simply discovered a limit to a particular community or area of agreement, and not a warrant to force cooperation. It is here that one also discovers a fundamental equality among all persons. If no hierarchy of values can be established as canonical, then individuals cannot be subordinated one to the other outside of the agreements of particular communities, or the wishes or actions of the person subordinated (e.g., as a part of just punishment). Moreover, the right of all persons to refuse to participate in any particular community makes each person equal to any other in the right to be left alone and to seek to fashion a community with willing others.

By appealing to the minimum notion of ethics as a means for peaceably negotiating moral disputes, one can disclose as a necessary condition for ethics the requirement to respect the freedom of the participants in a moral controversy. Since moral controversies can in principle encompass all moral agents (and, as we shall see, *only* moral agents), one has a means of characterizing the moral community as the possible intellectual standpoint of persons interested in resolving moral controversies in ways not fundamentally based on force. This view of ethics should not be seen as grounded on a conditional concern for peaceableness. It is not simply based on an interest in establishing the peaceable community. It should, instead, be recognized as a disclosure, to borrow a Kantian metaphor, of a transcendental condition, a necessary condition for the possibility of a general domain of human life and of the life of persons generally.[50] It is a disclosure of the minimum grammar involved in speaking rationally of blame and praise, and in establishing any particular set of moral commitments, other than through force.[51]

Since this is a very radical suggestion, it is worth putting it yet another way. If the expected means for establishing the correctness of a particular moral viewpoint fails, then without some new approach one will not be able (1) to establish *a* particular moral viewpoint as *the* proper moral viewpoint, and therefore (2) one will not be able to establish public policy bodies or individuals as having the moral authority to impose any particular moral points of view by force. Morality would, in fact, lack rational authority, and could at best have authority with a bar sinister, an authority based on force. The foregoing arguments suggest that circumstances are indeed this disparate. The hope of establishing through general secular arguments the moral probity of any particular concrete moral viewpoint appears unfounded. The monotheistic presumption has in short collapsed. However, if authority cannot be acquired through sound arguments, or through the conversion of all to a single moral viewpoint, it can be acquired through mutual agreement. The moral world can be fashioned through free will, even if not on the basis of sound rational arguments with moral content.

Though moral authority does not rest on sound rational arguments establishing the content of the good moral life, the process has a rationality that can lead to the fashioning of a common moral fabric. The general will to have at least a minimum fabric for morality introduces the context of mutual respect and peaceable negotiation. If one is to have reasons for actions that all can accept, one must have reasons that all have endorsed. The use of will to fashion a place for reason in moral discourse is a condition for the possibility of a general and inescapable domain of the endeavor of persons: mutual respect. The foundations of the moral point of view are thus best expressed not in disinterest with respect to personal advantage but rather in terms of mutual respect. Even if one does not attain transcendent rationality, one obtains an immanent, indeed transcendental,[52] rationality for this procedure of will. There is, in short, a remaining means to acquire authority in a straightforward fashion for general secular ethics. If the authority of good arguments and common inspiration fails, the final possibility remains of deriving authority from the consent of those who fashion a community. There is still a generally understandable meaning to acting with moral authority—that is, with the consent of all those involved.

These points concerning the resolution of moral controversies with authority may benefit from a summary. Resolution by force carries no intellectual authority either with regard to (a) what viewpoint is correct, or (b) whether the correct viewpoint *may* be imposed by force. Authority in such cases simply means force to compel. Nor will appeals to conversion by grace suffice for a secular society, though they may for those who form a community of believers who *feel* the force of the grace of common conversion or who are committed to a particular moral sense or set of moral premises. Others outside the community will not. Moreover, grace of conversion or special commitment has no intellectual authority. Sound arguments would have authority, were they able to justify a particular moral viewpoint. However, it does not appear possible for them to secure a concrete view of the good life, though they may be able to establish certain general, abstract constraints. Differences in the ordering of goods and harms offer numerous competing moral possibilities among which one will not be able to choose on the basis of strong rational arguments.

The only remaining source for authority will be common agreement. That is to say, authority can be derived either from force or from peaceable means. The peaceable means include assent on the basis of rational argument or agreement. Where rational argument fails in principle, one is left with agreement. However, agreement can be either on the basis of the conclusion being accepted by all because of all sharing a common moral viewpoint or sense (e.g., through grace of common conversion) or through some form of negotiation. Thus agreement through conversion is a limiting and unlikely (at least for any large society) example of resolution through agreement. The resort to resolution by agreement (hereafter to mean resolution by agreement other than through conversion; resolution by agreement will usually be equivalent to resolution through negotiation) provides authority. One wills rationality and gives authority to the notion of a moral community in asking questions regarding blame and praise, and commits oneself to mutual respect as a means of gaining moral authority, namely, through mutual consent. The use of persuasion, inducements, and market forces is rendered rational as a means of making it worthwhile for individual persons to will to join in particular communal undertakings. Such manipulations, as long as they are peaceable, as long as they do not involve threats of force or unconsented-to interventions that make free choice impossible (this does not foreclose the possibility of peaceably inducing others to agree to make choice impossible— e.g., let's get drunk together, seduce each other, etc.), form part of the proper fabric of a peaceable community. One encounters a way in which rational agents can will on rational grounds (i.e., an interest in being able with reason to hold persons blameworthy or praiseworthy) a general means (peaceable negotiation) for a general community (*the* community of all peaceable moral agents), without presupposing rational grounds for directly justifying the concrete moral viewpoints of particular communities.

Mutual peaceable negotiation emerges as the lynchpin of public authority in general and of authority in health care in particular. With the advent of the Reformation (which is the historical metaphor for the unlikelihood of common conversion) and with the collapse of the Enlightenment hope of delivering a secular, rational justification of the authority of a singular concrete understanding of the good life (which is the historical metaphor for the failure of reason to establish a particular concrete view of the good life), one is still left with a process for peaceably creating such a concrete viewpoint.

Mutual respect, peaceable negotiation, and the way out of nihilism

By conceiving of a moral community and therefore of the possibility for a minimum content for moral language and for justified blame and praise, individuals afford a general intellectual standpoint through which they can yet save something for ethics and thus for bioethics. The moral community is the intellectual standpoint through which one envisages resolving issues in ways not based on force, and therefore potentially with authority. It is the general intellectual framework through which one can hold certain actions to be blameworthy (i.e., as actions against moral authority) or endorsable (i.e., as actions with moral authority). Every time one acts to protect the innocent against unconsented-to force, one appeals to the authority of this community. When one enforces contracts because the parties had agreed to such enforcement, one appeals to the notion of a moral community that has its roots in this general possibility of holding certain actions blameworthy (i.e., those employing some variety of unconsented-to force, including deception, in a contract). Since a particular community will have only that authority that the individuals who constitute it grant to it, insofar as one will wish to speak of secular moral authority, one will have to respect the freedom of each individual as a condition for the possibility of that general secular moral community's authority. Respect of the freedom of individuals is thus a constraint (but it is not necessarily a value pursued, i.e., individuals can consistently decide freely not to value freedom highly) on public policy as a condition for the possibility of moral authority and leads to the practice of acquiring free and informed consent in health care.

This point must be underscored. Even with the failure to establish generally the authority of a particular moral sense, one can still have authority for common actions in pursuit of particular moral goods. One can secure a justification for moral judgments for certain biomedical policies. The authority is that of common assent. There is general meaning in the assertions, "We may do this for all involved have agreed"; "No one may use force with authority against the unconsenting innocent, for they have not consented either directly or indirectly through refusing to forbear from the use of unconsented-to force against other innocents", "If individuals act against moral agents without their consent, their action is without authority and rational beings anywhere in the cosmos can see that such actions place those individuals outside of a community with moral authority. Such persons are then blameworthy in that one is justified in using force in defense against them. That is, they are worthy of having their wishes thwarted in such a circumstance." In short, a form of moral discourse is secured for secular ethics, even though a general justification of traditional concrete ethical viewpoints fails. One is able to establish a procedural ethic, based on respect of the freedom of the moral agents involved, even without establishing the correctness of any particular moral sense. One can see why one may not use unconsented-to force against the innocent, even if one cannot establish a particular view of the good life or of the canons of moral probity (i.e., such actions would be without authority and all interested in moral discourse, in resolving moral controversy in ways not fundamentally grounded in force, could justifiably employ defensive force). These conclusions have major direct implications for practices such as paternalism and truth telling in medicine. Health care professionals will need to determine that they are acting with authority, with the consent of those involved.

I am offering what could be seen as a transcendental argument for Robert Nozick's principle of freedom as a side constraint.[53] The principle of mutual respect is a necessary condition for the possibility of a major endeavor of persons: rationally justified blaming and praising. Just as certain conditions must be presupposed for the very possibility of scientific reasoning, so here one finds a basic, minimum presupposition of ethics.[54] As such, this analysis has the character of unpacking a tautology. Such circular reasoning (i.e., reasoning from the notion of ethics as the enterprise of resolving moral controversies without a fundamental recourse to force, to the principle of respecting the freedom of the participants in a controversy as the basis of ethics) is tolerable if it discloses the character of a major element of the lives of persons.[55] It provides a useful moral insight. It shows that although one will not be able to discover the lineaments of the proper concrete view of the good life, one will be able to indicate the rationale for its fashioning.

This analysis suggests also how to address a major modern quandary: the problem of establishing the authority for ethical claims ingredient in public policy. Within a secular, pluralist society, not only will one not be able to identify who has embraced the *true*, concrete view of the good life, but agreement to moral claims by simple pluralities of the individuals involved in a controversy, or by majorities of two-thirds or three-fourths, also will not provide authority, unless *all* can be presumed to have agreed in advance to such procedures. One might think here of individuals wishing to acquire contraceptives, have abortions, take hallucinogens, or end their own lives. Laws forbidding such, even if enacted by a majority of three-fourths of the populace, are not simply of dubious authority, but may properly be seen to be attempts to use unconsented-to force against the innocent. To see clearly that majority decisions do not of themselves have a moral force, one might consider here, as a heuristic example, the prospect of adopting a new amendment to the United States Constitution: "One year after the adoption of this amendment, all avowed atheists or known abortionists may be shot at dawn by local church committees. Trials will be held according to local church laws of evidence and procedure." Were such an amendment to be adopted, it would be as legal as the eighteenth amendment, or currently proposed amendments against abortion. The question would be the extent to which such an amendment would possess any greater moral authority than the moral propositions held by a large, impressive, powerful, well-organized, and self-righteous mob. These reflections on the authority of governments have implications not only for the government regulation of health care, but for the authority of health care establishments and professionals as well.

The early government of Texas provides an interesting example of how these ideas developed within one variant of the American tradition. In this, the Republic of Texas can be seen as having departed most completely from the Aristotelian view of the city-state with its common moral consensus. When the founders of the Texian republic came to conceive of the authority of the state, they were even more powerfully influenced by deist and anticlerical sentiments than were the founders of the American republic.[56] As a consequence, the Texas Declaration of Independence, in somewhat perfervid tones, denounced the priesthood as an eternal enemy of civil liberty, an

ever-ready minion of power, and a usual instrument of tyrants.[57] The Texians
are best interpreted not as denouncing simply a particular priesthood, but
any moral orthodoxy imposed by force. Further, the Texian Bill of Rights,
articulated in the Constitution of the Republic and repeated in the first Texas
State Constitution (1845), portrays the government as the creation of free
individuals, and fundamental rights as those prerogatives free individuals
can never be presumed to have ceded to a government.[58] Thus, section 1 of
the Bill of Rights outlines a right to revolution: "All political power is
inherent in the people, and all free governments are founded on their
authority, and instituted for their benefit; and they have at all times the
inalienable right to alter, reform, or abolish their form of government in such
manner as they may think expedient."[59] The final section exempts the entire
Bill of Rights from revision. If a Bill of Rights lists natural rights in the sense
of those prerogatives that have not been ceded to a government, such a
government would have no authority to amend or change them. Section 21 of
the Constitution of 1845 states: "To guard against transgressions of the high
powers herein delegated, we declare that every thing in this 'bill of rights' is
excepted out of the general powers of government, and shall forever remain
inviolate . . ."[60] The authority of the government is thus derived neither from
God nor from a particular vision of the good life, but from the uncoerced
consent of moral agents who fashion a common thing, a *res publica*. The
most general chracteristics that mark *good* public policy are not its goals but
the procedures for its fashioning. The state and other societal endeavors can
first and most generally be identified as having moral authority in terms of
their springing from the consent of those involved. Particular visions of the
good life must come through the consent of those involved.

One thus confronts a major shift from the myth of the authority of a
majority, which can now be at best understood as the *Realpolitik* of
respecting overwhelming social force, to the recognition of moral authority
in public policymaking as derived from the consent of particular individuals.
Instead of attempting vain measures to derive a moral authority for a group
in terms of its organization, control of a particular territory, or its aspirations
to a particular form of moral rectitude, one will need to explore the extent to
which the moral authority of public policy (here policy bearing on health
care) can reasonably be seen to be derived from the agreement of those
involved. Further, the attempt to establish such authority discloses at once
the limits of such authority. The moral limits on such authority can be
expressed through a list of individual, or "natural," rights, where "natural
rights" are those that one can never presume individuals to have ceded,
without threat of force, to a social organization. These rights (which are a
function of the fact that a moral universe is fashioned by the collaboration of
individuals) are indefinite and include such rights as the right to use

contraception, to have abortions, and to commit suicide. These rights are secure against majoritarian decisions. Even a vote of all save one for their abolition does not affect their moral standing. Such rights are reminders that a community's authority over an individual in his actions with himself or consenting others is radically limited because such actions are a private issue unless those individuals either violate the conditions of a peaceable community generally or agree to submit their private lives to a particular community's regulation. Thus, in general, women have a basic moral right to seek an abortion with the help of a consenting physician.

This view of the state may appear disturbing in that states and political theory have been so influenced by the Aristotelian ideal of a state that forms a morally cohesive whole. Aristotle had as his model the city-state, which as he argued should not be larger than can be taken in at a single view (*Politics* 7.4.1326b), that is, not more than one hundred thousand citizens (*Nicomachean Ethics* 9.10.1170b). It is ironic that Aristotle conceived of politics in this backward-looking fashion, though he tutored Alexander the Great for Philip of Macedon, who fashioned one of the first major large-scale states. The problem is that of fashioning a large-scale state spanning numerous moral communities that have analogies with city-states, but whose communities are not bound to a particular circumscribed geographical location. As a consequence, a large-scale state must act as a neutral vehicle for spanning numerous communities with often diverse views of the good life.

Since this view of public authority will appear to some to be a radical suggestion, it is worthwhile remembering why one is driven to accept it. One accepts this view because of the difficulty of giving a general secular argument to justify a particular concrete view of the good life, and therefore of any public endeavor fashioned to support it. In that ethics is a rational endeavor, one is seeking the most general rational foundation for morality. The governmental theory actually presumed in enterprises such as the Republic of Texas *in part* reflected the force of this post-Enlightenment problem. One is in search of a rational mode of resolving moral controversy with moral authority, though there does not appear to be a rational mode for discovering the concrete character of *the* good life. The core of secular morality will as a result be procedural and set within the constraints of mutual respect. The study of morality will involve examining the ways in which individuals can agree to courses of action and the extent to which they retain rights of self-determination. Such explorations will be central to understanding the moral character of the interactions of health care professions and their patients and clients. It will be central as well to understanding the proper role of governments in regulating health care. The approach offered here requires viewing moral controversies in biomedicine as public policy disputes that are to be resolved peaceably by agreeing to procedures for creating moral rules based on the principle that force cannot be used against the innocent without their consent. Authority in health care is therefore contractual. Since the web of explicit and implicit consent is usually very complex, it will often be difficult to chart exactly when consent has taken place. It will often not be at all clear what one ought to do or where obligations exist. However, one should do the best one can under prevailing circumstances. Anything worth doing well is worth doing poorly, if conditions do not admit of greater perfections.

The example of Texas is instructive. Unlike Athens, which can be taken as the metaphor for the political assumption that the concrete character of the good life can be rationally disclosed, and Jerusalem, which can be taken as the metaphor for the political assumption that the concrete character of the good is disclosed by God, Washington-on-the-Brazos (the first capital of Texas) presents the image of all-too-human persons acting within the political constraints of mutual respect to create a political fabric where each can, with willing others, fashion the concrete substance of the good life. The Texian Republic stood as an inheritor of the pagans who gathered in the Althing in A.D. 930 at Thingvellir, a site chosen by Grim Goat-Shoe, thirty miles east of Reykjavik. It is from that pagan tradition, of which the Icelanders were a part, that we draw our jury system and our respect for the rights of individuals. However, one does not need to choose among Athens, Jerusalem, and Reykjavik, for Reykjavik (or Washington-on-the-Brazos) affords a peaceable place for the pursuit of Athens and Jerusalem, which might otherwise be places of despotism.

The two tiers of the moral life

These reflections are not meant to suggest that one must conduct oneself as a patient or physician only within the sterile context of a secular ethic that neutrally spans numerous actual moral communities. It is only within a particular moral community that one will receive instruction about when it is worth stopping smoking for better health prospects, accepting amputation and aggressive cancer treatment for a better chance of a five-year survival, or playing an active role in the choice of one's treatment rather than letting the physician decide. It is only within the embrace of a particular community that one learns whether it is right or wrong, worthwhile or not, to do the things one has a secular moral right to do. The domain of secular ethics does not exhaust the universe of ethical reflection. Secular ethics is, after all, explored in order to resolve the quandary of facing numerous competing concrete moral viewpoints.

In this volume I will use *community* to designate a voluntary association of individuals through a common concrete view of the good. I will use the term *society* to designate the associations of individuals who do not share a common concrete view of the good, though they may pursue a number of important goals together. Thus societies in this sense may encompass individuals from a number of communities. One must note that, insofar as a society brings together various communities around common goals and tasks, a higher order community is created. A consensus is fashioned, even if limited. Societies are thus also communities. When I use the term *society*, I will be underscoring the areas where consensus does not exist.

It is within particular moral worlds that one lives and finds full meaning in life. There one is a Roman Catholic, an Orthodox Jew, or a Texian deist. It is only within such communities that life and its pleasures and sufferings can take on full significance. It is in such communities that one learns what promises one should make. Only on the general secular level can one discover that breaking promises to a patient is usually a form of using unconsented-to force against the innocent. Within a particular community, however, one can also learn whether it is better to suffer the pains of a prolonged fatal illness or to avoid this through suicide, whether it is better to raise with love a defective child or to prevent its birth through prenatal diagnosis and abortion, whether it is better to accept sterility or to hire a surrogate mother. Such choices can be made only against the backdrop of a concrete understanding of values. Indeed, what I have termed moral communities give instruction regarding a whole range of values other than simply moral values. They offer an articulated view of the meaning of things. In delivering health care, one will need to attend to the peculiarities of practice within particular communities: devout Irish Catholics in South Boston, Protestant Wends in central Texas, Jewish homosexuals in San Francisco.

It is within particular moral communities that one finds a full and concrete moral life. Only in terms of the values that direct such communities does one learn which moral and nonmoral goods ought to be pursued, at what costs, and for what goals. And again, it is in such value contexts that young physicians and nurses learn through "role models" a particular view of good health care. Particular moral communities show us possibilities for understanding goodness, evil, and meaning in life. One might consider, in fact, the various moral communities as experiments in the building of moral worlds. They are creative endeavors of the spirit to fashion a view of the good life. In their diversity they are instructive of the range of ways in which individuals can experience the good life and can understand the goods of health care. They express the creative power of the human spirit in appreciating meaning in human birth, growth, sexuality, health, sickness, suffering, and death.

Because the differences in the composition of moral goods in competing moral viewpoints are often aesthetic in nature, some being more beautiful, well composed, or alluring than others, one is frequently best instructed in their character through stories of heroes, legends of saints, novels, poems, and plays. To appreciate their virtues, one must see what it would be like to live a moral life of a particular kind.[61] Surely this is why role models are instructive with regard to the character of a concrete view of the good life or of good medical practice. It is here, in fact, that literature can play a major role in the education of health care professionals. It can play that role as well for persons generally who will be patients. Further, if there are no generally sustainable, secular arguments to establish a particular view of the good life, and as long as the ways of life under consideration respect the freedom of the innocent, then choices among them will appear, from outside any particular moral community, to be aesthetic choices. There will, in short, be a number of moral viewpoints unexcludable on the basis of secular moral arguments. For example, is it better to be a devout Southern Baptist, a Texian deist, or a homosexual San Francisco atheist? Each is likely to carry special risks or advantages with respect to future morbidity, mortality, and quality of life. Is it better to practice medicine as a cosmetic surgeon, an abortionist, or an internist? Is it morally better to practice with profit as a central motive, or instead as a part of a nonprofit church clinic? In many circumstances, secular arguments will give little or no guidance. From the outside, for the unconverted, the choice will not be a moral choice in the strict sense of a choice one could hope to universalize. Instead, one can best understand someone's choice as a choice of that view of the good life, which, according to his sentiments, is the richest and most encompassing and appropriate. However, such choices cannot, as was shown earlier, be decisively demonstrated to be morally authoritative on the basis of sound arguments.

There will be a possibly strong contrast between the understanding of a particular moral community from within that community versus that from without. From within a particular religious group, it may appear self-evident that it is wrong, through a wrongness sustained by the Deity's disapproval and the very essence of being, to commit suicide, even when faced with the final weeks of debilitation due to cancer. Those who live in such a moral community will see their position as one that all *ought* morally to embrace, but they will not have general moral arguments to sustain their viewpoints. They can at best hope to convert through persuasion, not to resolve the issue on the basis of sound arguments. Rather, as my arguments suggest, since respect of freedom is core to the grammar of secular ethics, individuals will have a general, rationally defensible right to commit suicide. From the outside, then, an individual contemplating the moral instruction provided by a religious community that forbids suicide will properly attempt to assay how all of its commitments congeal into a coherent and full moral life. In the end, the outside observer may conclude that such a particular way of life provides in sum the best of lives and endows even one's death with meaning, so that it is clear that one ought not to commit suicide. However, that judgment will not be the assent of the true believer, moved by the grace of religious conversion. (Nor will it be the conclusion of a decisive secular moral argument.) It would instead be the sort of judgment one might expect from an individual at home in a secular, pluralist society, who is seeking to develop an understanding of life that will provide meaning and community.

Such choices are often made by individuals in many of the world's urban centers, where one has the opportunity to "shop" for intellectual and moral insights from various religious and cultural "traditions." One might think here of the ways in which Catholics, Protestants, Jews, and Moslems in cities such as Atlanta, London, Hong Kong, Istanbul, and Berlin have come to depart from their "traditional" orthodox views regarding contraception, abortion, and artificial insemination by donor, by incorporating moral viewpoints with roots in classic pagan times and in contemporary philosophical reflections. Or even more, one might think of how the religiously half-believing piece together from various quarters a sense of the meaning of pain, suffering, and disease. To the true believer, such attempts to assemble in an eclectic fashion a moral view may appear often shoddy, shallow, and lacking in true commitment. Such is the price of the peaceable tolerant community.

For the true believer, or for the person who would wish to be a true believer, the situation may be frustrating, if not intolerable. One is bereft of the opportunity for total and unrestrained commitment to one's belief. One is restrained from believing so firmly as to intrude into the freedoms of others. Perhaps many of the middle-class children who join revolutionary groups do so as part of a metaphysical quest for such an allconsuming dedication. They experience their lives as empty, or lacking a meaning that only selfless and unrestrained commitment could provide. The balance—the tolerance, the *sophrosyne* required by secular pluralist societies—is empty, insipid, and effete in comparison to the consuming commitment that can be felt as a member of the Baader-Meinhof gang, of the Communist party, of the National Socialist party, of the Inquisition, or for that matter of any religious or ideological group ready for consecration of self and of all to what is felt to be the truth. Such individuals seeking total commitment usually find themselves in a society with muted tones of dedication. A peaceable secular pluralist society of necessity speaks in material terms that can reach across particular communities of belief. It may be too difficult for such individuals to take inspiration from the virtues of temperance and *sophrosyne,* from the balanced worship of many gods and goddesses. They do not feel able to pursue their goals within moral enclaves as do the Hasidim or Amish, aspiring at most to convert through witness, never coercion. They are not content to live peaceably, as others worship strange gods.

Yet one is morally constrained to acquiesce in what one might term the triumph of the polytheistic presumption. Though one may not be committed to the worship of many gods, or to acknowledging that other gods are better perhaps than one's own, one is committed to acknowledging that there are other gods, radically different construals of the good life, and that in a secular pluralist society, individuals will be free to be influenced by their allure. The significance of medicine and its advances will differ greatly from moral community to moral community, and strong moral grounds to disallow a particular moral viewpoint often will be lacking.

Here again, one must realize that secular ethics, and therefore secular bioethics, is an enterprise in public policy making. Secular bioethics is not the attempt to live within, or appreciate the implications of, a particular view of the good life and of the canons of moral probity. It is rather a solution to the problem of common action by individuals drawn from diverse moral communities with competing views of the good life. Since it is an attempt to secure moral authority and purpose for common action across moral communities, it always presupposes the existence of a number of competing moral viewpoints and the richness of the moral life they contain. Taken by itself, secular bioethics would be an empty framework.

We are left with a dialectical understanding of the nature of ethics. While on the one hand recognizing an absolute though abstract grammar of ethics, one must recognize as well the plurality and relativity of concrete moral viewpoints. Though much of ethics is irremediably subjective and relative, there is as well an objective and absolute conceptual core. There is an intersubjective fabric to ethics in virtue of the very understanding of ethics as an alternative to the resolution of disputes through force. For example, though there will not be a generally defensible moral view regarding whether the use of abortion to prevent the birth of a fetus with Down's syndrome is morally exemplary or morally evil, it will be clear that women will have the right to have abortions, given the availability of willing abortionists. It will be a right sustainable in general, secular ethics, though within particular moral communities it may be held to be wrong to exercise such a right.

Since our analysis of ethics shows a tension between ethics as a procedure and ethics as content, between ethics which at its conceptual core turns on respect for the freedom of moral agents and ethics which in its concreteness involves the pursuit of particular goods, it will often be sensible to say, "The patient has a right to do that, but it is wrong." The moral universe is complex; there will be no assurance of compatibility between respect of moral agents, and the concern to achieve particular goods. There will not necessarily be compatibility among the various competing views of the good life or of good health care. In fact, given the divergence of moral inclinations, one could expect with confidence that the tension among the various possibilities for a concrete moral life will lead one to make tragic moral choices. In choosing a particular moral viewpoint as one's own, one will have to exclude whole worlds of moral value. One might think of the small child seeking a model for a good Christian life. One might imagine his being sent to a compendium of the lives of the saints, where he comes upon stories about St. Francis and St. Olaf. How ought he to choose between pursuing the virtues of St. Francis of Assisi (1182–1226) in his loving and kind attention to all animals, human and nonhuman, or the virtues of the warrior Saint Olaf Haraldsson (995–1030), who died at Stiklestad on Friday, July 29, 1030, trying his best to slay enemies and defeat the allies of King Canute?[62] General secular arguments will not provide conclusive guidance for the choice of a particular moral viewpoint if one presumes Olaf did not employ unconsented-to force against the innocent.

The moral life is lived within two tiers or dimensions: (1) that of a content-poor secular ethics, which has the ability to span numerous divergent moral communities, and (2) the particular moral communities within which one can achieve a contentful understanding of the good life. The first is defensible in terms of general moral arguments regarding the nature of ethics. This tier offers some absolute and universal moral conclusions, even if they are content poor. The second tier offers competing visions of the good life, including concrete accounts of virtues and vices. Here arguments are not conclusive and often, if not usually, require accepting certain basic premises that cannot be secured by argument. It is the first dimension that can establish a patient's right to know the truth about his illness and to be fully informed prior to treatment. It is the second dimension that will indicate whether it is better to try to know all about one's own treatment, or whether it is better instead to repose one's trust in one's physician.

Physicians, nurses, and other health care workers, as a consequence, come to pay complicated moral roles. First, as the foregoing shows, they must live their moral lives within two moral worlds, or within two moral dimensions or tiers. The first is that of the moral community from which they draw their concrete understandings of the good life, and within which they conduct their contentful moral undertakings. It is in terms of that world that they know what commitments they ought to make, what promises they ought to bind themselves to keep, what things are worth living and dying for. It is within such a moral context that one learns about concrete virtues and vices and is instructed in the formation of a good character, within a particular under-standing of that term. However, insofar as they recognize that the moral presuppositions that structure their own concrete moral world cannot sustain that moral worth with a general moral authority for all, they must recognize the possibility of the neutral lingua franca of a secular pluralist society. Even if they practice medicine or nursing within a Seventh Day

Adventist community and hospital, or in a devout Catholic community and hospital, they must recognize that they have created, and are sustaining, a special moral exclave. The more they come in contact with others who do not share their moral presuppositions, the more they will be forced to recognize recurringly that they live not only within their own moral community, but also within a secular pluralist moral fabric that reaches across communities and binds together individuals of disparate moral communities in common moral presuppositions. For instance, the Roman Catholic gynecologist who is opposed to contraception and abortion will need to come to terms with the fact that women will have a secular pluralist moral right to an abortion, although abortion is morally wrong in the eyes of that physician. The physician will need to develop means of warning patients about the range of services provided and of referring patients to other physicians when there is a conflict of moral intuition.

In giving such warnings, health care professionals take on the role of quasi-bureaucrats who remind patients of their rights and regarding circumstances under which their rights may come to be compromised. This metaphor of the health care worker as bureaucrat can illuminate the role that physicians and nurses must play when they may meet patients as moral strangers (a point we will explore in chapter 7). Where one in fact does not share the moral presumptions of those with whom one works, one must seek ways of protecting against misunderstandings. Bureaucratic rules and formulations are inevitable in such circumstances. They provide formal guidance where informal understandings cannot be presumed. They are attempts to meet the goal of protecting rights when individuals meet as moral strangers, as they characteristically do in large-scale secular pluralist societies. Here one might think of various stylized rules for obtaining free and informed consent (e.g., Institutional Review Boards and consent forms). Such are needed when it is not clear that those involved share the same assumptions regarding what best interests concerning health and well-being are to be secured by medical interventions and research.

Physicians and nurses will also play the role of geographers of values and rights. They will come to know, through their experience, what it is to be sick with particular diseases, or to be dying in particular ways. It will be they who can inform patients about the consequences of different choices of treatment, and with respect to the likely outcome of adopting particular illness or dying styles. To play this role as geographers, they will need to know the moral fine texture, not only of the secular pluralist moral framework, but also of the particular moral communities of particular patients. To do this, they will need to learn to take seriously divergent views of the good life. In living their moral lives on two tiers, they will need to be geographers within two dimensions of the moral life.

This chapter began with the case of a thirty-six-year-old woman seeking amniocentesis to determine whether her fetus had Down's syndrome, with a view to obtaining an abortion in the event that it did. This chapter leads to a complex understanding of such quandaries and their solutions. There will be no straightforward yes or no answer. One will instead be left with an understanding of the woman's rights within secular, pluralist moral terms, while recognizing that within particular moral viewpoints, her action may be seen as either morally opprobrious, or in fact a moral obligation, not simply a moral option. Within the geography of some particular moral viewpoints, her decision to carry a child with Down's syndrome to term may be seen as an unfair disregard for the best interests of other children she already has, and whose thriving may be harmed if that fetus is allowed to become a person. In short, these reflections support the judgment that she has a secular moral right to choose her course of action, even if within particular moral viewpoints her action may be seen to be wrong.

As the next chapter shows, such geographies of bioethical quandaries also reveal major points of tension within the moral life not simply between dimensions of the moral life, but between the major principles of morality: autonomy and beneficence. Physicians and nurses are recurringly confronted with the conflict between respecting the freedom of patients and doing that which is in their best interests. As geographers of values and rights, health care workers will need to become expert in introducing patients to the character of these tensions and to their moral consequences. Thus, one might add to the case of the pregnant woman the fact that she suffers from mitral valve disease, with the consequence that the pregnancy would entail a risk to her health, and perhaps to her life. If she wished to carry the pregnancy to term, in secular (and in fact within certain religious) contexts one would have a major conflict between what was in her best interests and what she had freely chosen. It is to this sort of conflict that we will turn next.

Notes

1. Hook reports the estimated prevalence at birth of Down's syndrome in maternal age group twenty years as .06 percent; twenty to twenty-four years as .11 percent; twenty-five to twenty-nine years as .29 percent; thirty to thirty-four years as .31 percent; thirty-five to thirty-nine years as .40 percent; forty to forty-four years as 1.27 percent; and forty-five years as 4.15 percent. See E. B. Hook, "Estimates of Maternal Age-Specific Risks of a Down-Syndrome Birth in Women Aged 34–41," *Lancet* 2 (July 1976); 33–41.
2. English estimated in 1975 that each of the 4,000 mongoloids born annually requires about $250,000 worth of care in his or her lifetime. See D. S. English, "Genetic Manipulation and Man," in T. R. Mertens (ed.), *Human Genetics: Readings in the Implications of Genetic Engineering* (New York: Wiley, 1975), pp.

95–108. Joseph Fletcher puts the implications of this point somewhat strongly. "It is cruel and insane to deprive normal but disadvantaged children of the care we could give them with the $1,500,000,000 we spend in public costs for preventable retardates." See "Costs and Benefits, Rights and Regulation, and Screening," in T. Mappes and J. Zembaty (eds.), *Biomedical Ethics* (New York: McGraw-Hill, 1981), p. 476.

3. In a study carried out under the auspices of the National Institute of Child Health and Development, two false negatives were reported among a total of 1,040 participants. Maternal cell contamination was suspected as responsible for this finding. No false positives were reported. See U.S. Department of Health, Education, and Welfare, *The Safety and Accuracy of Mid-Trimester Amniocentesis* (Washington, D.C.: National Institute of Child Health and Human Development, 1978, DHEW Pub. No. (NIH) 78–190), pp. 12, 38, 44. One could, however, envisage such false positives occurring through laboratory error in labeling samples.

4. Or as Kant said, "The principle of the analogies is: Experience is possible only through the representation of a necessary connection of perceptions." A176 = B 218, p. 208. Also, "The conditions of the *possibility of experience* in general are likewise conditions of the *possibility of the objects of experience.*" Norman Kemp Smith (trans.), *Immanuel Kant's Critique of Pure Reason* (New York: St. Martin's Press, 1964), A158 = B197, p. 194. Though my exegesis of the categorial conditions for knowledge and morality has a highly Kantian accent, they could in principle be recast with benefit in more Hegelian terms. A Hegelian categorial account would place the argument fully within the terms of reason and avoid the Kantian difficulty of mediating between the sheer givenness of the object and the predicament of the finite knower. Here is not the occasion to show how the concerns of the finite knower can be placed within a general categorial understanding. The reader may wish to consult sections 445 through 450 of G. W. F. Hegel's *Encyclopaedia of the Philosophical Sciences* (1830). See also Klaus Hartmann, "The 'Analogies' and After," in L. W. Beck (ed.), *Proceedings of the Third International Kant Congress* (Dordrecht, Holland: Reidel, 1972), pp. 47–62; and "On Taking the Transcendental Turn," *The Review of Metaphysics* 78 (December 1966): 223–49.

5. As Kant stated: "Hitherto it has been assumed that all our knowledge must conform to objects. But all attempts to extend our knowledge of objects by establishing something in regard to them a priori, by means of concepts, have, on this assumption, ended in failure. We must therefore make trial whether we may not have more success in the tasks of metaphysics, if we suppose that objects must conform to our knowledge." *Kant's Critique of Pure Reason,* B xvi, p. 22. "We can know a priori of things only what we ourselves put into them." Ibid., B xviii, p. 23.

6. In Kant's words,

It [the transcendental unity of apperception] is indeed the first principle of the human understanding, and is so indispensable to it that we cannot form the least conception of any other possible understanding, either of such as it is itself intuition or of any that may possess an underlying mode of a sensible intuition which is different in kind from that in space and time. (B139, p. 157) We can therefore have no knowledge of any object as thing in itself, but only in so far as it is an object of sensible intuition, that is, an appearance.... (B xxvi, p. 27)

7. With certain qualifications, there is no conflict between my position and that of Kant. He is reasonably to be understood as reconstructing the ways in which we experience reality through sensible intuition. He never considered that there might be, as in astrophysics and in quantum physics, modes of understanding other than Euclidean and Newtonian. Kant, however, realized that our mode of intuition need not be unique.

   This mode of intuiting in space and time need not be limited to human sensibility. It may be that all finite, thinking beings necessarily agree with man in this respect, although we are not in the position to judge whether this is actually so. But however universal this mode of sensibility may be, it does not therefore cease to be sensibility. (B72, p. 90)

8. For an interesting study on this point, see Ludwik Fleck, *Entstehung und Entwicklung einer wissenschaftlichen Tatsache. Einführung in die Lehre vom Denkstil und Denkkollektiv* (Basel: Benno Schwabe, 1935); the English translation is *Genesis and Development of a Scentific Fact*, ed. T. J. Trenn and R. K. Merton, trans. F. Bradley and T. J. Trenn (Chicago: University of Chicago Press, 1979).

9. See, e.g., G. W. Hegel, *Wissenschaft der Logik* (Stuttgart-Bad Cannstatt: Friedrich Frommann, 1965), part 1, pp. 61–5. My view of Hegel presumes a nonmetaphysical interpretation as developed by Klaus Hartmann in "Hegel: A Non-Metaphysical View," in Alasdair MacIntyre (ed.), *Hegel: A Collection of Critical Essays* (New York: Doubleday Anchor, 1972), pp. 101–24. See also Klaus Hartmann (ed.), *Die ontologische Option* (Berlin: Walter de Gruyter, 1976).

10. One might think here of the closing passage of Hegel's *Philosophy of Nature* where he notes that in studying nature we will find the mirror of ourselves and the reflection of spirit. See *Philosophy of Nature*, ed. and trans. M. J. Petrie (London: Allen & Unwin, 1970), vol. 3, sec. 376, Zusatz, p. 213.
   One might recall also Hegel's passage on toleration in which he argued against "Physician," and "Precepts."

11. See, for example, "The Art," "Decorum," "Law," "Physician," and "Precepts."

12. See, e.g., Samuel A. Cartwright, "Synopsis of Medical Etiquette," *New Orleans Medical and Surgical Journal* 1, 2 (1844): 101–104; and Medical Association of North Eastern Kentucky, *A System of Medical Etiquette* (Kentucky: Maysville Eagle, 1839). For a study of the development of American codes of medical ethics, see Donald E. Konold, *A History of American Medical Ethics, 1847–1912* (Madison, Wis.: The State Historical Society of Wisconsin, 1962).

13. *Code of Medical Ethics Adopted by the American Medical Association at Philadelphia in May, 1847, and by the New York Academy of Medicine in October, 1847* (New York: H. Ludwig, 1848).

14. As Tony Honoré indicates, the Greeks in close-knit city-states did not draw a sharp contrast between custom and law; *nomos* meant both. In contrast, Latin possesses *mos* (manner, custom, fashion) and *consuetudo* (custom, habit, usage) set apart from *jus* (right, law, justice) and *lex* (law). See Tony Honoré, *Tribonian* (Ithaca, N.Y.: Cornell University Press, 1978). The distinction among customs, codes of etiquette, and law becomes necessary as one is brought to act across communities of belief. A Greek city-state attempted to encompass one community. In contrast, Rome attempted to embrace various communities in one impartial system of laws. Rome also, with its developed polytheism, endeavored to embrace various religions, thus requiring further distinctions between what was law and what fell within particular customs.

15. One might think here of Hegel's view of the state as a neutral matrix of freedom

spanning numerous communities, which embrace different views of the good life. One might think also of Hegel's passage on toleration in which he argued against the anti-Semites of his day by holding that Jews should have full civil rights in the state. The state should not be Christian or Jewish, but a neutral framework that can peaceably embrace various communities of belief. Hegel argued:

> The fierce outcry raised against the Jews from that point of view (that they should be considered a foreign race) and others, ignores that fact that they are, above all, *men;* and manhood, so far from being a mere superficial, abstract quality, is on the contrary itself the basis of the fact that what civil rights rouse in their possessors is a feeling of oneself as counting in civil society as a person with rights, and this feeling of selfhood, infinite and free from all restrictions, is the root from which the desired similarity in disposition and way of thinking comes into being.

See Hegel, *Philosophy of Right,* trans. T. M. Knox (London: Oxford University Press, 1965), sec. 270, p. 169. This view of the state as a neutral matrix spanning communities is suggested also in the passage in which Hegel characterizes civil servants as the universal class. See *Philosophy of Right,* sec. 303.

16 As of June 1981, only twenty-five states (Alaska, California, Colorado, Connecticut, Delaware, Hawaii, Illinois, Indiana, Iowa, Maine, Massachusetts, Nebraska, New Hampshire, New Jersey, New Mexico, New York, North Dakota, Ohio, Oregon, Pennsylvania, South Dakota, Vermont, Washington, West Virginia, and Wyoming) apparently placed no restrictions on consenting adults engaging in oral intercourse. In contrast, other states may impose anywhere from six years maximum penalty (see, e.g., Nev. Rev. Stat. 201.190 [1973]) to twenty years maximum penalty (see, e.g., Ga. Code Ann. 26-2002 [1972]; Mont. Rev. Codes Ann. 94-5-505 [Spec. Crim. Code Pamphlet 1976]) for consensual sodomy. One should note also that the state of Virginia, which emblazons on bumper stickers "Virginia is for Lovers", under its code forbids as a felony "crimes against nature—if any person shall carnally know in any manner any brute animal, or carnally know any male or female person by the anus or by or with the mouth, or voluntarily submit to such carnal knowledge, he or she shall be guilty of a Class 6 felony." See Code of Virginia, sec. 18, 2-361.

17. Morton Hunt, *Sexual Behavior in the 1970s* (Chicago: Playboy Press, 1974), pp. 198–199. Later studies continue to support these findings, noting further the increased frequency of oral intercourse reported by married males and females. See Carol Tavris and Susan Sadd, *The Redbook Report on Female Sexuality* (New York: Delacorte Press, 1976), p. 88; and Anthony Pietropinto and Jacqueline Simenauer, *Beyond the Male Myth* (New York: Times Books, 1978), pp. 201–202.

18. Jehovah's Witnesses refuse blood transfusions on the basis of their reading of the passages of the Bible that forbid eating blood or meat full of blood. See Deuteronomy 12:22–23; Leviticus 19:26. Such restrictions appear to survive in the New Testament as well; see Acts 15:20. These passages in the Old Testament are the basis of Jewish laws of kosher, but they are interpreted by the Jehovah's Witnesses as also forbidding transfusions.

19. Catholic Theological Society of America, *Human Sexuality: New Directions in American Catholic Thought* (New York: Paulist Press, 1977), pp. 114–128. A more radical approach would be to find the changes not in human understandings alone, but in the rules embraced by God.

20. I use *metaphysics* to identify general a priori accounts of the character of reality, which are rationally defended but are transcendent in the character of the explanations they offer. They are accounts that at best recommend themselves,

one over the other, in terms of parsimony, elegance of explanation, and vision. Here one might think of accounts of the nature and existence of God or of an immortal soul. I use *ontology* to identify accounts of the basic concepts through which reality as we experience it must be understood. Were there space to develop a more categorial understanding of ontology, one would need to expand the concept of experience and allow of a categorial reconstruction of more than the Newtonian realm of experience to which Kant turns. Ontology, as I will use it here, provides the general concepts through which experienced reality exists and is known, or through which general and inescapable human practices are constituted. I have in mind claims concerning the nature of causality or of persons, which can be decided among in terms of which best accounts for the general character of experience or of a general human practice. Ontological accounts, in contrast to metaphysical accounts, appeal to empirical facts or the character of human practice, and do not refer to transcendent realities. Disputes regarding ontological accounts can be settled by showing that claimed basic concepts are not presupposed by and ingredient in experience or in the practices for which they are advanced in explanation. Thus, a claim that infants are persons as adults are persons is clearly false. *Person* here should be understood as identifying a general category of experienced reality and therefore as being an element of an ontological account. The claim that both infants and adults have souls would be either a metaphysical or a religious claim, depending on whether speculative or religious considerations were advanced to support the claim.

21. Paul Ramsey, *Fabricated Man* (New Haven, Conn.: Yale University Press, 1970), p. 133.

22. N. R. Hanson, *Perception and Discovery* (San Francisco: Freeman, Cooper, 1969)

23. I. Lakatos and A. Musgrave (eds.), *Criticism and the Growth of Knowledge* (Cambridge: Cambridge University Press, 1970); the work of Fleck with regard to the history of syphilis is also pertinent (see n.8). One should note as well that this volume influenced Thomas Kuhn, *The Structure of Scientific Revolutions* (Chicago: University of Chicago Press, 1962).

24. For a study of the laetrile controversy, see H. T. Engelhardt, Jr., and A. Caplan (eds.), *Scientific Controversies: A Study in the Resolution and Closure of Disputes Concerning Science and Technology* (Cambridge: Cambridge University Press 1985).

25. This is a well-discussed problem. Philosophers from A. J. Ayers in *Language, Truth, and Logic* (London: Peter Smith, 1935) to Charles Stevenson in *Facts and Values: Studies in Ethical Analysis* (Westport, Conn.: Greenwood Press, 1962, reprinted 1975) have raised the issue in modern times of whether moral claims can in any sense be true or false or whether they simply express emotions or function as ways of persuading others to join in common action.

26. J. Cook, *Captain Cook's Journal 1768–71,* ed. Capt. W. S. L. Wharton (London: Elliot Stock, 1893), pp. 91–95.

27. Colin M. Turnbull, *The Mountain People* (New York: Simon and Schuster, 1972), p. 135.

28. Henry Sidgwick, *The Methods of Ethics,* 7th ed. (London: Macmillan, 1907), pp. 338–342.

29. Roderick Firth, "Ethical Absolutism and the Ideal Observer," *Philosophy and Phenomenological Research* 12 (1952): 331–341.

30. Richard B. Brandt, *A Theory of the Good and the Right* (Oxford: Clarendon Press, 1979).

31. John Rawls, *A Theory of Justice* (Cambridge, Mass: Harvard University Press, 1971), pp. 17–22, 126–142. An exposition of the original position in more timeless terms is found in the chapter entitled "The Kantian Interpretation of Justice 'as Fairness'" (pp. 251–257). See also pp. 195–201 for an exposition of the relationship between the original position and the framing of constitution and laws. One should note that the strong similarity between ideal observer theories and hypothetical contract theories is appreciated by Robert Veatch. He states that "an ethic rooted in a social contract is, with these emendations, not at odds with the view that the moral order can be discovered. ... The model of contractors trying to discover the moral order is not very different from the one where contractors create or invent the moral framework." Robert M. Veatch, *A Theory of Medical Ethics* (New York: Basic Books, 1981), p. 124. This coincidence between ideal observer and social contract approaches derives from the fact that Veatch does not have real individuals participating in his social contract, but rather model contractors, that is, individuals to whom he can impute the proper moral sense and whose actual freedom he does not need to respect.

It is in terms of these presuppositions that Veatch develops his triple contract theory of medical ethics, which includes a basic social contract, a contract between society and the medical profession, and the contract between the individual professional and the patient. Ibid., p. 138.
32. As Rawls puts it, "... persons in the original position have no desire to try for greater gains at the expense of the equal liberties" (*Theory of Justice.* p. 156).
33. For Rawls, an acceptable amount of the primary social goods should be that amount distributed in accord with the two principles of justice. See, in particular, his formulation of the Second Principle, part (a), p. 302, in *Theory of Justice.*
34. Ibid., p. 137.
35. Ibid., p. 302.
36. For an interesting account of the BaMbuti, see Colin Turnbull, *Forest People* (New York: Simon and Schuster, 1961); and *Wayward Servants: The Two Worlds of the African Pygmies* (Westport, Conn.: Greenwood Press, 1965).
37. Rawls at times suggests the limited nature of this endeavor. He states, for example, at the end of *Theory of Justice:*

It is perfectly proper, then, that the argument for the principles of justice should proceed from some consensus.... Certainly, the argument for the principles of justice would be strengthened by showing that they are still the best choice from a more comprehensive list more systematically evaluated. I do not know how far this can be done. I doubt, however, that the principles of justice (as I have defined them) will be the preferred conception on anything resembling a complete list. (Here I assume that, given an upper bound on complexity and other constraints, the class of reasonable and practical alternatives is effectively finite.) Even if the argument I have offered is sound, it only shows that a finally adequate theory (if such exists) will look more like the contract view than any of the other doctrines we discussed. And even this conclusion is not proved in any strict sense. (p. 581).

38. Bruce A. Ackerman, *Social Justice in the Liberal State* (New Haven, Conn.: Yale University Press, 1980).
39. Robert Nozick, *Anarchy, State and Utopia* (New York: Basic Books, 1974). Consider, for example, Nozick's summary of his maxims of justice, "From each as they choose, to each as they are chosen" (p. 160).
40. The actions of the International Military Tribunal during the Nuremberg trials presuppose the notion of natural law. Though the character of the tribunal, in describing war crimes, crimes against peace, and crimes against humanity does

not explicitly make mention of natural law or of the *ius gentium*, it is the most
reasonable way to understand the full authority of the tribunal. In article 6, the
tribunal clearly states that it will not be a defense against charges of crimes
against humanity that the actions were "not in violation of the domestic law of
the country where perpetrated." "Charter of the International Military Tribunal
II, Art. 6c," *Trial of War Criminals* (Washington, D.C.: U.S. Government
Printing Office, 1945), p. 16. Though in the "Report of Robert H. Jackson to the
President," published as a preface to the *Trial of War Criminals,* an attempt is
made to justify the jurisdiction on the basis of past treaties, the author as well
appeals to Hugo Grotius's distinction between just and unjust wars, a distinction
drawn from natural law arguments.

41. As Gaius states, "Quod uero naturalis ratio inter omnes homines constituit, id
    apud, omnes populos peraeque custoditur uocaturque ius gentium, quasi quo
    jure omnes gentes utuntur." *Institutes of Gaius,* trans. Francis De Zulueta
    (London: Oxford University Press, 1976), p. 3, vp. 1.

42. In Justinian's words, "The law of nature is that law which nature teaches to all
    animals. Though this law does not belong exclusively to the human race, but
    belongs to all animals..." Flavius Petrus Sabbatius Justinianus, *Institutes of
    Justinian,* trans. Thomas C. Sandars (Westport, Conn.: Greenwood Press, 1922,
    reprinted 1970), Book I. 2, p. 7.

43. Blackstone speaks of the laws of nature that one is able to discover through the
    faculty of reason. These laws of nature are

    the eternal, immutable laws of good and evil, to which the creator himself in all his
    dispensations conforms; and which he has enabled human reason to discover, so far as they
    are necessary for the conduct of human actions. Such among others are these principles:
    that we should live honestly, should hurt nobody, and should render to every one his due; to
    which three general precepts Justinian has reduced the whole doctrine of law.

    See William Blackstone, *Commentaries on the Laws of England,* ed. St. George
    Tucker (New York: Augustus and Kelly, 1969), vol. 1, p. 40. One should note
    that the laws of nature so put are extremely abstract. The nature of honesty is not
    specified nor the nature of harm to others, much less what is due to another.

44. For historical accuracy, one must note that during the Middle Ages there were
    disputes regarding whether the pope or ecumenical councils possessed the final
    authority to resolve disputes. An endorsement of the preeminence of conciliary
    authority is found in the statement of March 30, 1415, by the Council of
    Constance, which affirmed that the authority of the council was in fact superior
    to that of the pope. It held that the council "had authority directly from Christ,
    and that everyone of whatever status or dignity, even if he were the pope, is
    bound to obey it in that which pertains to faith." *Conciliorum Oecumenicorum
    Decreta* (Basil: Herder, 1962), p. 384 (author's translation). Popes generally took
    the opposite view. In fact, the views of the conciliar movement were explicitly
    condemned. See, for example, the bull "Exsecrabilis" of January 18, 1460.
    Henricus Denziger (ed.), *Enchiridion Symbolorum,* 33d ed. (Rome: Herder, 1965),
    p. 345. A good overview of this dispute is provided by Heido A. Oberman et al.
    (eds.), *Defensorium Obedientiae Apostolicae et Alia Documenta* (Cambridge,
    Mass.: Harvard University Press, 1968). The issue of papal supremacy was then
    finally articulated by the First Vatican Council on July 18, 1870, when the
    doctrine of papal infallibility was promulgated.

45. Traditional Catholic doctrine, as it developed, saw reason as able to disclose the
    fundamentals of natural law or the *ius gentium*. See, e.g., the encyclical of Pope

Pius XII, "Summi pontificatus" of October 20, 1939. This point is also made by the First Vatican Council.

This Catholic doctrine has deep roots in Christian tradition. One might consider, for example, chapter 2, verses 12 to 16, of St. Paul's Epistle to the Romans, where Paul argues that the Gentiles have known the ordinance of God, even if they did not benefit from the written law of Moses. In this argument, Paul anticipates a long tradition of Christian natural law theory concerning the accessibility through reason alone of the laws of God.

46. As an example, here one might think of Thomas Paine's critique of Christianity in the *Age of Reason*.

47. One must appreciate that in the Middle Ages it was accepted that heretics, in particular heretics who would not repent or who had lapsed for a second time into heresy, were to be killed. This view is clearly enunciated in St. Thomas Aquinas's *Summa Theologica* II Q. xi Art. 3 and 4. As already noted, it also is reflected in the constitutions of the Fourth Lateran Council (1215), which held that "Catholics who truly take up the cross and give themselves over to the extermination of heretics, shall enjoy the same indulgence, which is given by sacred privilege to those who go to the Holy Land." *Conciliorum Oecumenicorum Decreta*, p. 210 (author's translation).

Who counted as a heretic became more complex after the Reformation, in that not only the Roman church but the various heretics, having now established churches in their own rights, proceeded to exterminate heretics. One must remember that the use of the writ "de haeretico comburendo" (the writ issued for the burning of a heretic) continued into the seventeenth century. No doubt such a writ would have been issued by the authorities of those times against both the author of this volume and many of its readers.

48. An excellent assessment of the consequences of the collapse of the Christian and Enlightenment hopes is provided by Alasdair MacIntyre in *After Virtue* (Notre Dame, Ind.: University of Notre Dame Press, 1981). I, unlike MacIntyre, hold that there is a vindication for a shred of the Enlightenment dream: the rationality of resolving moral controversies through agreement. However, MacIntyre makes a major contribution in outlining the modern predicament, which is defined in part by the remnants of its predecessors' cultures. It is the monotheist presumption of both the Christian synthesis and the Enlightenment, which has misled ethics into a search for definitive rational grounds for establishing a particular concrete moral viewpoint as morally authoritative.

49. I am very much in debt to Tom L. Beauchamp for his article, "Ethical Theory and the Problem of Closure," in Engelhardt and Caplan (eds.), *Scientific Controversies*, pp. 27–48.

50. I use *transcendental* here to identify an argument that lays out the conditions for the possibility of a major domain of human experience of action. As defining conditions, they are a priori. Here I am influenced by Kant, who underscores morality's presupposition of freedom (e.g., *Critique of Pure Reason*, B xxviii–B xxix; *Critique of Practical Reason*, 31, 43f, 46), but who failed to distinguish between freedom as a value and freedom as a side constraint. I too underscore the presupposition of respect of freedom as the necessary condition for the possibility of the rationality of morality, and therefore of blame and praise. Justified blame and praise (e.g., blame and praise that is due another, not just useful to assign) presupposes grounds for showing some actions to be right or wrong. The minimum rationality required for this moral nexus is provided by respect of the

freedom of the members of a moral controversy. That principle provides the minimum coherence of morality.

51. Think here of Ludwig Wittgenstein's remarks relating grammar and ontology: "Essence is expressed by grammar." *Philosophical Investigations,* trans. G. E. M. Anscombe (Oxford: Basil Blackwell, 1963), sec. 371. Or, "Grammar tells us what kind of an object anything is" (sec. 373). In this sense, grammar shows the possibility for the coherence of a dimension of human meaning. For a consideration of transcendental arguments in Wittgenstein, see Stanley Cavell, "Availability of Wittgenstein's Later Philosophy," in George Pitcher (ed.), *Wittgenstein: The Philosophical Investigations* (New York: Doubleday, 1966). Cavell states, for example, that "we could say that what such answers are meant to provide us with is not more knowledge of matters of fact, but the knowledge of what would count as various 'matters of fact'. Is this empirical knowledge? Is it a priori? It is a knowledge of what Wittgenstein means by grammar—the knowledge Kant calls 'transcendental'" (p. 175).

52. Kant restricted transcendental claims to areas of theoretical knowledge rather than morality and did not extend it to claims about morality. "I entitle *transcendental* all knowledge which is occupied not so much with objects as with the mode of our knowledge of objects in so far as this mode of knowledge is to be possible *a priori.*" *Kant's Critique of Pure Reason,* A11 = B25, p. 59. However, there is no reason so to restrict the realm of transcendental arguments. See especially Klaus Hartmann, "On Taking the Transcendental Turn," pp. 224–25. See *The Critique of Pure Reason,* A12 = B25. Here I extend the notion to the sphere of moral experience.

53. Nozick's presentation of freedom as a side constraint is inadequate. It is offered in his account somewhat as a given. Here, I have attempted to show its rationale and necessity, to show the central and essential warrant for its place in moral reasoning, by casting it in a radically different context—that of a transcendental argument.

54. My account of ethics portrays it as one of a number of major domains of possible experience and action. Unlike Kant, I underscore the transcendental conditions for morality, not just those of experience. Even in Kant's writings there are some suggestions as to how to proceed with regard to giving a transcendental account of morality. In addition to the ways in which one might regard Kant's writings concerning ethics, one should note that in the preface to the second edition of the *Critique of Pure Reason* Kant notes that we can have a priori knowledge either through determining the object of our knowledge or through making the object actual (B ix–x). What is provided in this chapter is an account of the necessary conditions for the possibility of fashioning a moral world. Whatever strengths or weaknesses transcendental accounts may possess in other areas, at least here they offer a means for understanding how the very conditions of morality are grounded in our character as persons. For an account of some of my views regarding the development of transcendental arguments, see *Mind-Body: A Categorial Relation* (The Hague: Martinus Nijhoff, 1973). See, e.g., *The Critique of Pure Reason,* A783 = B811 through A790 = B818; and A808 = B836.

55. One might think here of Hegel's argument that philosophy justifies itself within a circle of thought. The more encompassing the circle, the more powerful the explanation. See, e.g., *The Encyclopedia of the Philosophical Sciences* (1830), sec.17.

56. The Texas Declaration of Independence, March 2, 1836, in Ernest Wallace (ed.), *Documents of Texas History* (Austin: Steck, 1963), p. 98.

57. The phrase reads in its entirety, "the army and the priesthood, both the eternal enemies of civil liberty, the ever-ready minions of power, and the usual instruments of tyrants." Ibid., p. 98.

58. The Constitution of the Republic of Texas, March 17, 1836, and the Texas Constitution of August 28, 1845; *Documents of Texas History*, pp. 100–106, 146–159.

59. The Texas Constitution of August 28, Article 1, sec. 1, ibid., p. 149. This passage in the Constitution of 1845 is taken from the second right in the Declaration of Rights of the Republic of Texas (ibid., p. 105). This passage occurs as well, with only slight alterations, in the current Constitution of the State of Texas.

> All political power is inherent in the people, and all free governments are founded on their authority, and instituted for this benefit. The faith of the people of Texas stands pledged to the preservation of a republican form of government, and, subject to this limitation only, they have at all times the inalienable right to alter, reform, or abolish their government in such manner as they may think expedient.

See, Constitution of the State of Texas, art. 1, sec.2.

60. The Texas Constitution of August 28, 1845, art. 1, sec. 21, *Documents of Texas History*, p. 150. This passage exists as well in the current Constitution of the State of Texas. See art. 1, sec. 29.

61. Stanley Hauerwas, *A Community of Character: Toward a Constructive Christian Ethics* (Notre Dame, Ind.: University of Notre Dame Press, 1981).

62. Sigvat is quoted by Snorre Sturlason in the *Heimskringla* as giving the following characterization of Olaf Haraldsson:

> Some leaders trust in God—some not;
> Even so their men; but well I wot
> God-fearing Olaf fought and won
> Twenty pitched battles, one by one,
> And always placed upon his right
> His Christian men in a hard fight.
> May God be merciful, I pray,
> To him—for he ne'er shunned the fray.

Olaf Haraldsson is now regarded by Catholic and Protestant churches alike as the patron saint of Norway. See Snorre Sturlason, *The Heimskringla,* trans. Samuel Laing (London: Norroena, 1906), vol. 2, p. 645.

3

The Principles of Bioethics

At the very roots of ethics there is a tension. It springs from the difference between respecting the freedom and securing the best interests of persons. This tension is recurringly reflected in health care. Patients frequently choose to engage in behaviors that physicians and nurses know to be dangerous, possibly disabling, and in the end perhaps lethal. Out of respect for those persons, physicians and nurses must often, if not usually, tolerate noxious lifestyles or failures to comply with treatment. Yet physicians and nurses, in joining the health care profession, have consecrated themselves to achieving the best interests of patients. The discussions in the last chapter suggest that this tension is a radical one. This chapter will sustain that suggestion by elaborating two conflicting ethical principles: that of autonomy and that of beneficence. It is in terms of the contrast between these two principles that the moral tension felt in many choices regarding abortion, treatment compliance, or refusal of health care is to be understood. Autonomy and beneficence are principles in two senses. First, they summarize under two headings a range of moral problems and concerns. But they are also principles in the sense of indicating two different roots for the justification of moral concerns in health care.

Autonomy and beneficence: the conflict at the roots of bioethics

The will to morality and the problem of intersubjectivity

As the last chapter shows, there are major problems in reaching a rationally justified resolution of bioethical quandaries in secular pluralist societies.

66

When the premises held in common are insufficient to frame a concrete understanding of the moral life, and if rational arguments alone cannot definitively establish such premises, then reasonable men and women can establish a common fabric of morality only through mutual agreement. The concrete fabric of morality must then be based on a will to a moral viewpoint, not upon the deliverances of a rational argument. The moral point of view in its most generally definable sense will be that intellectual standpoint from which one understands that conflicts regarding the propriety or impropriety of a particular action can be resolved intersubjectively by mutual agreement, and which viewpoint one then embraces in order to enable an inter-subjectively grounded practice of blaming and praising, of mutual respect, and of moral authority. The moral fabric sustaining the various forms of the moral life is then a general practice that is as unavoidable as is the interest in resolving moral disputes.

One can find a similarity with the practice of intersubjectively establishing empirical knowledge claims. Though one cannot guarantee that the principles of induction will succeed in the future, if one is interested in the intersubjective establishment of knowledge claims, one can then in general terms provide the canons for justifying particular empirical knowledge claims, should such ever be possible.[1] Insofar as such knowledge claims can be established intersubjectively, they will presuppose approaches that can be described as inductive. One can without any metaphysical presuppositions or assurances indicate the necessary conditions for a very general and human practice: the development of empirical generalizations.[2] So, too, one need not be sure that an actual moral community will ever be formed. However, one can sketch its necessary conditions while recognizing that actual interests in intersubjectively fashioning a moral world will be required so that both the necessary and sufficient conditions of morality can be satisfied.

For a will to a moral viewpoint to be more than an inclination toward a particular moral viewpoint, it will need to be a will to a moral fabric as general as the very concept of morality itself. Yet an actual ethical life will require a particular concrete moral sense. In being tied to the notion of morality itself, the process of establishing a concrete morality by mutual agreement gains general rational justification in the sense of being coexten-sive with a generally available rationale that is ingredient in the very commitment to resolving moral disputes without recourse to force. If the practice of ethics is to be at least the endeavor of establishing the propriety of actions in ways other than through force, and if the moral senses of individuals are divergent, then the cardinal moral principle will be that of mutual respect in the common negotiation and creation of a concrete moral world.

Since moral fabrics gain particularity by commitment to a particular ordering of the goods of human life, the characterization of *the* moral fabric cannot provide the specification for such a particular ordering. If it did, it would lose its generality. On the other hand, the more the characterization of *the* moral fabric is tied to the very enterprise of being a person, the more firmly it can be generally justified. This is the case, for in asking a question about morals as a philosophical question, one is seeking a rational reply that is, as far as possible, inescapable. One is seeking a clincher to a dispute concerning which of the possible ways one can live life or practice medicine one *ought* to choose, where the sanction for violating the "ought" is not a threat of force or a feeling of guilt, but irrationality, worthiness of blame, or the failure to realize the goods one wishes to achieve. In seeking a characterization of the fabric of morality tied to the fabric of rationality, one is unlikely to secure content to characterize the concrete nature of the moral life.

With the arguments to this point, one can understand why physicians should not treat, experiment on or handle a competent patient without that individual's permission. One has established the basis for strong duties of mutual respect in health care. However, no duties of beneficence have been established. One does not know what goods one ought to pursue, only where one's authority ends. For example, ought one to provide health care for those who cannot pay for it? What are the noncontractual obligations of individuals and societies to do good, not just to refrain from unauthorized actions involving others? What is the good that ought to be done? Obligations to act with beneficence are more difficult to justify across particular moral communities than the principle to refrain from unauthorized force, in that one can have the possibility of coherent resolution of moral disputes by agreement without granting the principle of beneficence. The principle of beneficence is not required for the very coherence of the moral world. It is in this sense that this principle is not as basic as what I will term the principle of autonomy. The principle of beneficence is not as inescapable. One can act in nonbeneficent ways without being in conflict with the minimal notion of morality.

How Kant smuggled concreteness into moral principles

The difficulty of finding a general justification for beneficence is appreciated if one examines Kant's attempt to justify morality. He endeavors to show that to act morally is to act rationally in the sense of acting in ways that are not selfcontradictory.[3] In this fashion, Kant can show that one cannot speak consistently of self-respect and of oneself as worthy of blame or praise (i.e., worthy of happiness or unworthy of happiness) without regarding similar entities with similar respect. Kant elaborates an ethics of respect for persons. However, an appeal merely to self-contradiction does not provide a justification for a principle of beneficence. In fact, as Hegel[4] and Alasdair MacIntyre[5] following Hegel show, Kant does not have an argument that can provide content for ethics. Kant attempts to gain content for his ethics through arguments that depend for their success on (1) a failure to distinguish between freedom as a value and freedom as a side constraint (by securing respect of persons, Kant thinks he has secured the obligation to value autonomy), and (2) an appeal to a form of contradiction, which can be termed a contradiction in will. Under the latter he includes actions, the affirmation of which does not involve a conceptual contradiction (affirming the notion of the peaceable community, while at the same time deciding to use force against the unconsenting innocent, would involve a conceptual contradiction), but which Kant believes one could not in fact will for others without later willing the contrary for oneself (e.g., a refusal to be beneficent to others, though in the future one might wish such beneficence to be shown to oneself).

As to the first point, Kant's principle of respect for his moral law is not simply a constraint on acting against persons without their consent. It affirms freedom as a cardinal value and thus steps beyond the support of his actual arguments, insofar as they are based on the strict fabric of rational argument. The argument would require an appeal to a particular moral sense. Since Kant's arguments require such an appeal, Kant does not allow suicide, though in the case of a competent person there is surely consent.[6] As the preceding section showed, to make any value, including the value of freedom, the cardinal value is to endorse a *particular* ethic. One is doing more than elaborating and justifying the fabric of morality itself by valuing freedom. One can consistently treat all persons as ends in themselves while affirming as a moral maxim that individuals may freely decide when to cease to be free by choosing suicide or a term in the French Foreign Legion. Respect of freedom as the necessary condition for the very possibility of mutual respect and of a language of blame and praise is not dependent on any particular value, or ranking of goods, but requires only an interest in resolving issues without recourse to force. When one has distinguished between freedom as a condition for morality, and freedom as a value, one loses the basis for duties to oneself as well. Or to put it another way, one can freely release oneself from one's duties to oneself, if such duties were to exist.[7] In not highly valuing freedom for oneself, one acts within the constraint of not using unconsented-to force against the innocent. In contrast, a bioethics based on Kant's assertions would lead one not to respect the choices of patients unless they affirmed a contentful principle of autonomy. Patients would not be free to choose in ways that did not affirm freedom as a value (e.g., by committing suicide).

As to the second point, by claiming one cannot without contradiction will to abandon what I term the principle of beneficence, not because of any formal contradiction, but because of a contradiction in one's will, Kant also seeks further content for ethics.[8] Indeed, Kant acknowledges that arguments for duties of beneficence are based not on the impossibility of thinking their opposite. He claims, instead, that one cannot consistently will not to respect the principle of beneficence. To underscore, Kant sees here a contradiction in will, not in logic. This difference marks duties of beneficence, as he acknowledges, not as strict duties, but as meritorious duties. Kant portrays the sentiments of someone who would take this position in the following way: "What concern of mine is it? Let each one be as happy as heaven wills, or as he can make himself; I will not take anything from him or even envy him; but to his welfare or to his assistance in time of need I have no desire to contribute."[9] In response, Kant argues that though one can consistently conceive such as a universal law of nature, it would still be impossible to *will* that such a principle should hold everywhere as a law of nature. "For a will which resolved this would conflict with itself, since instances can often arise in which he would need the love and sympathy of others, and in which he would have robbed himself, by such a law of nature springing from his own will, of all hope of the aid he desires."[10] It is in this sense that Kant relies on a contradiction of will rather than a conceptual contradiction in order to ground a principle of beneficence.

This suggestion by Kant is heuristic. The moral world can be divided into one dimension admitting of strict justification in that it is tied to the notion of the rational life, and a second tied to a notion of sympathy. If one recasts Kant, matters can be put this way: one can regard the misfortune of others and consistently hold that the principle of beneficence as grounded in the notion of ethics spanning various moral communities does not provide strict moral obligations, but only a reasonable moral ideal. This is the case in that nonbeneficent actions do not conflict with the notion of the peaceable community, but rather only with that of the beneficent community. As a consequence, the use of force against peaceable nonbeneficent individuals is without authority, for it is against the notion of the peaceable community, which is the core of secular ethics. In fact, it would render those using such force blameworthy in terms of the core of morality itself. The principle of beneficence is exhortatory, whereas the principle of autonomy is constitutive. As a result, it is easier to determine international standards for free and informed consent in terms of respect of persons, but harder to establish a criterion for an international, decent level of health care.

The principle of beneficence can at least suggest that it would be good to support the provision of goods to persons in need, even if the principle cannot justify the use of force against the nonbeneficent. Thus, it is good for physicians to provide health care free to indigent patients who, for example, are not covered by insurance or Medicaid. Its violation can at least justify the withdrawal of beneficence not owed out of contract or agreement. The principle reminds one of what the moral life can be about—fashioning webs of sympathy through a commitment to providing goods to fellow persons in need. Yet what should count as needs generating moral claims can be determined only in a particular context and often only by multilateral agreement. The obligations of physicians become more substantial, once all members of a medical society have agreed that physicians should attempt, where practical, to provide free care.

One could be tempted to read Kant as unwittingly making a point of prudence in defending his principle of beneficence.[11] However, the issue is more forcefully and more consistently to be understood as a reminder of the necessary condition for the possibility of understanding morality as a reciprocal web of sympathy. The moral life is not exhausted by an account of it as the fabric of a peaceable community. It is also the fabric of mutual sympathy. The question is, how inescapable is this second understanding?

The sanctions for immorality

One should note here the moral sanctions for misconduct. Morality lacks the sanctions of the law and of religion. It cannot of itself execute, imprison, fine, or damn to hell. Morality can demonstrate that certain ways of acting are incompatible with rationality, justify blameworthiness, or impede the realization of the goals of the actors. Morality can also show that defensive or punitive force is justifiable.[12] But in itself it has no physical force. The sanctions of morality are tied to its justification. To use unconsented-to force against the innocent is incompatible with holding that others are wrong in using such force against oneself, or meaning anything more by terming another wrong or blameworthy than that one dislikes the other's conduct and wishes that he and others would refrain from it.[13] In short, the notion of the peaceable community as fashioned by the principle of mutual respect is a cardinal element in the lives of persons. One embraces it as soon as one attempts to talk about morality across moral communities. Not to adopt it is to lose the basis for coherent moral discourse in a secular, pluralist society. The sanctions are intellectual. To raise an ethical question is to raise an intellectual question regarding justifications for action.

The case for beneficence depends not on the coherence of morality, but on the need for content. Unlike the principle of autonomy, which justifies the process for generating content, the principle of beneficence identifies the content of the practice of morality. The principle of autonomy shows that patients may not be used as means merely; the principle of beneficence supports the concrete moral goals to which medicine ought to be directed. However, particular moral senses establish competing rankings of the goods of life. The principle of beneficence in its most general form simply signals the fact that moral arguments center on questions of what is good or proper to do. The difficulty with the principle of beneficence lies in the fact that any specific ranking of goods depends on a particular moral sense and is, therefore, not able to reach across moral communities. This indeed is the core of the difficulty. For example, under what circumstances, and to what extent, do obligations to aid others outweigh the good of having free time at one's disposal to pursue one's own goals? To put things more concretely, how much of one's office practice ought one to devote to free care for the indigent? Ethical disagreement regarding beneficence separates communities of moral commitment because there are no conclusive rational arguments to establish a particular moral sense. The problem of justifying any particular view of beneficence is under such circumstances insuperable.

Insofar as a general portrayal of ethics is possible, which in its generality marks it as integral to the endeavors of persons, then that account of ethics is justified in being an inescapable element of the rational life. It is in this fashion that the principle of autonomy has been justified: it is the necessary condition for the possibility of resolving moral disputes without force and for sustaining a minimum ethical language of praise and blame. It is in this sense formal. It provides the empty process for generating moral authority in a secular pluralist society through mutual agreement. It can show that abortion, contraception, and suicide may not be forbidden with moral authority, but it cannot show that it is good to pay for abortion and contraception for the indigent or to assist rational individuals seeking to commit suicide who need aid. One may contend that the rational life is in addition concerned with the common pursuit of the good. But unlike the appeal to mutual respect through the principle of autonomy, the principle of beneficence requires specification within the terms of a *particular* moral community in order to be of any practical use.

The principle of beneficence is, as a result, more qualified than the principle of autonomy for yet another reason. If someone asks, "Why ought I to do to others their good?" one will not be able to respond, "Because if you don't, you will deny the very possibility of imputability or of moral authority, for you will have denied the principle of respect to persons generally, including yourself." Instead, one can at best retort, "If we do not do to others their good, we will not have affirmed the possibility of what could be termed the kingdom of beneficence, or the beneficent community." The principle of beneficence reflects an interest in the common pursuit of the good life and of mutual human sympathies. It is the ground of what might be termed the morality of welfare and social sympathies.

Humans are social animals, and consequently they tend to conceive of goods socially. However, if some do not, what can one say of them beyond the obvious fact that they are not sympathetic persons?[14] What, in terms of morality, is the sanction for lack of sympathy or beneficence? In the case of violation of the principle of autonomy, the sanction is blameworthiness to the point of losing grounds for objecting to retaliatory force. The individual who violates the principle of autonomy is placed outside the peaceable community. Anyone who uses defensive force against such a guilty person does not violate moral authority, for guilty persons cannot consistently appeal to a principle they have rejected in order to condemn the users of force. The sanction is thus a major one. But if one fails to be beneficent, one has at most cut oneself off from the beneficent community. It is true that one cannot be unsympathetic and consistently claim the sympathy and support of beneficent persons—unless they have contracted to supply such support. In that case, their support would be grounded, not in the principles of beneficence, but in the principle of autonomy. Rejecting beneficence as a principle leads to an essential impoverishment of the moral life, not to its full rejection. Moreover, most will not reject the principle of beneficence outright, but rather only wish to substitute *their* principle for someone else's.

With these reflections in hand, one can now reappraise the sanctions for immorality. First, as has been noted, philosophical arguments will not deliver the sanctions available through certain religious arguments. Philosophers will not be able to demonstrate that particular forms of immorality will lead to eternal torture. Nor does philosophy have the sanctions of the law. It cannot provide fines, imprisonment, or the lash. The arguments examined earlier show that acting against the very notion of the peaceable community makes one blameworthy in the eyes of rational beings anywhere in the cosmos. As a result, one loses any ground for protesting against their defensive, punitive, or retaliative force. As soon as one is interested in ethics as an alternative to the resolution of moral disputes through force, one has committed oneself to mutual respect. And, if one rejects the principle of mutual respect, one cannot rationally protest when others respond with force. Since the questions regarding the sanctions for immorality are intellectual, the sanctions are intellectual. They pronounce outlawry upon the offending individual, a charge against which that person cannot consistently protest as long as he continues in affirming the immoral action. Reflections on autonomy lead to the justification of a morality of mutual respect, whose sanctions are the loss of the grounds for respect and for protest against certain actions by others. Reflections on the morality of beneficence, however, focus on the morality of common welfare. To affirm the morality of beneficence is to affirm the enterprise of the common good, of the fabric of mutual sympathies, which fashions the morality of welfare. To reject beneficence outright is to lose all claim to the sympathies of others. However, to reject a particular principle of beneficence is only to lose claims to the sympathies of others within a particular context or community. In summary, violations of the principle of autonomy justify circumscription of the autonomy of the offender. Violations of the principle of beneficence eliminate claims by the offender to the kind of beneficence rejected for others.

Giving authority and content to the principle of beneficence

What, then, can be said of the principle of beneficence? Must a physician who runs an abortion clinic provide a free abortion for a woman who otherwise would not have funds or means for securing the abortion (we will imagine that state or federal laws have removed public funds)? Does the answer to the question depend on how busy the physician is? Does it depend on whether the woman lives in the physician's local community, or in an adjacent city, or in an adjacent state? What if the physician, though not Australian, had trained in Australia, has an Australian medical license, lives now in Alabama, but is vacationing in Canberra and could at a local clinic run by a friend perform a free abortion for such a woman, who would otherwise not have access to the abortion she wishes? What if, by performing the abortion, the physician misses a visit to an important art museum, a religious shrine, the arrival of the pope in Australia, or a drinking party with friends? When and under what circumstances is the physician obliged because of regard for the principle of beneficence to provide treatment? Does the answer to the question depend on the strength of the need or desire? How does one compare the risk of major social costs (e.g., the woman is single and headmistress of a staid girls' high school; aside from one sexual affair and a willingness to secure an abortion, she is, even in terms of the school's professed criteria, an excellent administrator, and her affair and its consequences are, as of the time of the dilemma, unknown to others; the pregnancy, if continued, would ruin her career) with a risk of death to the woman? What if the woman is married and another child would significantly compromise the family's lifestyle (i.e., they would not be able to afford a modest yearly vacation, a second car, private university education for their children, or two beers a day for the husband and wife)? The difficulty lies in determining when it becomes obligatory to be beneficent, not just praiseworthy. There appears to be no clear answer in the abstract. The range of goods to be achieved and harms to be avoided for humans, as well as other animals, is wide and complex. The correct ordering is in dispute, as well as the point at which needs and desires impose particular obligations. It is important to note that this leads to two major difficulties with duties and rights of beneficence. One must establish (1) their content (which will depend on a particular view of the good life), and (2) their authority (i.e., the authority to require one, rather than another, view of beneficence, including the significance of the circumstances under which inconveniences or contrary inclinations properly excuse one from discharging a duty of beneficence).

The bonds of beneficence, if they are to be established, must be framed through mutual understandings, both implicit and explicit, which establish both content and authority. Only in particular social contexts, within the embrace of particular moral communities, can one discover what are in fact the bonds of beneficence. The bonds of beneficence that tie individuals in special roles of friend, colleague, spouse, parent, child, patient, and physician are *in part* contractual. By this I do not mean to suggest an explicit contract, but a web of usually implicit understandings. Some attempt to impart a special distinction to such understandings by employing the term *covenant*. They undoubtedly wish to suggest a quasi-religious meaning, though the biblical sense of covenant itself is derived from the notion of a treaty, usually made with a conquering force.[15] In any event, one fashions a web or nexus of commitments and understandings, both explicit and implicit, which sustain a fabric of moral understandings. These understandings are usually open to revision.

One can, in many circumstances, choose other friends, colleagues, patients, physicians, or HMO. One can even disown one's parents or children, or adopt children. One can emigrate or move to a new social group with which one has more substantial agreement. Though history, culture, and circumstance constrain such choices, life in a world containing a plurality of moral communities in intimate contact demonstrates daily the possibility of such fashioning and refashioning of social bonds. However, the principle of beneficence at stake here is not one sustained only by a particular moral community. Within a community of BaMbuti, Ik, Patrician Romans of the Republic, or contemporary Orthodox Jews or Mennonite Christians, there is a web of moral understandings that sustains concrete, though often complex, principles of beneficence. In terms of such principles, one is able to sketch in detail the obligations of beneficence of physicians to patients within such particular contexts. However, a principle of beneficence that would span such a diversity of communities could not support a particular ordering of goods, but only the provision of goods in general to persons in general. The principle can at best indicate that special roles of beneficence should characterize such relations. The principle of beneficence is in general simply the principle of doing good.

Because of the divergent understandings of what should count as actually doing the good, one cannot understand the principle of beneficence as the Golden Rule. If one does unto others as one would have them do unto oneself, one may in fact be imposing on others against their will a particular view of the good life. The Golden Rule can thus be (and in fact has been) the basis for the tyrannical imposition of particular concrete understandings of the good life. To avoid such tyranny, one will need to phrase the principle of beneficence in this positive form: Do to others their good. However, insofar as one attempts to do to others what they would hold to be their good, not what one or one's own moral community would hold to be their good, the sense of obligation weakens. First, one's own understanding of beneficence within one's own moral community will set standards for when one is obliged to shoulder what burdens to do good to others. Second, one will need to transfer that view of the proper exchange of burdens for the benefits of others to doing good to an individual in another moral community with a different view of the hierarchies of goods and harms and of the boundary between obligatory and supererogatory actions.

Consider a physician in community A, which holds that access to abortion on request by the indigent is a good that should be supported through all qualified physicians' volunteering to attend at a local abortion clinic once a month. In addition, that community holds that there is no obligation to save the lives of Down's syndrome children with intestinal abnormalities. Hence, no one provides services or feels obliged to provide services or funds to the indigent who might want to save their Down's syndrome children under such circumstances. In fact, community A may hold that saving the lives of such children is a nonbeneficent act to those children and to the community as a whole, which must then support and care for them. Then consider community B, which holds that it is an obligation to provide sufficient funds to save the life of Down's syndrome children born with intestinal abnormalities. However, community B does not hold it obligatory to use noncommunal resources to provide abortions for the indigent. In fact, community B holds that such provision would be nonbeneficent, because having as many children as possible is considered a good for individuals and the community. What are the obligations of the physician in community A to the indigent in community B? Is the physician obligated to provide funds or services to the Down's syndrome children? Should the physician attempt to convince the indigent in community B that it is better to have abortions and to accept funds for the acquisition of same?

Expressing the principle of beneficence in the maxim Do to others their good recognizes that any talk of the best interests of others presupposes a particular judgment about what constitutes those best interests. When one speaks across moral communities, different judges of best interests with different moral senses are presupposed. Moreover, the morality of mutal respect gives to individuals the right to veto the provision of a good they do not want. The more individuals are moral strangers, the more acts of beneficence become supererogatory rather than obligatory. The more individuals share a moral community and a single moral sense, the more clearly defined the moral obligations of beneficence become, and the more there will be an agreement between the giver and the receiver regarding the nature of the good.

An individual may also properly claim not to be obliged to provide a benefit to another because it would more seriously harm others or because it would in fact harm the individual seeking aid. The second case involves an instance of the principle of nonmaleficence, a special application of the principle of beneficence. It underscores the fact that one will not be obliged to provide to others a service one finds clearly and unequivocally to be a violation of the principle of beneficence. Here I use the principle of nonmaleficence as not doing to another a harm to which the individual does not object (and to which the individual presumably consents). Consider a college sophomore who at the end of a passionate love affair reads Goethe's *Die Leiden des jungen Werthers* and comes to the house of a friend to borrow a 16-gauge shotgun with which to commit suicide. Though the principle of mutual respect would not forbid the provision of the shotgun on request, the principle of nonmalefience would. Medical examples may include requests for unjustified surgical procedures, drugs, or other treatments. It will be obligatory or supererogatory to do to others their good, as long as the provision of that good in terms of one's own moral sense is not seen to be a harm. On the other hand, it will be neither obligatory nor supererogatory to provide to another that which one holds to be a harm, unless greater goods will flow to the recipient or to others. (Permission here is presupposed on the part of the recipient.) As an illustration of this point, consider a heterosexual psychiatrist treating homosexuals and holding that heterosexual lifestyles are preferable to homosexual lifestyles. He is willing to agree that a great number of homosexuals indeed want to remain homosexuals and do not wish to be transformed into heterosexuals, and that trying to force them to become heterosexuals will do more harm than good. The psychiatrist might hold that, given the balance of goods over harms, it is not only praiseworthy, but in fact obligatory, to help homosexuals who wish to remain homosexuals to adjust as well as possible to their homosexual lifestyle. On the other hand, he might find it not only blameworthy, but a violation of moral obligations, to comply with a request by a heterosexual who wishes to be "treated" in order to convert to a homosexual lifestyle, because of a supposed contrary balance of benefits and harms.

Other cases will lead to different conclusions. For example, consider the physician who is convinced that the only proper treatment for carcinoma of the breast is radical mastectomy. If that physician is confronted with a patient wanting a surgical excision of the carcinoma, followed by radiation and chemotherapy, may the physician comply, even if he or she does not believe this maximizes the patient's good with respect to survival? The answer here can be yes, in that the physician may also recognize the patient's concerns with function and cosmetic appearance, and may hold that the patient simply has a different hierarchy of values within which she balances maximal life expectancy, maximal cosmetic appearance, maximal use of her arm, and maximal realization of liberty values. The physician may regard the act of providing to the patient the treatment she requests, given its full context, as beneficent. The same may be the case when a fifteen-year-old girl seeks contraceptive information from a physician who does not believe that sexual activity among teenagers is good for them. One might even grant that the physician would hold that the provision of the information might increase the likelihood of adolescent sexual activity. Still, the physician might properly judge that the consequences of an unwanted pregnancy make the provision of contraceptive information and materials on balance a beneficent act.

Here again one must remember the context for the discussion of these moral principles: the attempt to reach across particular moral communities. Just as one must seek a foundation for moral authority across moral communities, one must also seek a characterization of moral content across such communities. The principle of autonomy signals, for example, the need for free and informed consent. So, too, the principle of beneficence, one would hope, would signal across moral communities what is proper to do for patients, such as providing minimal health care or free abortions for the indigent. This does not appear to be possible, at least in any concrete fashion. One is left, rather, with the principles of autonomy and beneficence, which contrast as a general principle of authority and a general principle of the good. As principles spanning particular moral communities, they possess only a minimal content. This circumstance makes the principle of beneficence a general concern for providing others with the goods of life. Even if it is somewhat vacuous, the principle of beneficence is central. Moral quandaries are not just quandaries about who has the authority to resolve moral disputes; they concern as well the character of the goods to be pursued. Indeed, a concrete understanding of the good life presupposes an ordering of goods and harms, as much as any peaceable moral community presupposes authority from its members. As a consequence, morality in a secular pluralist society is the practice of doing the good within the bounds of moral authority across communities with disparate moral visions.

The necessary conditions for the possibility of a *particular* moral community are, then, (1) an interest in pursuing the good and avoiding harm within (2) the constraints of moral authority. Goods and harms take on a concrete moral significance within the context of a community with a particular moral vision. The principle of autonomy marks the very boundary of all moral communities. To violate it is to be an enemy of moral communities generally. However, to honor it is not quite yet to be a member of *a* moral community. This is the case, in part because the principle of autonomy is a principle of forbearance only. It is a negative principle. The principle of autonomy is not beyond, but it is before, any concrete good or evil. It is only through the positive principle of beneficence that content is acquired for the moral life. Thus, not being beneficent is not to be an enemy of the moral community, but neither is it to be a member of *a* moral community. An individual who, as an egoist, pursues his own solitary good, but without violating the rights of others, falls thus into a sort of moral limbo. It is only in affirming the principle of beneficence that one commits oneself to the enterprise of fashioning *a* moral community and to giving content to beneficence.

For bioethics this means that an understanding of the restraints due to mutual respect is central, but insufficient for an account of proper health care. One must ensure free and informed consent, one must forbear from preventing access to abortion and contraception, and one must respect the rights of individuals to refuse lifesaving treatment. However, this necessary web of duties of forbearance will be insufficient for a picture of the moral life. One will need in addition to determine the obligations of physicians and society to provide care and support to patients.

Justifying the principles of morality

The justifications that have been offered for this principle of morality are not simply psychological claims regarding dispositions to be respectful or sympathetic. Rather, they are conceptual points regarding what it means coherently to think of ourselves within particular inescapable conceptual frameworks. Here it may help to develop this point through a characterization of similar principles. For example, to ask how to determine the causes of cancer or whether a berry is poisonous is to ask a question presupposing points of relative permanence, changes according to patterns or rules, and a reciprocity among the points of permanence and change. Here one should recall Kant's arguments regarding the necessary conditions for the possibility of experience.[16] Asking about (or thinking about) the nature of empirical reality (or even having a coherent experience) commits one to such a set of presuppositions regarding empirical coherence. Such principles are so inescapable that to reject them would be tantamount to endorsing a psychosis with full-blown autism.[17] Experience has a set of presumptions that are conceptually statable because it is the experience of a rational being.[18]

So, too, thinking about blaming or praising with justification presupposes a framework in terms of which there can be a criterion or authority for evaluation. The minimal condition for this possibility is mutual respect, which grounds both a sense of moral authority and a justification for blame and praise. To establish a more concrete moral sense, one would need premises that would be very difficult if not impossible to secure in general secular terms. Such premises would require committing oneself to a particular community with its already accepted metaphysical, religious, or ideological presuppositions. Mutual respect is barely sufficient, but still quite sufficient for a general justification of the practice of blaming and praising— in short, for the minimum grammar necessary for the world of mutual respect. The principle of autonomy as a summary of the core of the morality of mutual respect must be embraced insofar as one coherently thinks of oneself as making claims to respect, or regarding persons in terms of their worthiness of blame and praise, or as able to recognize moral authority in a secular pluralist context, that is, a context where special religious, metaphysical, or ideological premises are not granted. If one does not participate in this world of mutual respect, then one is left with using force without even a purported justification, or with an alleged justification (i.e., in terms of special religious, metaphysical, or ideological assumptions), which is in fact not secured for rational persons generally who do not grant those premises. Hence, persons anywhere in the cosmos interested in giving general justifications for respect, worthiness of blame or praise, and moral authority would have grounds for recognizing as immoral persons who employ such unjustified force. The morality of mutual respect, through the principle of autonomy, gives the boundaries to morality generally. It discloses those who are outlaws from that morality and therefore cannot protest against defensive or punitive force. It discloses one element of the grammar of morality. As such, it is a restraining principle.

The morality of welfare and social sympathies, which is summarized under the rubric of the principle of beneficence, discloses the nisus of morality, the interest in securing the good of persons and of sentient beings generally. To understand morality is to understand that it is concerned with achieving the good for persons. (1) The general limits on the capacity of reason to disclose a justified concrete view of the good and (2) the restraints due to the morality of mutual respect (expressed in a negative principle of autonomy) set limits to morally justified actions on behalf of beneficence. However, if one were to understand bioethics only within these restraints, one would have forgotten why one had decided to engage in health care to begin with, namely, to achieve a set of important goods for patients and potential patients. Significant concern about free and informed consent makes sense only if there is something important to achieve, the means regarding which are the subject of free and informed consent. The principle of beneficence for its part indicates a dimension of the grammar of moral concerns directed toward the goods of persons.

The principle of beneficence is as unavoidable as the question regarding what is good or bad to do, considered not just from my perspective but from as generally attainable a perspective as possible. To be interested in an intersubjective answer to such a question is to presuppose a concern for the good of persons and sentient beings generally. To raise the question of the good and the bad is to attempt to take a reasoned perspective, an anonymous perspective, one that belongs as much to all as it does to any particular person. It involves stepping away from particular personal interests and advantages so as to judge which lines of conduct should rationally be affirmed as good and which should rationally be condemned as evil. To answer such a rational question is, after all, not to determine what is true for me, but what is true for rational inquirers generally. The rational perspective is one that steps away from bias, prejudice, and personal distortion, toward anonymous appreciation, which is intersubjective.

Because of the unlikelihood of a general agreement about what is the proper concrete understanding of the good life, the question of what is good or bad to do cannot receive a concrete answer. The question rather becomes heuristic: it aims individuals toward as rationally justifiable an account as possible of good and bad consequences. However, such accounts will vary, as different individuals accept different hierarchies of benefits and harms. The best one can do is to articulate the principle of beneficence, Do to others their good, in the concreteness of particular moral communities. Particular understandings of good and harm must be pursued, while not forgetting the absoluteness of the general concern for doing good and avoiding evil. The principle of beneficence is thus dialectical. It speaks of a goal that cannot be directly articulated: a true and final understanding of what is good or evil to accomplish. The principle reminds one that even when absolute answers are not available, relative ones will still be of importance to those who live within a particular moral community. The contradiction is overcome in a realization of the earnestness of the task of living a concrete understanding of the good life.

The principles of autonomy and beneficence ground and summarize two central moral points of view: (1) that in terms of which one considers what it means to act with authority, within one's rights, and (2) that in terms of which one considers what it means to do good and avoid evil. Each is justified through being tied to an inescapable element of meaning. The principle of autonomy is inescapable, insofar as one asks the question whether one (or another) has acted rightly in the sense of with moral authority. The principle of beneficence is inescapable insofar as one asks a question regarding the good one ought to achieve or evil one ought to avoid for others. The principles express the fact that the moral point of view is one of beneficence within constraints of respect for persons.

The tension between the principles

Neither the principle of autonomy nor that of beneficence is justified in terms
of its consequences. They are rather summaries of unavoidable areas of
personal conduct. They are in this sense deontological principles, in that their
rightness is not defined in terms of their consequences. However, concrete
rules of beneficence are likely to be teleological in being justified in terms of
their consequences. Concrete applications of the principle of autonomy, in
contrast, bind, even if they have negative consequences for liberty. The
principle of autonomy, which is justified in terms of the morality of mutual
respect, does not focus on freedom as a value, but on respect for freedom as
the possibility for general moral authority and justified worthiness of blame
and praise. It is not goal or consequence oriented (i.e., teleological).
Physician–patient agreements (e.g., a physician's agreement to keep a
patient's disclosures confidential) bind in terms of the principle of autonomy,
independently of their consequences. Rules for free and informed consent
that are based on mutual respect also bind independently of their consequences. The sphere of the principle of autonomy, in its application, remains
in its core deontological. It grounds rights and obligations independently of
concerns for achieving what is good and avoiding what is evil. The sphere of
the principle of beneficence, in its application, becomes teleological. It
grounds particular rights and obligations in terms of their achieving what is
good and avoiding what is harmful (though the general principle is not so
justified). A particular rule of beneficence that caused more harm than good
would lose its justification. Thus, a rule for distributing health care resources
on grounds of beneficence would be defeated if it failed to provide more
benefits than alternative rules. The two principles thus lead to contrasting
spheres of moral discourse: one deontologically oriented, the other teleologi-
cally oriented.[19]

These dimensions of morality appear to be sufficiently distinct so as to
allow for an important form of tension. An act can be justified within one
dimension of morality but not within the other. Thus, one has conflicts of the
general sort, "*X* has a right (obligation) to do *A* but it is wrong." One might
advance as an example of this general formula, "Physicians have a right to do
what they want to with their spare time, even when they could easily
contribute a small portion of that spare time to aiding indigent patients, but
it is wrong not to use some of that time to aid those patients." One has a
conflict between the morality of mutual respect and the morality of welfare.
Still, one cannot specify the morality of welfare without appealing to mutual
agreement and therefore to the morality of mutual respect.

The principles of autonomy and beneficence are thus both mutually supporting, as well as the root of ineradicable conflicts in the moral life. Goods and harms become moral goods and harms in the embrace of a community with a moral vision. However, such a community can have moral authority only through respecting the principle of moral autonomy. Yet the principle of autonomy requires acquiescing in the choice by others of harms they hold to be goods, which may be at odds with the views of the moral community, for example, a young man deciding to commit suicide after sustaining nonfatal but disfiguring burns or individuals choosing within the rules of a medical insurance system in ways that will in the end subvert that very system through escalating costs. Respect for freedom and interest in the good will conflict.

Since views of the good are divergent, there will be no moral authority to stop persons from peaceably pursuing their view of the good life alone or with consenting others. One might think of a community attempting to bring its members to realize a higher level of health and to lower certain health care costs by stopping smoking and engaging in exercise programs. What of the sedentary smokers who do not judge that such is worth the effort? The achievement of the communal view of the good will often fall prey to the free choice of individuals not to aid its prospering. Such dissenters from an orthodox vision of the good can be characterized as having valued personal freedoms higher than other goods or as having embraced a different view of the good life with a different schedule of the relative significance of costs and benefits. As such, they remind us of the community's lack of authority to constrain individuals from such deviance. Such dissenters also underscore the tension between respecting freedom and acting benevolently, especially on a social level.

Dissenters not only underscore the tension between the principles of autonomy and beneficence, but in so doing they also indicate how a community can fragment into numerous communities, each with its own view of the good life. The arrangements can be complicated. Communities can in various areas overlap and separate. Consider how reform and orthodox Jewish physicians and patients may commonly presuppose certain views about the goods proper to the practice of medicine and still disagree regarding others. This fragmentation of the view of the good life leads, as has already been noted, to the tensions expressed in the application of the principle of nonmaleficence. Unlike other analyses, this volume supports the reduction of the principle of nonmaleficence to the conflict between the general and particular perspectives within the principle of beneficence.[20] This tension is exemplified when a physician is asked by a patient to achieve for the patient what the patient holds to be a good but what the physician holds to be a harm.

The moral life is lived across tensions, grounded in the conflicts between autonomy and beneficence, and among the various understandings of beneficence. There is both diversity and unity. We will return to this point in the subsection, "A right to do what is wrong." (See p. 87.) Respect of the principle of autonomy binds all persons together in the moral life. Respect of particular principles of beneficence separates communities. Respect of the general principle of beneficence reminds individuals from different moral communities of the common commitment to doing the good, even when the visions of the good diverge.

The principle of justice

Most appeals to the principle of justice can be understood as being at root a concern with beneficence. Principles of justice that support the distribution of goods under a particular moral vision will here be interpreted as a special instance of attempting to do the good. Justinian in his *Institutes* character-ized justice as "the constant and perpetual wish to render every one his due."[21] The problem, of course, lies in what is due to whom and why. On the one hand, autonomy-based understandings of justice, such as Robert Nozick's, construe just distributions as those that occur without violence to the free choices of owners.[22] In contrast, there are views of justice based on appeals to ideal distributions of goods. These presuppose particular views of the good life. As we shall see, these disparate foundations for claims about justice undergird major moral conflicts concerning the distribution of both privately and commonly owned goods.

These disparate foundations are at the root of complex claims such as those presented in the following statement: "It is your right to use your own private funds for the health care of those you choose and no others, but it is wrong in the sense that it shows no acknowledgment of the needs of others." The first clause, in its appeal to rights, signals the limits of public authority. It appeals to the principle of autonomy. The second clause, in its notion of wrongness, appeals to a particular moral vision of the good life and of just distributions. It appeals to a particular principle of doing good, of being beneficent. This same conflict can recur in the allocation of commonly owned goods: "I know that we voted according to commonly agreed-to procedures regarding the ways in which we would invest our common resources. However, investing them as agreed, primarily in the development of good vineyards rather than in health care research and care, is wrong." The first clause appeals to a view of the good as fashioned through common agreement. The second clause appeals to a particular view, not so sanctioned, regarding the proper use of resources. In short, an examination of the principle of justice reveals the principles of autonomy and beneficence, each grounding its own sphere of claims.

The principles of bioethics

In approaching the problems of moral judgment in bioethics, we have then two major moral principles. Their character reflects the fact that they are principles for resolving moral disputes among individuals who do not share a common moral vision. They have their place through sustaining the ethical fabric of a secular pluralism. They sustain the possibility of moral discourse in secular pluralist societies where no one moral sense can be established. They function also as guides for tracing the lineage of supposed authority for public policy. Public policy that lacks a morally justified authority is without moral force. One might think here of laws forbidding aiding and abetting the suicide of competent individuals.[23] Such laws are without moral authority, at least as long as the individuals have not explicitly ceded their right to suicide (e.g., one might imagine that officers in the armed forces might be required to relinquish that right under specified conditions as a condition for their commission). On the other hand, laws protecting human research subjects against being used in experimentation without their consent carry moral authority in that they are grounded in the very notion of protecting the peaceable community. They spring from the notion of the morality of mutual respect.

Other areas of public policy have less certain moral authority. It will be clear how to use commonly owned resources in ways that support the common good. The provision of a mix of preventive and primary health care out of common funds would appear reasonable. However, arguments can reasonably be advanced for various mixtures, including a major preponderance of either preventive or primary health care. The actual character of public health policy will thus have to be created by common agreement and will not be discoverable by an inspection of the principle of beneficence in isolation. One will need to appeal to the principle of autonomy as the basis for the common fashioning of particular programs of beneficence. In most cases, one finds both principles intertwined. These two principles are principles in the sense of being *principia*. They indicate foundations for major elements of the moral life. (Further derivative principles will be introduced in chapter 4.)

PRINCIPLE I. THE PRINCIPLE OF AUTONOMY

Authority for actions involving others in a secular pluralist society is derived from the free consent of those involved. As a consequence,
  i. Without such consent there is no authority.
  ii. Actions against such authority are blameworthy in the sense of placing a violator outside the moral community in general, and making licit (but not

obligatory) retaliatory, defensive, or punitive force by members of any particular moral community.

A. Implicit consent: individuals, groups, and states have authority to protect the innocent from unconsented-to force.

B. Explicit consent: individuals, groups, and states have the right to enforce contracts.

C. Justification of the principle: the principle of autonomy expresses the fact that authority for resolving moral disputes in a secular, pluralist society can be derived only from the agreement of the participants in the disputes, since it cannot be derived from rational argument or common belief. Therefore, consent is the origin of authority, and respect of the right of participants to consent is the necessary condition for the possibility of a moral community. The principle of autonomy provides the minimum grammar for moral language. It is as inescapable as the interest of persons in blaming and praising with justification and resolving issues with authority.

D. Motivation for obeying the principle is tied to interests in acting in a way i) that is justifiable to peaceable persons generally, and ii) that will not justify the use of defensive or punitive force against oneself.

E. Public policy implications: the principle of autonomy provides moral grounding for public policies aimed at defending the innocent.

F. Maxim: Do not do to others that which they would not have done unto them, and do for them that which one has contracted to do.

G. The principle of autonomy grounds what can be termed the morality of autonomy as mutual respect.

PRINCIPLE II. THE PRINCIPLE OF BENEFICENCE

The goal of moral action is the achievement of goods and the avoidance of harms. In a secular pluralist society, however, no particular ordering of goods and harms can be established because that would require a particular moral sense for justification. As a result, within the bounds of respecting autonomy, no particular moral sense can be established over competing senses (at least within a peaceable secular pluralist society). Still, a commitment to beneficence characterizes the undertaking of morality, because without a commitment to beneficence the moral life has no content. As a consequence,

    i. On the one hand, there is no general contentful principle of beneficence to which one can appeal.

    ii. On the other hand, actions against beneficence are blameworthy in the sense of placing violators outside the context of any particular moral community; such actions place individuals beyond claims to beneficence; insofar as one rejects only particular rules of beneficence, grounded in a particular view of the good life, one loses only one's own claims to beneficence within that particular moral community; in either case, petitions for mercy may still have standing. Actions against beneficence constitute moral impropriety. They are against the content proper to the moral life.

A. Implicit contract: content for a principle of beneficence is acquired by fashioning a community with a common view of the proper ordering of goods and harms.

B. Explicit contract: content for duties of beneficence can be derived as well from explicit agreements. In this case, as in the previous case, the content of a duty of beneficence is grounded in the principle of autonomy.

C. Justification of the principle: the principle of beneficence reflects the circumstance that moral concerns encompass the pursuit of goods and the avoidance of harms. Since such disputes can be resolved in secular pluralist societies only by an appeal to the principle of autonomy, the principle of autonomy is conceptually prior to the principle of beneficence. One can know when one is violating the morality of mutual respect, even when one cannot know, because of its lack of content, whether one is violating the principle of beneficence. However, recognition of the principle of beneficence provides the minimal characterization of the content required for moral concerns.

D. Motivation for obeying the principle is tied to interests in acting in a way: i) that is justifiable to beneficent persons generally, and ii) that will not justify one in being characterized as an unsympathetic individual who may be excluded from a particular or any community's beneficence.

E. Public policy implications: the principle of beneficence provides the moral grounding for refusable welfare rights drawn from common holdings.

F. Maxim: Do to others their good.

G. The principle of beneficence grounds what can be termed the morality of welfare and social sympathies.

In light of these two principles, one can appreciate better the character of conflicts in health care. The conflicts are often deep, if not intractable, because they reflect profound tensions within the project of morality itself. Concerns with mutual respect and concerns with common welfare appear sufficiently distinct so as not to allow a means for a mediation of their tensions.[24] At best one will be able in particular communities commonly to agree to particular ways for understanding claims of beneficence. Yet even under the best of circumstances, such agreements will not be sufficiently complete or detailed to avoid tensions between the rights and obligations of individuals within the morality of mutual respect versus what appears right or wrong to do within the morality of common welfare.

Rights and obligations[25]

A right to do what is wrong

In order to appreciate the force of conflicting assertions regarding rights and obligations, one should attend with great care to the justificatory lineage of all claims with regard to rights and obligations, as well as to what is right or wrong to do. One should act as if all such claims came with footnotes to their justification. For a claim such as "young children have a right to organ transplants to save their lives," one should add a subscript under "right" that marks the genre of justification for such a claim. This inspection of justifications will allow one to know how seriously one should take claims with regard to obligations of persons, or the wrongness of particular acts. Conflicts also occur because moral discourse occurs not only within the domain of general secular ethics, but within particular moral languages as well. Thus, one can have a number of interpretations of the general formula

X has a right to do *A,* but it is wrong.

In some cases this formula captures the tension between the morality of mutual respect and the morality of beneficence. This occurs in the statement

Doctor X has a right to charge *Y* amount for *Z* procedure in all cases, but it is wrong that the physician does not make exceptions in order to treat some patients who could not otherwise afford such services.

We will presume here that the claim of the physician's right is based on the physician's autonomy rights to dispose of time as he or she sees fit. The claim for wrongness, we will presume, is supported by some general secular considerations of beneficence, such as some form of a utilitarian argument.

Conflicts between a physician's rights and what is wrong to do can also occur, as we have seen, when there is a tension between two levels of moral discourse. Consider

The physician has a right to perform the abortion at the woman's request, but it is wrong.

The claim of the physician's right may be based either on considerations of respecting autonomy or on considerations of beneficence. The claim of wrongness, let us presume, is in contrast embedded in a particular set of religious, moral, and metaphysical considerations, such as the current Roman Catholic position regarding abortion. Such claims of wrongness may either be beneficence-regarding considerations or turn on special claims of irreducible wrongness.

As these conflicts of moral claims show, the universe of moral claims is complex and heterogeneous. Numerous claims with regard to rights and obligations, and with regard to the rightness or wrongness of actions, can be generated on the basis of different elements of secular morality (i.e., autonomy-regarding morality versus beneficence-regarding morality), as well as in terms of conflicts between secular philosophical ethics and moralities based on particular religious or moral viewpoints. In addition, considerations regarding beneficence are themselves complex. There appears to be a number of competing reasonable accounts of what it means to be beneficent, to act to support a web of mutual sympathy, to support the common welfare.

Different ways of articulating concerns to achieve the good or avoid evil will lead to different claims regarding what is good to do. This includes the circumstance that different lexical orderings of goods will produce different views of what it means to act beneficently. Which is more important, to control pain fully but at the risk of addiction, or to avoid any substantial risk of addiction, but at the price of substantial pain? One might think of the conflicts that occur between financial interests and concerns to achieve optimal health, or optimal chances of curing disease and restoring function. Such conflicts exist both on a societal level as well as for individuals. As we have noted, there are conflicts between interests in maximizing the chances of cure and prolonging life expectancy, versus risks of pain and suffering that confront a patient in choosing among various means for treating cancer. How does one compare a lower chance of a five-year cure for cancer of the larynx with a greater chance of maintaining acceptable vocal function? Or how does a woman compare various five-year survival rates for cure of breast cancer with various degrees of disfigurement and impairment that will result from different therapeutic approaches? When one examines the principle of beneficence, one finds it fragmenting into a number of senses of beneficence. There is no single sense of what it is to do the good, for the goods open to persons are multiple and often incompatible. As a consequence, different rules for acting beneficently will conflict.

It is by no means clear how one can discover a way of ordering these goods and possible harms so as to know which trade-offs are rational and which are irrational. At least within a large range, there appears to be no consensus in these matters. One encounters rationally irresolvable conflicts that must often be resolved by what is tantamount to an arbitrary choice. Even in other areas where a greater consensus can be found regarding what ought to count as rational choices, one still confronts deep conflicts of values. Consider the comparability of concerns to maximize health and longevity versus interests in living a relatively unrestricted, unfettered existence. One might term this the mountain climber's quandary. At what point does it become irrational to risk one's life in order to be the first to scale a particular face of a mountain in a particular season of the year? Similar questions arise for the homosexual whose lifestyle exposes him to a greater risk of AIDS, or for the individual with chronic obstructive pulmonary disease who wishes to continue to smoke a little, or for the individual with hypertension or diabetes who wishes not to be fully compliant with a physician's suggestions regarding optimal treatment. These "mountain-climber" cases present a conflict between various liberty and other values and the values of health and longevity.

One finds as well conflicts between interests in health and short-range concerns to avoid anxiety that occur when patients choose to deny that they have a disease and pretend instead that they are well. Such choices lead to the noncompliance of patients with hypertension and similar diseases. One can surely list other conflicts as well. Consider a woman who deeply wants a child and chooses not to interrupt a pregnancy that threatens her health. Medicine is an arena for conflicts of values, which in many circumstances appear even to a great number of rational and prudent individuals to be incommensurable. A lexical ordering does not appear discoverable. It does not appear possible to disclose a general rational hierarchy of such goods and harms so as to indicate in general what choices should be made by rational and prudent individuals.

This is not to say that a careful analytical examination of choices and their consequences will not be helpful. The more one is able to display for individuals the consequences of their choices, the more they will be enabled to choose rationally. One should, as far as possible, play the role of a geographer of values, mapping the various consequences of placing oneself at a particular place in the terrain of possible outcomes. Such a geography will obviously be complicated. One will need to chart a multidimensional world of various possible outcomes tied together by various probabilities. Most choices in medicine do not lead to a particular outcome with a probability of 1. This will itself raise issues in value theory. How does one compare a very high probability of a very disastrous outcome with a low probability of a very disastrous outcome? As the stakes come close to being those of life or severe impairment, the usual assessment of what counts as prudent bets appears to change. Thus, an individual might be willing to accept fifty thousand dollars in order to expose himself to a one in a thousand chance of being killed in a risky experiment, but he is unlikely to agree to being killed for fifty million dollars outright. However, in terms of straightforward objective calculations, the two "bets" are comparable. That this does not seem plausible to many individuals makes even more difficult a general calculation of the best interests of others.

To find one's way around the moral world defined in terms of interests in respecting free choice, and interests in achieving the goods of persons, one will need to attend carefully to these complexities. One will need to recognize in addition that the conflict between concerns for respecting the free choices of individuals and concerns with achieving the best interests of individuals is complicated not only by numerous senses of best interests, but also by the fact that moral concerns are framed within a secular dimension, as well as within numerous particular religious and other communities. The moral world fragments into numerous tiers and dimensions. To find one's way around in a multitiered, multidimensional moral universe, one will need to fashion as best one can accounts or geographies of the terrain of moral rights and obligations, of right-making and wrong-making conditions. How patients and physicians see the proper trade-off between control of pain and risk of addiction will be influenced by their particular views of the character of the good life and of rational choice. Though it will be difficult to fashion uncontested geographies of moral relations in many cases, some guidance still will be better than none.

It is to this end that I have already suggested the importance of indicating the basis for claims regarding rights and obligations, or regarding the rightness or wrongness of actions, by making reference to the morality of mutual respect and the moralities of welfare. As has been suggested, this distinction itself is a complicated one, since various senses of well-being constitute our notions of welfare or best interests. Further, the elaboration of the principle of autonomy and of the principle of beneficence places concerns with liberty as a good under the rubric of beneficence. The principle of autonomy concerns the rights of individuals to choose freely even when that freedom is directed, not to valuing freedom, but trading liberties for other goods. Finally, as has been argued in some detail, we live our moral lives in part with reference to a set of arguments we attempt to fashion in order to bridge particular moral communities. This I have termed the secular tier of moral discourse. I have contrasted it with those contexts in which we live our concrete moral lives informed by particular religious and/or other metaphysical and ideological understandings that provide us with a concrete portrait of the good life (e.g., as a politically liberal Methodist).

Particular secular communities will need to create a commonly shared moral understanding. Since it will be a moral understanding fashioned by individuals maintaining certain individual rights, it will need to be a vision from which individuals can freely exempt themselves in their private lives. One might think here of medical welfare rights. In fashioning plans for using common resources to support the health of citizens, one will need to create particular entitlements and particular rules for qualifying for those entitlements. Which is to say, when one actually owns goods in common, and no prior common understandings exist, there is no way to act rationally and peaceably in distributing those goods, save by majority rule directed by the best intentions to achieve the common good of all, or of as many as possible. This will lead where possible to fashioning complex entitlements, specified according to explicit rules (often bureaucratic rules). Further, autonomy rights will allow competent individuals to refuse such welfare, since rights to be left alone exist unless individuals have individually ceded them. One finds excellent examples of such rights and their refusal in the instance of Jehovah's Witnesses and Christian Scientists.

By assigning footnote markers or subscripts to claims regarding rights and obligations, and regarding right and wrong conduct, one can help physicians, patients, and society generally to become oriented in the moral world. Such subscripts, by indicating the kind of argument supporting the claim, place it within a particular dimension of morality (e.g., autonomy-oriented or welfare-oriented morality), as well as locating it within a particular dimension of morality (e.g., secular moral claims versus claims made within a particular religious or special moral context).

One also will need to note that the issue of common cooperation will create a special genre of rights involving circumstances in which the general community, out of prudential interests, will not use force to stop what can in general secular terms be shown to be wrong or to violate the rights of particular parties. Thus, a physician's failure to save the life of a patient to whom he owes no particular fiduciary obligation, when it would cost a trivial amount of time and effort, and when the physician recognizes that out of considerations of beneficence he is bound to help the patient, may still not be recognized as grounds for actions against that physician (e.g., ostracizing him through removal from a local medical society). It may be recognized that it is simply too difficult to demonstrate that a physician has failed to discharge a positive duty of beneficence to an individual under such circumstances. Thus one will need to add to the mapping of conflicts an additional interpretation of the formula.

X has a right to do A but it is wrong. Here "has a right" can identify the right of the physician not to accept a patient for treatment. "Has a right" will mean that such actions are licit in the sense that, because of prudential interests, such actions will not be hindered by communal interventions. Wrongness will be grounded in general considerations regarding duties of beneficence.

Fundamental and concrete rights and obligations

With these distinctions at hand, one can now fashion a number of summary headings in order to display the relations among rights and obligations. The obligation to do to others their good is a fundamental one. However, the obligation as such is abstract. Only in concrete contexts can one determine the extent of the obligation, and how to rank the various goods that can be at stake. The general obligation not to use force without authority has a greater concreteness in that it can be clearly disclosed in particular situations without an appeal to anything more than the understanding of the individual who would be subject to such force. Thus, the right not to be treated without one's consent gains concreteness at once from the wishes of the possible patient. It is enough for that individual to refuse in order to indicate that the authority of the physician does not extend to him or her. In contrast, the claim that one should out of beneficence support someone's health care costs rather than give the funds to friends for a trip to Nevada to gamble, eat well, and drink, requires an argument about the relative importance of these goods. A final answer to such a question will require an appeal to a particular view of the good life.

Rights to do with oneself or with consenting others as one chooses are not only fundamental, but function without an appeal to a particular social understanding. This is because such rights are justified in terms of the perspective of moral agents in general, that is, persons interested in resolving disputes without recourse to force. It is this perspective that justifies the morality of mutual respect. No particular view of the good life is presupposed. In addition, as has been argued, there is the point of view of moral agents interested in achieving the good. This is the intellectual standpoint in terms of which one grounds the morality of mutual welfare and social sympathies. However, particular rights and obligations of beneficence presuppose a particular moral viewpoint.

It is because of these differences in justification that fundamental rights to beneficence and fundamental rights to forbearance thus contrast. The former require a particular community's understandings and agreements for the obligation of doing to others their good to have sufficient authority and concreteness to support actual, particular rights to beneficence. However, obligations to forbearance do not require a community's concurrence, but only the dissent of the individuals about to be subjected to force. The individual's refusal is sufficient to give concreteness. Of course, things are never simple: particular notions of particular boundaries support special rights to forbearance and often will require the particular understandings of particular communities. Still, there will remain a general range of actions where the presumption will reasonably be that the person about to be subjected to force must first be asked for permission, because they cannot be presumed already to have consented. Here one will need to list circumstances involving possible imminent loss of life, mutilation, or compromise of bodily or psychological function. Standing community assumptions can defeat these general rational presuppositions. Going to the dueling grounds under particular circumstances and behaving in a particular way can be sufficient to communicate to all concerned that one is prepared to risk one's life in a good-faith duel. To walk up in a line of persons receiving vaccination and proffer one's arm can be enough to constitute consent, but not enough to create a right to the vaccination. In short, a difference between duties of forbearance and beneficence derives from the fact that another's refusal is sufficient to create an obligation of forbearance, whereas mutual agreement is required for a concrete duty of beneficence. Rights and obligations to forbearance as a result possess a greater absoluteness, a greater capacity to hold in a transcultural fashion, than do rights and obligations to beneficence. It is easier to establish the claims that women have a right to refuse an abortion than that they have a right to have others pay for that abortion, should they not be able to afford one.

Absolute rights and obligations

Absolute rights would hold without qualification and without reference to a particular cultural context. With regard to autonomy rights, these can be articulated in an absolute fashion, but only if they are put very generally: "Do not use unconsented-to force against the innocent"; "The innocent have a right not to be the subject of unconsented-to force." This obligation–right pair is absolute and fundamental in being a general articulation of the basic principle of the morality of mutual respect. The pair expresses what it means to treat persons with respect. Since it turns on the concept of the peaceable community in general in a way that focuses on particular individuals and their rights to respect, it sustains a general obligation for all who use force to be clear about their authority. As a consequence, this obligation–right pair leads to an indefinite series of basic or fundamental rights in the sense of opportunities for persons to bring into question the authority of others, including the community, to use unconsented-to force. In this sense, there are fundamental rights to commit suicide, to be aided in suicide or abortion by consenting others, to have access to pornography produced by consenting others, and not to be a subject of experimental manipulation without one's consent. Obligations of beneficence require both content and authority for that particular content (i.e., to bind all parties to that interpretation of concreteness). For example, consider the obligation to provide a decent level of health care for those in need. Since it requires a definition of what will count as "decent", and of the limits of the burdens that must be borne by those being beneficent (e.g., providing decent health care), it remains empty and abstract outside particular cultural contexts. Still, just as some diseases are more culture independent than others, the concern for certain goods shows a certain independence of culture and society, such as concerns for food, basic medical care, and money as a means of realizing preferences. However, a claim on my beneficence (e.g., "Help me! I need treatment for my malaria") will not be as clear and unequivocal (e.g., "My obligations to aid others in need of treatment for malaria are defeated when they constitute significant interference with my life and the use of my private resources, and significant interference for me is. . . ") as the right of others to my forbearance ("Don't touch me!"), because the latter requires no appeal to my particular hierarchy of values or my particular agreement, but depends on the very notion of morality. The fact that autonomy rights are more absolute (i.e., less culture relative) is thus tied to their being more fundamental.

Derivative rights and obligations

All actual concrete rights and obligations regarding beneficence will, as a consequence of the foregoing considerations, need to be created through mutual agreement; they will have a derivative or fashioned character in contrast to the rights that have been termed absolute or fundamental, and that tend to be discoverable by an examination of what is meant by mutual respect. Of course a range of rights grounded in the morality of mutual respect will be created as well. Here one might think of contractual rights.

Prima facie rights and obligations

Certain circumstances sustain an onus for or against particular lines of conduct. Activities that are likely to annihilate a person or significantly circumscribe that person's capacities must be presumed to be forbidden until consent is established, because in most circumstances consent cannot be presumed. Thus, one must presume that consent is necessary in order to use persons as subjects of research. Certain social circumstances may set aside these first-blush, or prima facie, expectations. A physician who has been treating a patient for a particular disease can reasonably presume the patient's continued consent to such treatment. Recognizing particular obligations and rights as prima facie obligations and rights reminds us where we should look for justification in order to shoulder the burden of proof. Moreover, where one can in fact show that prima facie rights and obligations give way to other considerations, one has the opportunity rationally to disclose a hierarchy of rights and obligations so as to direct human behavior in a morally justified fashion.

Deontological versus teleological rights and obligations

As has already been indicated, the claims made within the morality of mutual respect are deontological in character. They are justified not in terms of their maximizing the good, but in terms of the very practice of understanding worthiness of blame or praise. They focus on worthiness of happiness or unhappiness, worthiness of having desired goods, or worthiness of losing those goods. In contrast, the morality of welfare and mutual sympathy focuses on achieving and maximizing those goods. The principles of autonomy and beneficence support a sharp contrast between obligations to respect freedom of persons and the moral interests in achieving their good. This contrast obviously leads to conflicts. Such moral conflicts are surely nowhere more poignant or painful than in medicine, where respecting the freedom of patients may lead to tragic failure on the part of patients to comply properly with medical treatment or to avoid disease-inducing lifestyles. Respect of freedom and the concern to achieve best interests contrast and conflict as two major and distinct roots of morality. As a consequence, the price for respecting freedom is often the tragic (but morally unavoidable) loss of important goods.

Utilitarian and other schemes for determining rights and obligations

One should attempt to secure as maximal a balance of benefits over harms as possible through forethought and careful calculation and within the constraints set by the morality of mutual respect. The question will then arise as to what counts as the best understanding of the proper balancing of benefits over harms. Should it be understood in terms of maximizing average utility, or in terms of the advantage of the least-well-off class? The considerations we have already explored regarding the principle of beneficence suggest that an answer can be found only within a particular community. Though there may in the end be rational arguments to tip the balance in favor of rule utilitarianism over act utilitarianism, there is likely to be a wide range of positions, from rule utilitarian understandings of beneficence to Rawlsian understandings, depending on how risk aversive one judges rational persons ought to be. The more risk aversive one's image of the rational person is, the more one will move to a Rawlsian view in order to benefit the least-well-off class, should one turn out to be a member of that class. However, the more one sees a certain amount of risk taking as a part of the rational life, the more one will move to a utilitarian posture and maximize the greatest good for the greatest number and take the risk that one will be a member of the least advantaged class.[26] These points can also be phrased altruistically in terms of risks to others.

One will be able to decide what is a proper mode for distributing scarce resources, including medical resources, only when one has given content to the notion of a rational person, so that one can know how much risk one ought to take. However, such a contentful understanding of the rational person will require a particular moral sense. Only in such a context will one know whether one should invest health care funds in research programs that, over the long run, will maximize the greatest good for the greatest number, or instead balance one's investments so that one is always careful to advantage the health prospects of the least well-off class. The proper answer can be divided only within the context of an articulated view of the good life and of the proper way to act beneficently.

Positive versus negative rights and obligations

It is often argued that negative rights and duties are stronger than positive rights and duties. Thus, it is held that the duty not to kill and the right not to be killed without one's permission are stronger than the duty to provide resources to save a life or the right to have access to resources in order to save one's life. Thus, for example, the duty of physicians not to kill patients in human experimentation is usually held to be much stronger than their duty to provide sufficient care and resources in order to save lives. This view is supported here, at least when persons meet as moral strangers. One need not know anything about another in order to know that one may not kill that person without permission. However, when one meets a stranger in need of expensive health care to whom one has not made prior commitments, the issue is not as clear. (How much trouble are we obliged to go to?) General negative duties based on mutual respect hold clearly without any special agreements or understandings. Thus, one has prima facie obligations to obtain consent for the use of human subjects in medical research, wherever one might be engaged in such endeavors. Contractual obligations to provide a good or service (e.g., expensive medical treatment) can be just as strong, but they require a special prior understanding (an insurance policy, a health maintenance organization's commitment to certain levels of care, and so on). Consider the difference between a physician vacationing at a posh hotel in Calcutta and the same physician on duty in an HMO. While in the hotel the physician has a less defined set of obligations (if any) to patients in need in Calcutta than to patients of his HMO. Obligations of beneficence appear to depend on special contractual agreements and/or special interpretations of the principle of beneficence. The principle of beneficence, it should be noted, generates negative duties, as well as a duty not to harm others, even with their permission. Thus, physicians ought not to provide treatment they judge to be harmful, unless liberty or other interests of the patient outbalance the harm. These negative duties will have the same imprecision as positive duties of beneficence.

Conflicting rights and obligations

As has already been argued, the moral world is complex and its elements are often in tension with themselves. It will not be possible to decide in many circumstances which obligation or right ought to be honored. If one is attempting to distribute goods in a beneficent fashion in health care, how does one rank the needs of individuals in end-stage renal failure versus the needs of those who have a high likelihood of being exposed to measles or polio and have not been vaccinated? How does one compare the claims of preventive medicine and specialty care medicine, or claims of those wishing to treat cancer and those wishing to treat arthritis or the everyday aches and pains of living? Ranking obligations of beneficence is, as has already been acknowledged, extremely difficult.

Further, what does one do in cases where there appear to be conflicts of promises and contracts? One must, as carefully as possible, draw out the geography and genealogy of rights and obligations to see which likely have precedence. Consider the case of a couple seeking counsel regarding the possibility of having a second child with an inherited recessive birth defect. If tests indicate that in fact the husband cannot have been the father of the first child, what obligation does the physician have, and to whom, and why, regarding a disclosure concerning the risks of future children with the disease for that couple? May the physician simply reassure the couple that they have no risk of having another child with the disease and privately inform the woman of the risks of further reproduction with the lover who sired the child in question? Must the physician inform the husband that he is not the father of the first child, especially if raising the child will entail special financial, psychological, and social costs?

One of the ways to approach an answer would be to determine with whom the physician has the primary patient–physician relationship, the husband or the wife. Such priority could perhaps be determined by who contacted the physician first, or by who is paying the physician. Is the matter changed in any way if the physician is reimbursed through a third party? What if the third party is the government? Must one instead turn to the ways in which the physician agreed initially to aid the couple? At times, perhaps, the physician will be lucky enough to have the relationship so structured that the lines of obligation are clear. Perhaps the physician is the woman's obstetrician, with primary obligations to her. In other cases, the issue may be irresolvable. Important moral questions may have at times no clear resolution.

TEYKU: the opacity of some problems to moral reasoning

Classic examples of moral quandaries can be found in Western religious texts. Consider Judas Maccabaeus' solution to the disposition of the stones of the altar of the Second Temple, which had been desecrated by the Hellenic Syrians during their occupation. Since he could not determine how to dispose of these holy but desecrated stones, he ordered them to be placed on the Temple hill until a prophet should come and indicate what should be done with them (1 Maccabees 4:44–6). The unresolved problem in moral reasoning has been underscored in the Talmudic notion of TEYKU. TEYKU problems involve disputes regarding the law that do not admit of resolution, in that the arguments on either side balance each other. TEYKU problems stand indefinitely in a state of insolubility. Or as some of the mystical literature suggests, Elijah, the herald of the Messiah, will come to solve the TEYKU problems.[27] One is left with an appreciation of the fact that some important moral problems may in fact be insoluble, either due to the unclarity of the facts of the situation, or due to unclarities regarding moral principles themselves.

To recur to the case of the child with the genetic disease, it may be unclear in principle whether one's obligations of beneficence to the husband or to the wife are stronger. In questions of moral conflict where issues are truly TEYKU, one is surely free to flip a coin, follow one's inclinations, or choose on the basis of prudential self-interest. However, there are often differences in consequences. In such circumstances one should act so as to lose as few goods as possible and to violate as few rights as possible (the satisfaction of rights grounded in mutual respect will have first claim). Since medicine is a discipline practiced in tragic circumstances where all patients die and most suffer illness before death, physicians are often faced with choices where not all rights can be satisfied and surely not all goods realized, and where a definitive and all-encompassing hierarchy of rights and goods cannot be established.

I have used the concept of TEYKU to indicate the limits of reason in resolving moral quandaries. At times, it may not be clear what one ought to do. Here I should stress again that such unclarity will at times spring from the very tension within morality itself: between the concern to respect persons and to do the good. In most cases, it will be clear that individuals will not have authority to use force to achieve their view of the good against the protests of innocent persons. However, one might ask, what if the existence of a nation or of a corporation such as IBM or Texaco were at stake? Or for that matter the world, perhaps the cosmos? May one enslave one individual in order to achieve such an important beneficent goal? May one torture *one* unwilling individual to save the cosmos? When does the good at stake become so important as to override the very notion of a peaceable moral community? Would it be reasonable to shoot an innocent stranger to save one's family of three? What if one has a family of twelve? What if the lives of a hundred are at stake? Of ten million? Of ten billion? Of a hundred trillion? Such cases, perhaps, are not so much TEYKU as deeply tragic. An individual who violated the morality of mutual respect for such an important and beneficent good would surely be blameworthy. If the good at stake is so overwhelming, one should show special mercy and understanding. But one would still need to recognize that a violation of the moral order had occurred.

Principles

Discussion of moral principles and the classifications of rights and obligations cannot solve or illuminate successfully all moral conflicts and quandaries. However, such can be useful up to a point in displaying the geography of moral obligations and rights. In this sense. principles can function as chapter headings or indexes directing one to clusters of issues. In such cases, principles function as rules, perhaps as rules of thumb, which direct the inquirer to a particular approach to the solution of a problem. As such, principles are, even if not fundamental, at least useful. Principles can also function to indicate the sources of particular areas of moral rights and obligations. Principles can also be justificatory; in this sense they are *principia*: beginnings, commencements, or origins of particular areas of the moral life. Here they provide the fundamental bases for moral solutions, when solutions are accessible. In such circumstances, principles do not lead to a tyranny of principles, but rather to the clarification of moral quandaries and questions. Even if one were to have a college of pontiffs on the model of ancient Rome (the ten men, the *decem viri,* who decided legal cases), reaching resolutions to quandaries not on the basis of explicit rules, but on the basis of their wise capacities to pontificate equitably, *if* one is interested in knowing the justification for such actions of the ten men, *then* one will need to look for principles in the sense of bases for holding that the pontifices judged correctly and with authority.[28] Thus, if one had a group of ten wise physicians who seemed always to choose correctly, one would need to determine (1) if in fact they always chose correctly, and (2) by what standards they were correct.

The moral tensions in bioethics

These reflections have left us in a somewhat unhappy but inescapable position. The roots of the moral world are heterogeneous. Not only are they to be understood within two different dimensions—secular pluralist morality, and the particular concrete moralities of particular communities—but in addition, secular morality itself draws from two contrasting moral concerns, the first to respect persons and the second to accomplish their good. For bioethics, this means irreconcilable moral tensions. Though patients must be respected if they refuse to comply with health- and life-preserving medical treatment, one may often properly judge such noncompliance as wrong. The principle of the respect for persons leads one to a morally enforced acquiescence in the loss of important goods. There will be a wide range of instances where one will be able to judge in secular pluralist terms that individuals are treating themselves, their spouses, or children improperly, but will need to acquiesce. The exegesis of the phrase "X has a right to do B but it is wrong" has thus become very complex. The phrase can at times be understood in terms of a conflict between tiers of the moral life. In other circumstances, it must be understood as a conflict within the very roots of secular pluralist morality itself. There is an intrinsic tragedy to morality; bioethics provides one with grounds for understanding that others are acting improperly, in fact, even immorally, while yet often constraining one to acquiesce on moral grounds in such immoral actions.

The tragic nature of medicine is thus accentuated. Medicine treats individuals, all of whom will die, some of whom will suffer greatly, in circumstances where medicine can often not postpone death or greatly ameliorate suffering. The character of medicine is such that one must often make choices among alternative possibilities of different forms of suffering and death without knowing with certainty what will happen. One may choose to operate in order to save a life only to have the patient die of the anesthesia. One may give antibiotics to a patient only to have the patient develop a life-threatening allergic reaction. The character of the choices physicians must make carries the possibility of leading inexorably to unwanted painful outcomes. In addition, the character of morality through which one must make choices regarding approaches to treatment is itself flawed in the sense that the moral obligation to respect persons will often constrain physicians to acquiesce in patients' choices—choices that most likely will lead to the loss of important goods. In medicine, one is recurringly confronted with the loss of goods, both through the lack of sufficient knowledge and power, as well as through the restraints of morality itself.

Notes

1. Hans Reichenbach, *Theory of Probability* (Berkeley: University of California Press, 1949), pp. 470–82.
2. This view of inductive knowledge does make ontological presuppositions in the sense that its deliverances presume a general conceptual structure.
3. Consider the first formulation of the categorical imperative: "Act as though the maxim of your action were by your will to become a universal law of nature." Immanuel Kant, *Foundations of the Metaphysics of Morals,* trans. L. W. Beck (Indianapolis: Library of Liberal Arts, 1959), p. 39; *Grundlegung zur Metaphysik der Sitten,* Akademie Textausgabe (Berlin: Walter de Gruyter, 1968), vol. 4, p. 421. All citations to the German text of Kant's writings are from this edition.
4. G. W. F. Hegel, *The Philosophy of Right,* trans. T. M. Knox (London: Oxford University Press, 1965), sec. 135.
5. Alasdair MacIntyre, *A Short History of Ethics* (New York: Macmillan, 1973), pp. 190–8.
6. Karen Lebacqz and H. Tristram Engelhardt, Jr., "Suicide," in D. J. Horan and D. Mall (eds.), *Death, Dying, and Euthanasia* (Washington, D.C.: University Publications, 1977), pp. 669–705; Kant, *Grundlegung,* pp. 421f.
7. Marcus Singer, "On Duties to Oneself," *Ethics* 69 (1959): 202–11.
8. Kant, *Grundlegung,* p. 424.
9. Kant, *Foundations of the Metaphysics of Morals,* p. 41; *Grundlegung,* p. 423.
10. Ibid.
11. Kant generally does not see concerns of prudence to be truly ethical concerns. Indeed, he would not have acknowledged concerns with beneficence to be merely concerns of prudence.
12. What is offered here is an account of the basis of retributive justice. However, the

account is in a negative form. It shows simply when certain actions of punishment would not be forbidden. This understanding reveals similarities between ancient Germanic and Kantian theories of retributive justice. The criminal who acts against the very fabric of the moral community repudiates mutual respect, rejects the law of the peaceable community, and becomes an outlaw who can neither appeal to the peaceable community for protection nor consistently protest the use of defensive or punative force.

13. In such a circumstance one would be left with only an emotive account of ethics. Charles L. Stevenson, *Facts and Values* (New York: Yale University Press, 1967), esp. pp. 1–70.

14. For Hume, sympathy is the powerful principle in human nature that produces our moral sentiments. As he argues:

> Now justice is a moral virtue, merely because it has that tendency to the good of mankind; and, indeed, is nothing but an artificial invention to that purpose. The same may be said of allegiance, of the laws of nature, of modesty, and of good manners. All these are mere human contrivances for the interest of society. And since there is a very strong sentiment of morals, which in all nations, and all ages, has attended them, we must allow, that the reflecting on the tendency of characters and mental qualities, is sufficient to give us the sentiments of approbation and blame. Now as the means to an end can only be agreeable, where the end is agreeable; and as the good of society, where our own interest is not concerned or that of our friends, please only by sympathy: It follows, that sympathy is the source of the esteem, which we pay to all the artificial virtues. David Hume, *A Treatise of Human Nature* (Oxford: Clarendon Press, 1964), p. 577.

15. For an analysis of the biblical concept of covenant, see George E. Mendenhall, *The Tenth Generation* (Baltimore: Johns Hopkins University Press, 1973), and Diebert R. Hillers, *Covenant: The History of a Biblical Idea* (Baltimore: Johns Hopkins University Press, 1969).

16. Kant lays out the conditions of possible experience in general as that which is presupposed for the possibility of encountering objects. See *Critique of Pure Reason,* trans. N. K. Smith (London: Macmillan, 1964), A108 = B197.

17. Eugen Bleuler defined autism as "this detachment from reality, together with the relative as absolute predominance of the inner life." *Dementia Praecox or the Group of Schizophrenias,* trans. Joseph Zinkin (New York: International Universities Press, 1950), p. 63. The reality of which Bleuler speaks is the one we must acknowledge for common endeavors. This reality has similarities with Kant's phenomenal reality. Bleuler holds that there is no way to demonstrate the existence of external reality in itself. One must take it for granted as the necessary condition for the possibility of intersubjective activities. "But for the existence of the external world there are no proofs. That the table which we see has existence is only an assumption, even if of practical necessity. But if I once take for granted the existence of the table, and that of other people, and the external world, then this table can be shown to these other people. Like myself they can perceive it with their senses. *The reality of the physical world is therefore uncertain and relative, that is, it is not possible to prove it, but on the other hand, it is objectively demonstrable.*" Eugen Bleuler, *Textbook of Psychiatry* (New York: Macmillan, 1936), p. 8.

18. For the list of Kant's categories, see *Critique of Pure Reason,* A80 = B106.

19. I distinguish here between deontological principles as those that cannot be reduced to interests in the achievement of particular goods or values, and

THE PRINCIPLES OF BIOETHICS

teleological principles that can be so reduced. As John Rawls indicates, "A deontological theory [is] one that either does not specify the good independently from the right, or does not interpret the right as maximizing the good." *Theory of Justice* (Cambridge, Mass.: Harvard University Press, 1971), p. 30. In contrast, within teleological theories, "the good is defined independently from the right, and then the right is defined as that which maximizes the good." Ibid., p. 24.

20. For a treatment of nonmaleficence as an independent principle, see Tom L. Beauchamp and James F. Childress, *Principles of Biomedical Ethics,* 2d ed. (New York: Oxford University Press, 1983), pp. 106–47.

21. "Justitia est constans et perpetua voluntas jus suum cuique tribuens." Flavius Petrus Sabbatius Justinianus, *The Institutes of Justinian,* trans. T. C. Sandars (Westport, Conn.: Greenwood Press, 1970), Book I. 1, p. 5.

22. Robert Nozick, *Anarchy, State, and Utopia* (New York: Basic Books, 1974).

23. H. Tristram Engelhardt, Jr., and Michele Malloy, "Suicide and Assisting Suicide: A Critique of Legal Sanctions." *Southwestern Law Review* 36 (November 1982): 1003–37.

24. As Hegel would point out, this abstract conflict is mediated in the concrete ethical life, within *Sittlichkeit*; see *The Philosophy of Right*. Still, regarded abstractly, there is an antinomy in practical reason between the duties of autonomy and the duties of beneficence.

25. The terms *obligation* and *duty* carry no clear differences of meaning. Consider, for example, Richard Brandt's remark, "English . . . tends to confuse matters . . . by labouring distinctions without a significant difference. A prime example of this is the existence of terms like 'duty,' 'obligation,' and 'wrong.' . . ." Brandt recognizes that "some have argued that something is an obligation only if one has made a contract or promise. . . ." Richard B. Brandt, *A Theory of the Good and the Right* (Oxford: Clarendon Press, 1979), p. 8. I will rely on the suggestion that obligations depend on a community. Even the core obligation to respect the freedom of persons springs from a notion of the originary intellectual standpoint of the community of persons. I will therefore in most instances employ the term *obligation* in preference to *duty* in order to accent these circumstances.

26. For a critique of the Rawlsian avoidance of risk, see J. Harsanyi, "Can the Maximim Principle Serve as a Basis for Morality: A Critique of John Rawls' Theory," *American Political Science Review* 6 (1975): 594–606.

27. Louis Jacobs, *TEYKU* (New York: Cornwall Books, 1981).

28. Stephen Toulmin, "The Tyranny of Principles," *Hastings Center Report* 11 (Dec. 1981): 31–9.

4

The Context of Health Care: Persons, Possessions, and States

Not all humans are equal. Health care confronts individuals of apparently widely divergent capacities: competent adults, mentally retarded adults, children, infants, and fetuses. These differences are the bases of morally relevant inequalities. Competent adults have a moral position not held by fetuses or infants. In addition, there are social inequalities among competent adults as a consequence of disparities in wealth. The wealthy may buy goods and services not available to the less fortunate. These inequalities reach into the central fabric of health care decisions. Finally, special questions of equality and inequality among persons are raised by the existence of states. States frequently claim special moral prerogatives to regulate health care and to distribute health care resources. To come to terms with bioethical issues as they arise for patients and health care professionals within the embrace of states, one will need to know how seriously one ought to take the various moral and financial inequalities among humans and the supposed moral prerogatives of states.

The special place of persons

Persons, not humans, are special. Adult competent humans have much higher intrinsic moral standing than human fetuses or adult frogs. It is important to understand the nature of these inequalities in some detail, for physicians and medical scientists intervene in numerous ways in the lives of adult humans, children, infants, fetuses, and laboratory mice. There is a need to understand in some detail why obligations of respect or of beneficence vary according to the moral status of the entities involved.

Only persons write or read books on philosophy. As my arguments have already shown, it is persons who are the constituents of the moral community. Only persons are concerned about moral arguments and can be convinced by them. The very notion of a moral community presumes a community of entities that are self-conscious, rational, free to choose, and in possession of a sense of moral concern. It is only when these entities are interested in understanding when they or others are acting in a blameworthy or praiseworthy fashion that there comes into existence a sphere of moral discourse I have termed the peaceable community. The peaceable community exists both actually and potentially. It exists potentially as a moral standpoint in terms of which self-conscious rational entities can speak of blame and praise. It is an intellectual standpoint in the sense that once one understands what it means justly to blame or praise, one realizes that such activities presuppose entities worthy of blame and praise, beings that could have abided by the conditions for the possibility of a peaceable community. In terms of this possible moral standpoint, persons can at any time in any place conceive of themselves as belonging to, and being bound by the rules of the peaceable community. An examination of moral language reveals a very important intellectual standpoint: the *mundus intelligibilis* of Kant.[1] Competent physicians and patients of any rational species anywhere in the cosmos can participate in this moral standpoint, which embraces not only the staff and patients of terrestrial hospitals, but also ships' doctors and their patients on flying saucers, should such exist. It is in terms of this intellectual possibility or standpoint[2] that persons can think of themselves as free; as Kant put it, ". . . we think of ourselves as free, we transport ourselves into the intelligible world as members of it and know the autonomy of the will together with its consequence, morality . . ."[3] When persons actually deport themselves in accord with the notion of the peaceable community, they can come to live in a general moral community with real boundaries, so that those persons that act against the peaceable community are by their own choices moral outlaws of all and any particular moral community. In summary, all persons can envisage (1) the *notion* of *the peaceable (moral) community*. (2) Insofar as they act in accord with this notion they participate with others in *the peaceable (moral) community* (i.e., defined by general secular pluralist morality), and (3) have the opportunity to fashion with consenting others a *particular* moral community (defined in addition by its particular view of the good life).

By examining the foundations of morals, Kant offered what could be termed the grammar of a major dimension of human thought. It is impos-

sible for rational, self-reflective entities coherently to construe themselves
except as moral, responsible entities. To protest that they ought to have been
treated differently, to blame themselves or others for their actions, is to enter
the domain of moral discourse, and at once to place all entities that engage in
that discourse in a special light. The self-reflective character of our thought
commits us to certain ways of regarding ourselves and similar entities. We
cannot coherently regard ourselves solely as caused to do the things we do.
An entity that asserted that all of its assertions were simply caused, not
rationally affirmed, would at that point abandon any truth claim to that
assertion regarding determinism. It would be holding, instead, that it had
been caused to make that statement (i.e., "I am determined") independently
of considered reflections or rational bases for assent. The domain of morality
in which we think of ourselves as free and responsible is inescapable. On the
other hand, there is, as Kant also recognizes, the domain of scientific and
empirical reflections where we do indeed treat the world as determined. This
is for Kant a second standpoint, as equally unavoidable as the moral point of
view.[4] For Kant, persons are put in the peculiar predicament of having to
conceive of themselves as determined, caused to do the things they do, while
on the other hand conceiving of themselves and other persons as moral entities,
worthy of blame and praise and therefore free.[5] It is important to realize that
Kant is not advancing a metaphysical proposition. He is rather indicating
two major and inescapable domains of human reasoning and experience. Our
very notion of ourselves as self-conscious, rational entities requires us to treat
ourselves as moral agents, as persons, and as knowers.

As a consequence, persons stand out as possessing a special importance for
moral discussions, for it is such entities who have rights to forbearance and
who may not be used without their permission. This moral concern, it must
be stressed, focuses *not on humans but on persons*. That an entity belongs to a
particular species is not important unless that membership results in that
entity's being in fact a moral agent. This should be fairly clear if one reflects
on what it means to be a human, a member of a particular species. First one
must note that there have in fact been a number of human species within the
genus *Homo*. To identify an entity as a member of *Homo sapiens* is to place it
in a particular taxonomic locus. The genus *Homo* shares with the genera
Ramapithecus and *Australopithecus* membership in the family Hominidae of
the suborder Anthropoidea of the order primates of the class Mammalia. In
identifying an entity as human, one indicates that it possesses primate
characteristics, such as long limbs and pentadactyl hands and feet, along with
an increased specialization of the nervous system. With the family Hominidae one would want to note the development of tool-making capacities,
language, and other symbol-related or -dependent behaviour. If one were in
the future to possess a galactic study of rational species in the cosmos, one

would likely find that numerous, somewhat different biological bases lead to the ability to use tools, language, and abstract symbols. Humans would be distinguished primarily through their biological peculiarities as primates. But insofar as one characterizes the peculiar anatomical structures and physiological capacities of humans as primates, one advances a set of biological characteristics that take on moral significance only insofar as they support the special characteristics of persons, namely, their capacity to play a role in the moral community. It is because members of *Homo sapiens* are usually self-conscious, rational, and possess a moral sense that being a human is so significant.

As talk of angels and of gods and goddesses, not to mention current science-fictional speculation regarding rational, selfconscious entities on other planets, indicates, not all persons need be humans. The archangel Gabriel appearing to Mohammed in the desert, and E.T. going through a modern twentieth-century American town, provide examples of entities that are persons, though they are clearly not human. What distinguishes persons is their capacity to be self-conscious, rational, and concerned with worthiness of blame and praise. The possibility of such entities grounds the possibility of the moral community. It offers us a way of reflecting on the rightness and wrongness of actions and the worthiness or unworthiness of actors.

On the other hand, not all humans are persons. Not all humans are self-conscious, rational, and able to conceive of the possibility of blaming and praising. Fetuses, infants, the profoundly mentally retarded, and the hopelessly comatose provide examples of human nonpersons. Such entities are members of the human species. They do not in and of themselves have standing in the moral community. They cannot blame or praise or be worthy of blame or praise. They are not prime participants in the moral endeavor. Only persons have that status.

It is because of interest in morality that talk about persons as moral agents occurs. One speaks of persons in order to identify entities one can with warrant blame and praise, which can themselves blame and praise, and which can as a result play a role in the core of the moral life. In order to engage in moral discourse, such entities will need to reflect on themselves; they must therefore be *self-conscious*. They will need in addition to be able to conceive of rules of action for themselves and others in order to envisage the possibility of the moral community. They will need to be *rational* beings. That rationality must include an understanding of the notion of worthiness of blame and praise: *a minimal moral sense*. Sociopaths would cease to be moral agents (persons in the moral sense), only if they lost even the capacity to understand blameworthiness to the point that they could not blame those who might injure them. These three characteristics of self-consciousness, rationality, and moral sense identify those entities capable of moral discourse. These characteristics give to those entities the rights and obligations of the morality of self-respect. The principle of autonomy and its elaboration in the morality of mutual respect applies only to autonomous beings. It concerns only persons. The morality of autonomy is the morality of persons.

For this reason it is nonsensical to speak of respecting the autonomy of fetuses, infants, or profoundly retarded adults, who have never been rational. There is no autonomy to affront.[6] Treating such entities without regard for that which they do not possess, and never have possessed, despoils them of nothing. They fall outside the inner sanctum of morality. Just as this concern with respecting moral agents excludes some humans, it may in fact include nonhuman persons, should such exist. Though failing to treat a fetus or an infant as a person in the strict sense shows no disrespect to that fetus or infant, to fail to treat E.T. or a peaceable extraterrestrial at a *Star Wars* bar scene without such respect would be to act immorally in a fundamental fashion. It would mean that one had acted against the very possibility of *the* peaceable community.

What is important about us as humans is not our membership in the species *Homo sapiens* as such, but the fact that we are persons. This distinction between persons and humans will have important consequences for the ways in which one treats human personal life versus merely human biological life. Once these distinctions are clearly drawn, one can disclose some of the conceptual confusions that have plagued the moral debates regarding abortion. One will not be interested in when human life begins, unless one is attempting to determine when the human species evolved. Life, it would appear, is an unbroken continuum some four billion years old, and human life a phenomenon some two million years or more old. One is, or should be, concerned with determining when in human ontogeny humans become persons.[7]

In summary to this point: not all persons need be human, and not all humans are persons. In order to understand the geography of obligations in health care regarding fetuses, infants, the profoundly mentally retarded, and the severely brain damaged, one will need to determine the moral status of persons and of mere human biological life, and then develop criteria to distinguish between these classes of entities. Further, even if infants are not persons in the strict sense that E.T. would be, there still may be important reasons for according special rights to infants. In order to sort out and distinguish the obligations one holds to competent adults, infants, fetuses, and the severely brain damaged, one will need to assess the moral significance of different categories of human life.

Such categorizations require no metaphysical commitments or doctrines. Nor do reflections about the status of persons commit one either to affirming or to denying traditional religious or metaphysical views regarding the existence of the soul or its entrance into the human body at some particular point in human ontogeny. One must, rather, ignore such for the purposes of these considerations. In general secular reflections, one must presume that beings are rational beings whenever they show evidence of being rational. One will not assume that fetuses in some occult or hidden fashion are in fact rational beings. One will not assume that there is a rational soul in some fashion lying hidden and undisclosed. Persons are persons when they have the characteristics of persons, when they are self-conscious, rational, and in possession of a minimal moral sense. In anticipation of future distinctions in this volume, one should note that such entities are *persons in the strict sense*.

A bias in favor of persons?

Though this approach simplifies matters by freeing discussions of metaphysical quandaries, it begets some special problems and puzzles of its own. First, one might object that this way of construing things creates an unduly person-centered or person-oriented construal of the moral universe. This difficulty is inescapable. Since it is only persons who reflect on the world and fashion accounts of its meaning, all accounts will perforce be developed in the rational language of persons, such that rational beings and their concerns will recurringly be central to moral accounts. One cannot give a rational account of the nature of things except from the point of view of rational beings: persons. It is for this reason that respect of persons is so central to moral discourse.

This orientation marks the morality of welfare and social sympathies. It is persons who can define for themselves their own best interests. They can place themselves and their concerns in their own terms for any calculations made under the principle of beneficence. But for nonpersonal organisms, others must choose on their behalf. Others must determine for those entities what their best interests are. A competent adult patient can define in his own terms his own best interests. It is surely the case that rational individuals can make mistakes in such calculations. But their judgments about themselves have a cardinal significance in that persons can decide for themselves the ordering of costs and benefits that they wish to take seriously for their lives, including the risk they are willing to run. Persons are in this very important sense self-legislating. This is not the case in the instance of infants, the profoundly mentally retarded, and other individuals who cannot determine for themselves their own hierarchy of costs and benefits. Persons must choose for them. Since such choices will depend on the moral sense of the chooser, and since there is not one univocal moral sense to deliver a single authoritative hierarchy of costs and benefits, nonpersons will have imposed on their destiny the particular choices of particular persons or communities of persons. Both the morality of mutual respect and the morality of welfare and mutual sympathies are inextricably person-centered.

When persons must calculate the weight that should be given to the interests of persons versus nonpersons, it is quite likely that the position of persons will remain central. Persons can appreciate harm and good, pleasure and pain, in intricate, reflective fashions. It would appear likely that rational beings after careful reflection will hold that it is better first to test pain-killing substances on animals, even when such experiments will mean suffering for the animals, rather than to move directly to trials on persons. The greater good of persons will likely be seen as having a higher position in the hierarchy of goods than the good of experimental animals who will need to be sacrificed in the course of medical experimentation and research. The hunter will decide that the delectation of the hunt, and the refined recall of the kill in sharing stories with other hunters, is a good that outweighs the value of the life of the animal to be hunted and killed. The same will be the case for those individuals who plan to raise animals for food. There will be none but persons to adjudicate which goods are to be given greater weight. Moreover, when such arguments come to a complete standstill and fail to deliver a view as to which side ought to be given precedence, when the problem is TEYKU, then it is not unreasonable for persons to choose on the side of their intuitions. This is not a consequence of mere prejudice or idiosyncratic bias. It reflects what it means to give rational moral arguments in these circumstances and what as a consequence will appear as rational, defensible choices. Even animals who are not persons, and will never be persons, are thus placed inescapably within the bounds of a person-centered morality, dominated by person-centered interests.

One should note that prejudice in favor of persons is not like prejudice in favor of humans versus other possible rational species. If, for instance, we ever needed to compare the competing claims of humans and extraterrestrial persons, we could never morally use them merely as means, as one may use animals.

Potentiality and probability

What is one to make of those entities such as embryos, fetuses, and infants who will with great likelihood develop into moral agents? It might appear that one could in such circumstances appeal to a notion of potentiality in order to argue that since fetuses and children are potential persons, they must *eo ipso* be accorded the rights and standing of persons. This argument cannot succeed. This was already clear to the theologians of the Middle Ages who approached the issue of abortion within the compass of an Aristotelian world view and its commitment to a doctrine of potentiality. St. Thomas Aquinas argued that taking the life of an early fetus did not involve the evil of murder, even though the early fetus or embryo was potentially a person.[8] This view was reflected in Roman Catholic theology and in canon law from the time of St. Thomas until 1869, except for a brief period between 1588 and 1591.[9] During that time, taking the life of an early fetus or embryo was held usually to be a mortal sin, somewhat analogous to the mortal sin of contraception.[10] However, it did not involve the sin of murder. The Catholic church correctly perceived that human life developed only over time into the life of a person. It recognized that a sort of human life preceded the human life of persons. This issue surfaced in an interesting fashion in speculations regarding the doctrine of the Immaculate Conception of the Blessed Virgin Mary. If Mary's body only later developed into being a body for a rational soul, then the immaculate conception of her *soul* could only take place sometime after the physical conception of her *body*. "Before the creation of Mary's soul, that which was to become her body shared the common lot; but before the creation of her soul *Mary* did not yet exist."[11]

If X is a potential Y, it follows that X is not a Y. If fetuses are potential persons, it follows clearly that fetuses are not persons. As a consequence, X does not have the actual rights of Y, but only potentially has the rights of Y. If fetuses are only potential persons, they do not have the rights of persons. To take an example from S. I. Benn, if X is a potential president, it follows from that fact alone that X does not yet have the rights and prerogatives of actual presidents.[12]

Undoubtedly, the language of potentiality is itself misleading, for it is often taken to suggest that an X that is a potential Y in some mysterious fashion already possesses the being and significance of Y. It is therefore perhaps better to speak not of X's being a potential Y but rather of its having a certain probability of developing into Y. One can then assign a probability value to that outcome. Recent research concerning zygotes suggests that there is a great amount of zygote wastage. Since only 40–50 percent of zygotes survive to be persons (i.e., adult, competent human beings), it might be best to speak of human zygotes as 0.4 probable persons. In this fashion one can indicate that they are the kinds of entities likely with that probability to develop into full-fledged moral agents, without suggesting that they are in some mysterious fashion already persons.[13]

It follows from these considerations that one harms *no person* either by not conceiving that entity or by aborting the body from which it would develop. Though one is bound morally to respect persons in the sense of forbearing from unconsented-to harms against them and acting to aid them in achieving their good, it does not follow that one is bound to increase the number of such entities to which one has obligations. One might very well come to the reasonable conclusion that there are sufficient persons already to whom one has obligations. Reflections on the consequences of overpopulation may lead to the rational conclusion that it would be best if there were not more persons to feed, care, and respect. In addition, one might conclude that persons of a particular sort, such as those with severe physical or mental impairments, would create particularly severe moral obligations, which would be best avoided. In such circumstances, one might decide to prevent such obligations from coming into existence by using abortion. That zygotes, embryos, or fetuses are human rather than simian or canine would be of significance primarily in terms of one's interest in having more humans rather than more individuals of a different species. One might indeed imagine circumstances in which one would be very pleased regarding the high likelihood that a whooping crane embryo would go to term, but disvalue the likelihood that a human embryo (e.g., one likely to lead to the birth of a severely deformed infant) would go to term.

The value of animal life, which is not the life of a person, must be determined by other persons. Since in the case of such animals there is no person to respect, the issue is the value that must be imputed to the entity and the regard one must give to the pains and pleasures of that animal. The more an organism's life is characterized not just by sensations but by consciousness of objects and goals, the more one can plausibly hold that the organism's life has value for it. The more an organism can direct itself with appreciation and subtlety to certain objects and away from others, the more plausible it is that it has an inner life with some prereflective anticipations of values as values are understood by self-conscious free agents. Adult higher mammals enjoy their lives, pursue their pleasures, and avoid sufferings in elaborate and complex ways. Their lives in this very straightforward sense can have both value and disvalue for them. But since they are not persons, they cannot require that they be respected. They cannot as persons set moral limits to the extent to which they can be used by others. They cannot refuse with moral authority to participate in the results of comparisons of the value of being beneficent to them versus being beneficent to other entities. They are not members of the moral community but are rather objects of its beneficence. The value of an animal's quality of life is thus set by persons in two senses. First, if the animal has no developed conscious life, persons may find little intrinsic value in such life and the predominant value may be the value that the life has as an object for persons. Second, even if the animal has an inward life that in a prereflective sense has a value for that organism, persons must still compare that value with other competing values.

It is for these reasons that the value of zygotes, embryos, and fetuses is to be primarily understood in terms of the values they have for actual persons. Zygotes, fetuses, and embryos do not have the rich inward life of adult mammals. Thus, if the zygote promises to be the long-awaited child of a couple that has been struggling for years to have another child, it is very likely to be highly valued by the couple and by all who are sympathetic with the would-be parents' hopes. On the other hand, if the zygote is in an unwed graduate student for whom the pregnancy would mean a major disruption of study plans, the zygote will likely be highly disvalued by her and by all who are sympathetic with her plans. Or if the zygote has a trisomy of chromosome 21, not only will the parents and those close to the parents likely disvalue the zygote, but so will society, which will need to participate in the costs of raising a defective child, should the pregnancy be uninterrupted. Some value is likely to be assigned to the zygote simply because it is human. However, one must remember that the sentience of a zygote, embryo, or fetus is much less than that of an adult mammal. One might even develop a suggestion of the natural theologian Charles Hartshorne so as to argue that from the perspective of the Deity the intrinsic value of a human fetus will be less than that of an adult normal member of some other mammalian species.[14] One might still be concerned that the processes of abortion might cause pain to the fetus. But one must remember that the level of obligations one has to a fetus in this regard is the same as one would have to an animal with a similar level of sensorimotor integration and perception.

To put this into perspective, one must realize that circumcisions are routinely performed for ritual and so-called medical reasons on male infants without the benefit of anesthesia. The basis for this practice is the incapacity of the newborn infant to integrate experiences sufficiently so as to actually suffer. For suffering to occur, there must be some fairly well-developed frontal lobe connections to allow the entity not only to experience the pain, but to recognize the pain over time as a noxious quale that must be avoided.[15] The capacities of fetuses give no indication that they approach the capacities for suffering of adult mammals. As a result, one's moral obligations will simply be to make sure that the good pursued, such as avoiding the birth of a Down's syndrome child, outweighs the evil of the pain to the animal organism to be killed.

An excursus regarding animals

Some have found this assessment of the comparative standing of persons and animals to be improper. Robert Nozick speaks critically of the maxim "Utilitarianism for animals, Kantianism for people."[16] He speaks against the notion that "human beings may not be used or sacrificed for the benefit of others; animals may be used or sacrificed for the benefit of other people or animals, *only if* those benefits are greater than the loss inflicted."[17] This position derives from the Kantian moral contrast between persons and things. This moral position, in fact, is presupposed by the industry of medical research and investigation that first studies drugs through animal models. Persons are then used only after animal research has indicated that such a course is relatively safe. Such an approach is Kantian. Persons for Kant are subjects whose actions can be imputed.[18] There may be grounds for suspecting that certain nonhuman mammals are indeed not only animals but also persons as we are. If they are persons, then we owe them respect. However, the behavior of all but perhaps the higher apes shows no evidence of a rational appreciation of the moral life. Persons are moral agents, entities that can with justification be blamed and praised. They are entities that can be a part of the community of ends. In contrast, nonpersons are not worthy of blame or praise. As a consequence, "Every object of free choice that itself lacks freedom is therefore called a thing (*res corporalis*)."[19] For Kant one has duties to persons, and duties to persons regarding things, including animals.[20] This duty to other persons regarding animals is constituted in part out of an obligation to act in ways that will enhance and protect moral sensibilities. Thus, Kant argues that "tender feelings towards dumb animals develop humane feelings toward mankind".[21] Certain rules or practices of kindness and consideration toward animals work to the advantage of moral practices established to secure respect for persons.[22]

One must go beyond the Kantian perspective. One ought, in addition to recognizing duties to other persons regarding animals, recognize as well a duty directly to regard the pain and suffering of animals. One has duties of beneficence to animals, even if the strongest of such duties are usually simply negative ones of beneficence, that is, duties of nonmaleficence. Though one does not have duties of respect to animals because they fall outside the bounds of the morality of mutual respect, one has duties to them in terms of the morality of welfare and mutual sympathies. Here it might be useful to distinguish between persons, who ought to be objects of respect, and animals, which ought to be objects of beneficent regard. We owe to persons both respect and beneficent regard. To animals we owe only beneficent regard.

One can in part take account of Nozick's concerns and bring them within a reformed Kantian viewpoint in which one recognizes that it is only persons who are the judges of the relative significance of harms and benefits and the objects of our respect and beneficent regard, while animals are the objects of our beneficent regard. When persons are dealing with entities that are not persons, it is persons who will make the judgment regarding the significance of any exchanges of harms and benefits. It is persons who fashion actual moral communities with their particular moral senses, histories, and practices. Nonpersonal animals do not constitute moral communities, nor do they have a history. Moreover, there is no border of respect protecting organisms that are not persons. Animals are protected rather through a web of moral concerns regarding welfare and sympathies, which also protects persons. Respect of persons springs from the concern to act in ways in which persons can be justified as praiseworthy or blameworthy. In contrast, caring for animals springs from the concern to have a world that maximizes welfare and sustains a web of sympathies.

This web of sympathy binds us most tightly to those animals with which we can actually share sympathies—usually mammals and perhaps some birds. These bonds of sympathy are most fully drawn between humans and mature primates; they can also reach between human persons and human zygotes or fetuses. This web of sympathies justifies a wide range of beneficent action, not only to laboratory animals, but to human fetuses as well. Such concerns may influence the kind of abortifacient one might choose, all else being equal. They will as well have implications for the ways in which animals are treated generally. They strongly support policies of kindness and sympathy toward animals. However, they do not foreclose the raising of animals for meat or hunting, much less for use in research, whether it be medical research in the strict sense or even the testing of the safety of new cosmetics.

Infants, the profoundly retarded, and social senses of "person"

These conclusions raise a third and very vexatious difficulty. What is one to make of the status of infants, the profoundly mentally retarded, and those who are suffering from very advanced stages of Alzheimer's disease? Such entities are not persons in any strict sense. Yet we are concerned usually to accord such entities many of the rights normally possessed by adult persons. In the case of rules against maiming and injuring but not killing fetuses and infants, one can advance a justification of our moral concerns in terms of respect for the future person that such a fetus or infant will likely become. Even if one does not accord special moral rights to merely possible persons (e.g., the persons who could be conceived were the readers of this volume engaged in fruitful sexual congress rather than philosophical study) or probable persons (e.g., zygotes that would develop into competent persons, were the women carrying them not to seek an abortion in order to complete their graduate studies in theology), one can still understand the status of fetuses in the light of the standing of future actual persons. Future persons can have the standing of actual persons who we know will in the future exist. If one plants a bomb in the foundations of a grammar school with a timing device so that it will explode in fifteen years, one is intending to murder actual persons who will in the future exist. So, too, if one injures a fetus or infant, but does not kill it, one then sets in train a series of events that will in fact injure a future actual person.[23] In these terms one can secure certain moral protections (and moral grounds for the legal protection) of infants.

Considerations of beneficence protect animals, which are not persons, against being tortured uselessly, whether or not they are human. Considerations of the contingent rights of future persons protect entities that will become persons from being maimed. They do not protect infants, the profoundly mentally retarded, or those suffering from advanced Alzheimer's disease from being killed painlessly at whim. What one must seek are the grounds that may justify the practices through which infants, the profoundly mentally retarded, and the very senile are customarily assigned a proportion of the rights possessed by entities who are persons strictly, including being protected from being killed at whim. Here, perhaps, one can take a suggestion from Kant regarding the need to support practices that will, in general, lead to the protection of persons. To find grounds for protecting such entities, one will need to look at the justification for certain social practices in terms of their importance for persons so as to justify a social role one might term "being a person for social considerations." Since this sense of person cannot be justified in terms of the basic grammar of morality (i.e., because such entities do not have intrinsic moral standing through being moral agents), one will need rather to justify a social sense of person in terms of the usefulness of the practice of treating certain entities as if they were persons. If such a practice can be justified, one will have, in addition to a strict sense of persons as moral agents, a social sense of persons justified in terms of various utilitarian and other consequentialist considerations.

Most societies in fact have such a social sense of person, which is usually assigned to human beings at birth, or at some time soon after birth. In ancient Greek law an infant could be exposed with impunity up to the time it would be admitted into the family through a special ceremony, the *amphidromia*. After that the infant had standing and received some of the major rights of persons.[24] In other societies the line has been less clearly drawn. To take one example, a strain of Jewish interpretation holds that the death of an infant during the first thirty days of life should be considered a miscarriage. Such an infant had not yet been given the full standing of children that have survived beyond this point.[25] Even in contemporary American society one can note a greater acceptance of the cessation of treatment for severely defective newborns than would be the case with young children fully socialized within the role of child. It is as if the full conveying of social personhood does not occur immediately for many neonates.[26] As we shall see in chapter 6, this informal distinction between the treatment accorded to neonates versus other children has come under critical attack from some quarters.[27] In many societies, and to some extent in ours, there remain informal distinctions between the standing accorded to neonates and that given to infants who have been brought fully within the role of the child and accorded robust rights similar to those possessed by persons in the strict sense.

A social role of person can be justified for infants and others in terms of (1) the role's supporting important virtues such as sympathy and care for human life, especially when that life is fragile and defenseless, and (2) the role's offering a protection against the uncertainties as to when exactly humans become persons strictly, as well as protecting persons during various vicissitudes of competence and incompetence, while (3) in addition securing the important practice of child-rearing through which humans develop as persons in the strict sense.

Since the assigning of the status of person in the social sense on the basis of such concerns must be justified in terms of utilitarian and consequentialist considerations, the justifications will be somewhat different, depending on whether the practice concerns (1) humans who in the past were persons in the strict sense (e.g., individuals now suffering from severe Alzheimer's disease); (2) humans who are likely to become persons and have been brought within a social role giving them special social standing (e.g., infants); (3) neonates who could become persons, but who have not yet been brought within a social role giving them special social standing (e.g., neonates in an intensive care unit who have not yet been fully accepted by the parents); (4) neonates who, because of their serious handicaps, will not be accorded strong social rights; and (5) those humans who have not, and never will, become persons in the strict sense (e.g., the profoundly mentally retarded). There are likely to be somewhat different justifications for the protection afforded in each instance. In each case, one will find a special social role justified in terms of a set of important moral considerations sustained by a major social practice, such as child rearing.

Severely defective newborns: weakening the protections
of the social role of person

The moral claims of these practices of assigning rights to humans who are not persons will not be absolute. When one can advance a set of consider- ations to show clearly that suspending the practice will achieve a greater balance of benefits over harms, such an exception can be justified. One may want to require that such exceptions be generated only in terms of well- drawn rules for weighing the goods at stake. One may even require what is tantamount to a conflict between practices. In any event, there are moral grounds for not imposing undue financial and psychological burdens on those who are persons in the strict sense. First and foremost, persons have a right, unless they have agreed otherwise, to act at liberty as long as they are not employing unconsented-to force against other innocent persons, or imposing unjustifiable suffering on innocent organisms. Parents who judge that a defective newborn should either be allowed painlessly to die or be aided in dying painlessly offend against neither of these two constraints. Practices of protecting the interests of parents and guardians who are persons in the strict sense will conflict at times with practices of imposing duties on parents and guardians through fashioning a social role of persons for children. The obligations imposed by others in terms of the social roles of persons will thus be prima facie obligations, which can in particular circumstances be set aside.

A balance must be struck between the likely benefits and costs to be incurred by allowing parents to choose the circumstances under which they will become the guardians of persons (i.e., children who are persons in the social sense and who may become so in the strict sense). The greater the economic, social, and psychological burdens involved for the parents, the less affront is likely to be given to the practice of according personhood to infants, if exceptions are made under such circumstances. One must recognize that the parents are persons strictly, whereas infants accrue their significance as social persons in terms of the contribution of the practice of parenting to persons in the strict sense.

The concrete nature of the web of beneficence that characterizes the obligations to provide welfare, including care for severely defective newborns, is determined within a particular community through the judgments of those who are persons in a strict sense. There is likely to be a range of legitimate relativity. In addition, there is the issue of the extent to which families have committed themselves to the social constraints of the surrounding society so as to oblige them to treat infants against the choices of the family members. The more one takes the freedom of individuals seriously, the more one will need to take seriously as well the moral standing of the family as a free association of persons who have rights to judge regarding those of its members who are not persons in the strict sense. To force parents to treat a severely defective newborn may indeed count as imposing by force and without justification a particular view of beneficence.

The geography of obligations shifts as a family accepts an infant and assigns it the role of child, while accepting social support in various fashions for the child's care and development. The infant may then acquire a moral standing within both the family and society. It is before that point that matters are not clear. For example, under what circumstances might parents insist not only that they will not provide for the care of a severely defective infant, but moreover that that infant should (a) be allowed to die, or (b) be killed. We will return to these matters in the discussion of severely defective newborns in chapter 6. Here it is enough to note that defective newborns offer us an example of entities that may have a special attenuated standing as social persons, in contrast with those infants who have been brought fully within the social role of person. Infants, the profoundly mentally retarded, and the severely senile may accrue a moral standing through which they possess rights but no duties. There will be justifications in certain circumstances for withdrawing elements of that moral standing. For a rather clear example, discussed further in chapter 6, hopelessly severely senile individuals are often accorded the standing of social persons in an attenuated sense very similar to that of severely defective newborns, for whom also nothing but basic nursing care need morally be provided. Finally, the hopelessly comatose, and anencephalic infants, appear to have a moral standing, which imposes even fewer obligations.

Being a person: in the strict sense and in various social senses

Let me summarize where this leads us with regard to a number of senses of person important for medicine. By anticipation one can make the following distinctions. There is a sense of person as moral agent, which I have termed being a person in the strict sense (one might call this person$_1$), which contrasts with a social sense of person to whom nearly the full rights of persons strictly are accorded as in the case of young children (person$_2$). A social sense of person is accorded to neonates as well, but it is not yet as strong or as secure as that of infants generally (person$_3$). The status of the neonate changes to that of a young child once there is a commitment to that level of treatment. A social sense of person is also accorded to individuals who are no longer, but who once were, persons$_1$ and who are still capable of some minimal interactions (person$_4$), and a social sense of person is also assigned as in the case of the very severely and profoundly retarded and demented who never were and will never be persons in the strict sense (person$_5$). Some may also assign a social sense of person to certain severely damaged humans (i.e., severely and permanently comatose humans), who cannot interact in even minimal social roles. As we will see in chapter 6, the law should be changed so they can be declared dead (i.e., in that chapter I will defend a neocortical definition of death). I advance these distinctions to emphasize the many ways in which rights are accorded to humans.

There is unavoidably a major distinction to be drawn between persons who are moral agents and persons to whom the rights of moral agents are imputed. One can blame and praise adult competent patients, for they hold both rights and duties. They are moral agents. One cannot blame and praise infants. They are bearers of rights, but not of duties. One can at best act in their best interests. Persons who are moral agents have rights as a part of morality itself. The rights of persons in a social sense are created by particular communities. In addition, there are real distinctions between the moral standing of humans that can at least play a social role and those who cannot play such roles (e.g., the permanently comatose, or anencephalic children). These distinctions reflect a geography of moral presuppositions already well in place. Moreover, this geography of moral presuppositions accords with what can be justified in these areas.

What may at first blush appear to be exotic if not outrageous conclusions should under closer examination gain a certain familiarity. Though our language provides us with only one term for person, a close examination of the actual ways in which we deal with humans shows that we in fact have more than one concept of person. In dealing with competent adults, young infants, and newborn severely defective infants, we make decisions within moral practices supposing quite different senses of bearers of rights. Indeed, only persons in the strict sense are bearers of both moral rights and duties. Infants and the comatose have no moral obligations. One cannot avoid such distinctions among the moral statuses possessed by humans as persons in the strict sense, as infants brought within the role of child and as defective newborns not yet given such a social role.

These conclusions are not forwarded in order to weaken the status of children or infants. Rather, the very opposite is the intention. The goal has been to provide the strongest grounds, justified in terms of general secular arguments, for the moral standing of humans. It is because a careful examination of the practice of morality reveals a central importance for persons in the strict sense, but not for humans as such, that one is forced to elaborate secondary social senses of person in order to account for the moral standing of infants, the profoundly mentally retarded, and the senile.

Some may find it disquieting that the strongest rights claims that can be advanced in favor of humans who are not persons in the strict sense depend on consequentialist, if not indeed on utilitarian, considerations. These conclusions do not represent an assault on those who are not persons in the strict sense. The circumstances reflect the limits of secular philosophical reasoning. Only some of our prejudices can be justified. One should be pleased (perhaps, indeed, *relieved*) that at least the arguments available support strong deontological rights for persons in the strict sense. These establish strong claims of physicians and adult competent patients to be treated as free moral agents.

Those who are concerned that only a consequentialist, and most likely utilitarian, bulwark exists for the major rights possessed by infants, the profoundly mentally retarded, and the senile should recall that utilitarianism has been responsible for a great proportion of the liberal advances in personal rights.[28] The fact that the moral standing of infants, the profoundly mentally retarded, and the senile depends on consequentialist considerations that will in part vary given different circumstances, and that more easily admit of exceptions, does not mean that those entities will be treated capriciously, or immorally. But one can only do as best one can. Where stronger arguments are not available to support one's moral intuitions, one must recognize this circumstance, no matter how painful it may be.

Sleeping persons and the problem of embodiment

There is yet another major puzzle to face. What are we to make of the status of sleeping individuals? If being a person depends on being a moral agent, and if one does not have a metaphysical doctrine of the soul to explain where persons go when they are asleep, what is the moral standing of a sleeping person?[29] Do personhood and its rights go away while one sleeps? This puzzle can be answered without metaphysical assumptions concerning souls of similar substances, through an analysis of what it means to be a person, and to possess moral claims on the peaceable community of persons generally. This analysis depends on at least two major factors, the satisfactory resolution of either of which should dispel the puzzle sufficiently to give sleeping persons a standing tantamount to those who are persons strictly.

The first point turns on what it means to be an embodied person. Persons do not appear to themselves as discontinuous. They sew together their various episodes of wakefulness and presence within a single identity. Alfred Schutz has explored this in his phenomenological account of going to sleep and awakening. The very sense of a person includes its unifying various temporally discontinuous episodes into one life.[30] Of course these attempts can fail. John Hughlings Jackson was one of the first clearly to recognize that our integration as one continuous person is a precarious and difficult undertaking.[31] To be a finite, spatiotemporal, sensibly intuiting person is to have the task of constantly constituting temporally diverse experiences as one's own. This point is appreciated by Kant in his characterizations of person or subjects in terms of the transcendental unity of apperception, the capacity to unite experiences under an "I think," to make a diverse manifold of experiences one's own.[32] Those experiences that one can unite within one's unity of apperception under one's "I think," one's "I experience," become one's own. Persons, if they are not free of spatiotemporal extension (e.g., angels or gods), will be subject to the difficulty of integrating various experiences as their own. Sleep constitutes simply one example of such a problem for integration.

This can be better appreciated in terms of an understanding of the mind–brain relationship. To talk of minds that are finite, spatio–temporal, and sensibly perceiving presumes that they will span spatial and temporal extension as a part of their very being.[33] Their embodiment is their spatially and temporally extended place in this world. The integrative function of the brain must span brief pulsations of attention that are experienced in a single act of self-consciousness. As a result, what one can minimally mean by a person in such circumstances cannot be an unbroken godlike continuity of selfconsciousness. Rather it is a self-consciousness, as a recurring integration of experience spanning discontinuities. This analysis does not require metaphysical presuppositions or a doctrine of potentiality, such as that required for those who hold that since fetuses are potential persons, they should count as persons. The question is not whether to regard an entity that has never shown the capacities of a person, as if it were a person. The question is rather how to regard an entity that intermittently shows the full capacities of a moral agent. How should one regard that entity during a period of time when it is not showing those capacities, but when one believes it will again in the future demonstrate those capacities?

To begin with, there is a difference in kind between a body that *is* someone's body, and a body that *may become* someone's body. With respect to a zygote, fetus, or even young infant, one does not yet know the person who will come to be "in" (or perhaps better, in, through, and with) that body. With respect to a sleeping person, one knows whose body it is. One knows who is there. The person will again awaken, make judgments, and answer questions. The body with the full capacities of sensorimotor integration that are the physical expression of a person's life is that person in the world. The body's capacities are the capacities of a person. One will need to distinguish between the potentiality *to become* a person and the potentialities *of* a person. There is a difference in kind between knowing who is sleeping, in the case of an adult competent human, and knowing who a fetus will be.

The point is that the very meaning of a spatiotemporally extended, sensibly intuiting person involves the spanning of, and the integration of, temporal extension. The existence of such persons will therefore not be set aside by temporal discontinuities across which their identity can reasonably be presumed to span. Talking about persons as spatiotemporally extended entities will therefore mean regarding their intact embodiment as them, as long as that embodiment maintains the full capacities that are the physical substrata of moral agents.

This point can be put a second way. The very language of blame and praise presumes that moral agents span discontinuities of experience. If interruptions in attention or self-consciousness shattered the identity of persons, the minimum moral fabric of the peaceable moral community would be set aside. Given the discontinuous nature of finite, spatiotemporal moral agents, discontinuity would make the moral community impossible, if strict continuity were required. If one allowed moral agents who are fully self-conscious to exterminate without the permission of those innocent moral agents whose attention had temporarily waned, had become temporarily obtunded, or had fallen asleep, one would be allowing them to act against the peaceable moral community insofar as it exists. Since spatiotemporal persons fashion moral actions over time and across moments of attention and of sleep, they are the sort of entity, should they come into existence, that would need to be treated with respect even when they were inattentive or sleeping.

These considerations do not lead one to the position that one is morally obliged to bring moral agents into existence so as to continue the moral community as an actual community through history. Such an argument would turn the moral community into a goal to be pursued. Rather, what has been advanced is a sketch of the minimal conceptual conditions for the notion of a moral community of spatiotemporal persons. Insofar as we think of ourselves as moral agents, we must think of ourselves as acting across these discontinuities in self-consciousness that occur, though our brains, our embodiments, remain intact. It is a condition of understanding ourselves within the practice of morality. One cannot respect other moral agents, while willing to destroy their unique place in the world, their embodiment. To will to destroy the embodiment of actual persons is to will to act against the very morality of mutual respect. The very notion of mutual respect and of moral authority would have to be rejected. This situation contrasts with the killing of fetuses or infants. In the case of competent adults not only does one know whose embodiment is at stake (unlike fetuses and infants, whose bodies are not yet anyone's embodiment), but taking a view that would allow the killing of sleeping persons would make a coherent portrayal of a moral community of spatiotemporally extended persons impossible. Killing fetuses only prevents possible persons from becoming persons and therefore members of the moral community. Finally, if the embodiment of a person is so compromised as to preclude any future states of consciousness, the person has ceased to exist. The person has died. But beforehand the person perdures.

The reader may suspect that such reflections are the contemporary equivalent of the supposed medieval theological pursuit of a census of the number of angels dancing on the pins of Christendom. However, since moral questions are intellectual questions, they commit us to tracing out the implications of moral theories. The controversies regarding the moral significance of killing fetuses force us to explore the differences between actual moral agents (e.g., competent, adult patients) and fetuses, while paying attention to those borderline cases that might constrain us to reaccept a doctrine of potentiality, or even to speak of souls within the context of general secular ethics.

Split brains, transplanted brains, and the starship Enterprise

Some puzzles remain. There is evidence that each hemisphere of the brain has an at least partially independent sphere of consciousness. This independence is exaggerated when the right and left hemispheres are disconnected, as occurs with a transection of the corpus callosum.[34] Such questions regarding the unity of individuals go back at least to the nineteenth century and the reflections of Wigan[35] and John Hughlings Jackson.[36] These issues have spawned a considerable contemporary literature,[37] which is relevant here insofar as it raises the issue of what will count as *one* moral agent. What does one make of the moral responsibility of *a* particular personality of an individual with multiple personalities?[38] Who are the persons inhabiting the body of the "individual" with numerous personalities? What does one make of the standing of an individual who has lost all memory of the past? Does he start over as a new person? These questions focus more on the problem of personal identity and the grounds for the distinctions among persons, than on what will count as a moral agent. The issue is the identity of moral agents and the individuation of moral agents.[39]

Special problems of personal identity can be raised by fantasies in which one imagines being able to transplant the brain from the crushed body of a man into a woman's body that is intact, save for the fact the brain has been destroyed.[40] If John then awakens in the body of Mary after the operation and states, "I'm John. What am I doing in Mary's body?" what should one make of these circumstances? Let us presume that James was married to Mary and that Sally was married to John. Is Sally still married to "John," though he is now "in" Mary's body? What if Sally had promised to make love to John on his birthday, and John, now in Mary's body, still wants her to keep her promise? Since criteria not only of continuity, but also of memory and consciousness (the ability to continue uniting experiences under an I think) are satisfied, as are criteria of bodily continuity (John's brain in Mary's body is the same brain that was in John's body before the operation), it appears to be reasonable to say that John has survived the operation and that James's wife is dead. Moreover, Sally and John will now need to work out new understandings under unanticipated circumstances (yet circumstances that would have analogies to what would obtain were John to have an operation to change his phenotypic sexuality).

Even more exotic fantasies appear to be manageable within the usual criteria of personal identity. One might imagine a human with connected cerebral hemispheres being specially raised so that each hemisphere is equally linguistically competent.[41] At some point one could then imagine the hemispheres of this completely ambidextrous individual being separated and transplanted to two new bodies. Thus, John$_1$ would give rise to two subsequent Johns, John$_2$ and John$_3$, each of whom would have inherited the memories of the original John. Both of these Johns, one would assume, would have inherited half the obligations and half the property of the original John. (What of John's wife Sally? Does she now have two husbands?) Finally, if there were a way in the future to re-fuse John$_2$ and John$_3$ into one consciousness, one would have produced a John$_4$ with the memories and obligations of not only the original John but now of John$_2$ and John$_3$ as well.[42] These are relatively unproblematic examples in that continuity of memory and continuity of body remain.

Major puzzles arise when continuity of body is no longer preserved. One might consider *Star Trek*'s Captain Kirk of the starship *Enterprise*. If the captain and a group of his crew are dematerialized and transported to a nearby planet, do their physician–patient understandings with the ship's physician Dr. McCoy continue in place after they have been again dematerialized and rematerialized and returned to the ship? Are they the same persons they were beforehand? If bodily continuity is a criterion for personal identity, do the captain and his crew maintain their identity as the same persons during all of these transformations? Terence Penelhum has argued that if there is a resurrection of the dead, the people resurrected cannot be the same as the people who died, because of the absence of bodily continuity.[43] On the other hand, the captain and his crew, as well as the saints resurrected, have a continuity of memory. They continue to unite their experiences under an I think and to see their past and present as the past and present of the same individual. This may lead one to hold, pace Penelhum, that they are the same persons.

But what if the transmitting device (the transporter) malfunctions, as occurred in one episode of the television series, so that two Captain Kirks materialize, not one? What if God resurrects one saint and also creates an exact copy? Does the physician have a physician–patient relationship with both Captain Kirks? The two Kirks possess the same memories. We may be tempted to treat both Captain Kirks the same and to impute to both Kirks the life led by Captain Kirk before he was beamed down. (How could one, for example, tell the two Kirks apart? Could even God tell the two apart?) There is the additional consideration that in fashioning the copied person's brain, one has engaged in actions tantamount to ensuring that the past causal chains effective in the brain of the person copied determine the initial state of the brain of the copy. There is the equivalent of causal continuity. If we are at peace with such distinctions, what do we make of the case of God creating an exact copy with all the memory of the original saint, while the original saint is alive? Is the copy a new person? Or is it as if the old person had split into two, as would be the case with the individual with two fully competent cerebral hemispheres, separated and placed in two new bodies? If in the case of the separated cerebral hemispheres we held that when John$_1$ divided into John$_2$ and John$_3$, John$_2$ and John$_3$ inherited the obligations of the original John, should we say here that an analogous event has occurred with regard to the saint?

These are complex and intellectually interesting questions, for which there are no univocal answers. However, at least this much can be said. First, insofar as one regards persons as existing in terms of their unity of experience embodied in a particular assemblage of organized matter, it may be enough that the organization of the matter of the copy corresponds to the organization of the matter (especially that of the brain) of the person copied. If in creating the copy saint, God fashions a materially equivalent consciousness and embodiment, has God not created another instance of that person?[44] (Of course, as soon as the copy has new experiences, it begins to be distinguishable from the original saint.) Unless one wishes to assign an importance to the matter involved being a particular bit of matter (i.e., the matter in *that* saint), mere physical continuity would not appear to be that important. The copy would recognize himself as the true saint, as would the one who is a copy. The copy would have inherited through the process of being copied, the causal consequences of the events that shaped the original saint's life, so that the copy would have an equivalent continuity with the past life of the saint, as does the saint from which the copy is made. In short, the less significance one gives to a particular piece of matter, and the more significance one gives to the structure of matter and the unity of consciousness, the more one will decide that both saints inherit from the past of the original saint. These science-fictional reflections support the conclusion that we identify persons as the same persons because there is a continuity of memory and the capacity to unite past and present experiences under an I think (so that the individual can think "these are all my experiences"). In addition, there may be an important role for the criterion of causal continuity.

In considerations of personal continuity, one must distinguish between a person's *personality*, that is, the way in which that person handles the world with particular dispositions and capacities of wit and humour, and the *person* having the personality. Through tragedy or disease an individual may change from being optimistic and engaging to withdrawn and despondent. But as we have seen, there are important ways in which he or she can remain the same person, possessing a continuity of memories united under an I think, an "I experience all of these changes as mine." However, when there has been severe brain damage, one may in fact question whether the person continues. In cases where memory has been greatly impaired and past experiences lost, one may have grounds for holding that the same person is no longer there. The successor person who arises after the links of memory have been broken is perhaps best seen as a new person with some of the personality of the old person. However, with most of the senile elderly, some remote memory is preserved, along with the ability to unite past experiences under an I think. It will make more sense in such cases to say that one encounters the old person in a damaged condition, rather than that a new person has come into existence as a successor to the old.

Problems of the sort raised by the science-fictional examples are associated with reports of individuals with genuine multiple personalities. In such cases, one will need to confront questions such as those occasioned by the defective transporter in the starship *Enterprise*. In order to answer the moral question regarding which personality is responsible for what, one will need to determine as best one can which personality has what knowledge of which actions, and what control over them. One will need to determine the extent to which each personality is able to distinguish certain experiences as his and others as alien, that is, belonging to the other personality. Since bodily discontinuity cannot help in sorting out who is different from whom, the entire weight of such distinctions will need to be borne by the criterion of continuity of memory and the capacity to organize an experience as one's own.

These reflections show the importance of ontological considerations in medicine. What appear at first blush as exotic problems disclose a general challenge for persons (i.e., maintaining the unity of *a* person) and a challenge for philosophers (i.e., understanding what it is to achieve that unity). In order to understand how to treat patients as persons, one must at times seriously reflect on what one will mean by persons and their continuity. It is not merely the cases of disconnected cerebral hemispheres that raise questions regarding the continuity of persons.[45] Each individual faces the task of imposing sufficient unity and continuity on his or her life so as to make it all the life of one person.

Owning people, animals, and things

John Locke remarks, ". . . it seems to some a very great difficulty how any one should ever come to have a property in any thing . . ."[46] The difficulty is bringing things within a conceptual framework of possessions and possessors. Any particular system for speaking of possessors and possessions appears to be culturally relative and open to challenge by members of other societies with other conventions. One might think here of the conflict between the European immigrants to America and the Indian aborigines with regard to rights to land and the use of land. The resolution of such problems is central to understanding moral justifications for the allocation of scarce resources, in particular, scarce health care resources. One must understand who owns what and in what way in order to account for the rights of physicians, patients, and national and international authorities when they allocate medical resources.

Some have held that property rights exist only within a particular civil society. Others such as Immanuel Kant hold that full property rights can be realized only within a civil society.[47] Still others such as William Blackstone (1723–80), while recognizing the right to private property, acknowledge the diversity of theories regarding the origin of property rights. Blackstone notes the view of Hugo Grotius that property rights are founded on a tacit assent of all mankind that the first occupant of a piece of territory should become the owner, in contrast with Locke's view that there is no such implied assent, but that possession derives from bodily labor transforming a mere thing into a possession.[48] As will later be clear, I will side with Locke, but in a somewhat Hegelian fashion. Labor transforms an object from a mere object to an entity fashioned by the ideas and will of a person. By rendering the object a product, it is brought into the sphere of persons and their claims.

Hegel notes that we take possession of things (1) by directly grasping them physically, (2) by forming them, and (3) by marking them as our own. His paradigm example of possession is our possession of ourselves.[49] There is no place we more fully grasp, form, or use than ourselves. We render things ours by eating and devouring them, by incorporating them into ourselves. As a result, they become part of us, such that an action against them is an action against us as persons and therefore a violation of the morality of mutual respect. One's body, one's talents, and one's abilities are similarly primordially one's own. As Locke argues, "Every man has a property in his own person: this nobody has any right to but himself."[50] One's body must be respected as one's person, for the morality of mutual respect secures one's possession of one's self, and one's claims against others who would use one's body or one's talents without one's permission. Again, since spatiotemporally extended persons must occupy a space, to act against that space or place is to act against such persons themselves. Such unconsented-to interference would be an action against the very notion of mutual respect and the peaceable community.

The problem is how to account for other forms of ownership. How does one own tools or land? Owning other persons would appear to be more easily accounted for than the ownership of things. If others own themselves as we own ourselves, they can then convey title over themselves in whole or in part. Ownership rights in the services of other persons are based directly on the morality of mutual respect. Respecting other persons includes respecting the right they have to agree to perform certain services and to enter into special relationships of obedience. Thus, one can understand the rights of the military to order its personnel to submit to certain medical procedures. Indeed, various forms of indentured servitude, from joining the Marines or the French Foreign Legion, to entering a monastery, getting married, or, in some instances, becoming an intern, can be understood in terms of transferring to others in whole or in part rights one held over oneself. Certain special status relationships of being chattel can perhaps be understood in this way. Children, insofar as they remain unemancipated, fail to go out and support themselves on their own, remain in their parents' hands and are thus in part owned (or to recall the ancient Roman usage, they remain *in manu* or in parental *potestas*). In return for parental support, they can be seen as falling under the moral control and partial ownership of their parents. This holds only if the children or wards are persons in the strict sense, and can be regarded as having implicitly engaged in such an exchange of support for obedience. As a result, these considerations apply to the status of older children and adolescents, but not infants and very young children.

In short, indentured servitude provides the clearest example of notionally translucent ownership. One can own others insofar as they have freely transformed themselves into property. Their status as property is clearly understandable, because both owner and owned are persons, minds. That which is owned is not a thing in need of translation into conceptual terms in order to be appreciated as property. It is rather mind meeting mind in order to create a fabric of obligations. Again, examples of such indentured servitude abound. One might think here of the medical student who agrees to serve in the armed forces in return for financial support while studying medicine.

One also owns what one produces. One might think here of both animals and young children. Insofar as they are the products of the ingenuity or energies of persons, they can be possessions. There are, however, special obligations to animals by virtue of the morality of beneficence that do not exist with regard to things. Such considerations, as well as the fact that young children will become persons, limit the extent to which parents have ownership rights over their young children. However, these limits will be very weak with regard to ownership rights in human zygotes, embryos, and fetuses that will not be allowed to develop into persons, or with regard to lower vertebrates, where there is very little sentience. For example, it would appear very plausible that plants, microbes, and human zygotes can be fashioned as products, and be bought and sold as if they were simply things. In contrast, strong claims of ownership would cease, as children become persons and *sui juris,* self-possessing. This latter moral issue also arises with regard to normal adult nonhuman higher primates. It is much more plausible to suspect that higher, nonhuman primates are in possession of themselves than to suspect that such is the case with even one-year-old human infants. At the point that an entity becomes self-conscious, the morality of mutual respect would alienate the property rights of the parents over the children or other animals. New rights over the children could then come into being as the children submit to parental authority in exchange for parental support.

As to things, one need not hold that the matter itself is owned. Instead, one need claim only that the form imposed is an extension of the producer's self, and is that person's possession *in* the thing. As Hegel argues, in the ownership of things the right to the forbearance of others with respect to one's own body is extended to objects one has formed. Taking possession of objects is a process of fashioning them, forming them, transforming them in the image and likeness of one's ideas and according to one's will. It is a way of incorporating things within one's own domain. In this fashion, one increases the sphere of one's embodiment and extends the border of one's rights to the forbearance of others. Things that are untransformed by others one may freely transform for one's own purposes. Things that one has impressed with one's ideas will become one's own insofar as one has fashioned them and has not abandoned them through lack of use, and they may not be altered or changed by others without one's permission, except insofar as the others have some prior right in those objects. Insofar as animals are not self-conscious, and not able to regard themselves as under the moral law, they are in part things to be used, refashioned, or simply taken. As Gaius remarks in his *Institutes,* "... if we capture a wild animal, a bird or a fish, what we so capture becomes ours forthwith and is held to remain ours so long as it is kept in our control."[51]

This approach allows one to give an account of ownership. Unless one sees possession as a somewhat magical process by which emissaries of countries land on unclaimed regions and plant a flag, and thus take *possession,* one will need to account for how brute physical matter can be owned by persons. What I have suggested is that, insofar as an individual enters into a thing, refashions it, remolds it, and, to follow Locke's suggestion, mingles his labor with the object, the object comes into his possession. As Locke characterizes this, "Whatsoever then he removes out of the state that nature hath provided, and left it in, he hath mixed his labour with, and joined to it something that is his own, and thereby makes it his property."[52] One's possessions in the object would only reflect the outcomes of one's labor, or the labor of others one has received as a gift or in trade. Possession reflects the extension of one's own self or the selves of others. To seize, alter, or change without permission a substantial extension of a person is to act against that person. The morality of mutual respect thus protects not only one's immediate embodiment but also the objects in which one embodies one's will and energies. Embodiment in this world does not stop at the edges of one's body, but is extended into other objects marked by one's will. Rights of ownership are then derived from the fundamental right not to be interfered with without one's permission. Once such a right is acquired, it may then be freely sold or otherwise transferred to others, just as persons may transfer rights over themselves.

This approach will go a good way toward accounting for the ownership of products. The nagging difficulty is what to say of the brute matter itself, the stuff out of which the products are fashioned. As untransformed, it would appear impossible to be owned by any particular person. At most, it would appear possible to speak of the rights of all to have equal access to that matter. Similar considerations have led individuals such as Thomas Paine,[53] W. Ogilvie,[54] and Baruch Brody,[55] to hold that taxes are justified as a collection of rent on the matter used in products. One may also be able to collect taxes on the basis of the so-called Lockean proviso. Locke qualifies the right of individuals to take possession of material through mixing their labor with it, with the provision "at least where there is enough, and as good, left in common for others".[56] Taxes may then be collected on the basis of the extent to which an individual claiming a particular property through labor diminishes the opportunities of others to claim similar property through labor.

This approach solves problems not clearly soluble by Robert Nozick,[57] who also takes the morality of mutual respect seriously. Namely, how does one justify taxing individuals (e.g., to provide individuals with funds they could use to purchase health care) who have not in fact agreed to that tax— that is, agreed individually, each and every one. The answer is that objects cannot be fully possessed by individuals or particular groups of individuals (e.g., societies or states). Matter itself, the dimension of things that remains after the things are transformed into products, remains in common owner- ship. However, that common ownership is not the common ownership of a particular society or state, but of persons generally. This leads then to another difficulty. Taxes should be collected at an international level at the very minimum, and perhaps at an intergalactic level, if possible. However, those on other planets are plausibly due less since terrestrial use deprives them of little if anything on the basis of the Lockean proviso. Such a tax would need to reflect a fair rent on such material, apart from considerations of its status as a product. This tax might also include special costs to others of the nonavailability of the material for their use. Unquestionably, there would be much to clarify and to dispute with regard to setting tax rates. Nations would have no particular claim to being the proper tax collectors on such a general rent due on land. Here my view contrasts with that of Baruch Brody, who has argued for a negative income tax distributed on a national basis.[58] One would need to establish why nations would have a claim on the right to collect such a tax, since the tax involves at least the interests of all on the earth. Since rent-tax concerns at least the rights of all on the earth, it would best be collected and distributed on an international basis.

Taxation on property in order to reclaim for all their element of ownership in that property will not produce communal goods. Such taxation as rent on property would lead instead to a duty on the part of the taxing authorities to provide payments to all individuals in a form somewhat similar to a negative income tax. A general taxing agency would lack authority to earmark those resources for particular projects, without the permission of those involved. Picking any particular project to support through such rent-tax would entail endorsing a particular concrete moral sense. One further qualification must be noted that protects individuals from families that might aggressively reproduce in order to benefit from the international negative income tax (though one might note that individuals would not be due such payments until they become persons in the strict sense). Reproduction, when it leads to compromising access to resources and the environment, affects the opportunities of others by creating new individuals with entitlements to the negative income tax collected on the rent of material generally. Such reproduction thus constitutes an action against the rights of others for which a tax can be levied to cover such costs. When individuals are not able to pay such a tax, it would be permissible to prevent their engaging in further reproduction.

Funds for a community to apply to particular projects could be acquired only through common endeavors undertaken to produce such funds, or through gifts to the community for discretionary use. Governments can come into being and gain revenue insofar as they are constituted as the free, common endeavor of their citizens. There is a major difficulty in that most, if not all, current governments are coercive in constraining their citizens toward particular endeavors, including the remittance of funds under the rubric of taxation. Such endeavors are usually redistributive, rather than being a collection of rent on the material of the earth. As a consequence, they lack moral justification. Indeed, the ownership of common funds by multinational corporations would appear to be morally much less suspect than the ownership of common resources by governments, in that governments are much more coercive than most, if not all, corporations, national or multinational. Corporations do not draft individuals into service. It is much easier to change jobs from corporation to corporation than to change citizenship. The consent of stockholders or workers, whether or not represented by unions, appears to be less overborne by threats of force in the case of corporations than in that of governments.

Insofar as one fashions peaceable corporations or peaceable governments, and agrees jointly to engage in common endeavors, one can fashion common resources that are commonly owned and that need not be returned to the owners or participants in the corporation. Corporations and governments may charge for their services. Such resources may then be used in various general welfare endeavors that need not be paid out in the form of dividends or negative income tax payments. These reflections are of major importance in justifying welfare designated for health care. In the absence of strictly communal resources, one will only be able to provide a negative income tax payment as a return from rent-tax collections. To the extent to which such communal resources exist, they can be used to provide the poor with health care, rather than simply with funds with which they would be at liberty to purchase health care, food, or amusement. However, as already noted, the rent-tax (including that amount collected due to the Lockean proviso) would best be collected and distributed on an international basis, since it concerns at least the rights of all on the earth. Special funds for particular social groups and their projects would be available only insofar as one can trace the lineage of corporations or governments to peaceable agreements that produced the resources in question, and thus justify common ownership and common decisions with regard to investing resources in particular welfare endeavors or in the pursuit of the arts and the common subvention of the pleasures of their brief life.

There are then three forms of ownership: private, communal, and general. Things can be owned privately and communally, insofar as they are transformed into products. Even the use and care of rangeland can give it in part the character of a product, as can finding a precious stone. Its status is the product of a person's labor and will. However, since this transformation is never complete, a residual right is held by all persons individually. It is this last sense of ownership that I have termed general ownership. Communal ownership comes into existence only insofar as individuals enter into a joint endeavor with a view to creating a common fund for communal undertakings. Private and general ownership rights will provide individuals with private funds through which they will be at liberty to purchase health care. Socially supported positive rights to health care will come into existence only to the extent that common resources are available, and insofar as a common decision has been made to invest them in the creation of such rights. There should morally thus always be the opportunity to participate privately and communally in the purchase of health care. Insofar as individuals privately own things, there will always be a right to purchase health care services on a fee-for-service basis, unless all physicians have surrendered their right to sell their services privately.

These reflections can be encapsulated in what one may term the principle of ownership. This principle will be central to understanding the roles of public and private funding in health care, as well as the rights of physicians to exempt themselves from the constraints of national health services. Owning private property, insofar as such private ownership exists, will always permit patients merely to buy around the established system. So, too, having the right to own one's talents will permit physicians to sell around the constraints of the system. This can be tendentiously summarized as the basic right of persons to the black market.

PRINCIPLE III. THE PRINCIPLE OF OWNERSHIP

Ownership is derived from the morality of mutual respect. One respects claims to ownership insofar as the entity owned has been brought within the sphere of the owner, such that violating that ownership would be a violation of the person of the owner.

    i. Things are owned insofar as they are the products of persons.

    ii. Animals are owned insofar as they are fed and/or bred by persons, domesticated, and thus rendered products, or insofar as they are captured. Such ownership rights are limited by the principle of beneficence.

    iii. Young children and mere human biological organisms are owned by the people who produce them. Ownership rights may be limited not only by the principle of beneficence, but by the circumstance that the young child (or fetus) will become a person.

    iv. Persons own themselves and own other persons insofar as they have agreed to be owned. Such ownership includes contracts for the provision of services and the provision of products, as well as special relationships such as being a member of an army.

A. Ownership by implied contract: ownership of one's self, ownership rights in one's children and in one's products exist in terms of the morality of mutual respect, apart from any explicit rules. This form of ownership has similarities with what has been classically termed "natural modes of acquiring ownership."[59]

B. Ownership by explicit contract, or consent: such modes of ownership derive from formal, often stylized, forms of agreeing to provide services or a product. One might think here of stock in a corporation or commodity futures. Though these forms of ownership may presuppose natural modes of ownership, these have been dramatically transformed through highly developed social understandings common to a group of individuals.

C. Justification of the principle: one cannot act against an innocent person in the absence of his consent without acting against the very notion of a peaceable community. Insofar as persons (1) extend themselves to objects, make those objects *theirs* by transforming them into products, (2) acquire rights to the person of another through the consent of that person, or (3) have transferred to them an object that was made a product by another, or receive rights in another person by transfer, an action against that property is an action against the owner. It is a violation of the morality of mutual respect, insofar as persons extend themselves into their possessions.

D. Motivation for respect of the principle: one will be moved to respect the principle of ownership insofar as one is interested in the possibility of a peaceable community. Moreover, insofar as one embraces the morality of beneficence and wills to others their good, one must will them as well to have that which is theirs. Therefore, the motivation for respecting property rights will be the motivation for respecting the principle of autonomy and beneficence. However, insofar as there are persons with insufficient resources for their flourishing, there will be a conflict between the beneficent wish that each should have his own goods in his possession, and the beneficent wish that each should have goods sufficient for his flourishing. Since the principle of autonomy holds precedent, one should be moved to respect property rights even under such conditions of tension within the principle of beneficence (i.e., between giving to individuals their property and giving to others what is necessary for life).

   E. Public policy implications:

      i. Ownership cannot be totally communal. In addition to there being individual private ownership, the things of the world also continue in part to be in the possession of all persons. Further, insofar as persons in particular communities join in common endeavors, there will be the possibility of producing common resources.

     ii. Taxes may be collected to be distributed to all persons on the basis of the common ownership of material, and on the basis of the Lockean proviso in order to compensate all insofar as the possession by some does not leave like material available for others to possess.

    iii. Tax may also be collected insofar as it reflects a charge for the services of a community to individuals such as toward production of private property for and at the behest of those individuals.

    iv. There is a fundamental moral right to participate in the black market. No one has the right to forbid free individuals from exchanging their services or property for the services or property of other free individuals. This basic moral right justifies physicians in establishing fee-for-service practices alongside any governmentally established health service.

   F. Maxim: persons own themselves, what they make, or what other persons own and transfer to them; communities have property insofar as persons fashion such communities and transfer funds to common ownership, or insofar as groups create common wealth. Therefore: Render to all that to which all have a right; refrain from taking that which belongs to some or one alone.

States and their authority

The author of the Hippocratic text *The Law* remarks: "Medicine is the only art which our states have made subject to no penalty save that of dishonor."[60] Though there may have been no criminal sanctions, there were at least some civil remedies available in Greece for malpractice.[61] Currently, there is no question that the practice of medicine is controlled in many very important ways through law and regulation. Legal constraints exist with respect to the drugs physicians may prescribe for dying patients. Heroin is available in the United Kingdom for the control of pain, but not in the United States even in the terminal stages of cancer.[62] The ability of physicians to provide contraception, sterilization, and abortion varies from country to country. There are civil remedies through which patients can bring suits against physicians. The practice of medicine now, unlike the time of ancient Greece, is restricted to those licensed by the state. Indeed, even the purchase by hospitals of expensive medical devices, as well as the decision whether to treat defective newborns, has in various fashions been touched by law and state regulation. State authority is so ubiquitous and commonplace that its justification is rarely if ever brought into question other than in a piecemeal fashion.

To understand the position of physicians and other health care workers in heavily regulated societies, one must raise fundamental philosophical issues regarding the moral authority of the state. To what extent do states and their representatives have moral authority to regulate the character of health care? Is there any moral force to the mass of state regulation of health care? Or are violations of law or state regulations at most imprudent, considering the substantial risk of being discovered and punished? Aside from the obvious sanctions of criminal and civil punishment, does any moral blameworthiness attach to those who violate the law? May their actions be condemned as immoral? A decent intellectual answer to these very important questions can be secured only by examining the justification of state authority.

Do states possess any authority not possessed by individuals? If states derive their authority directly from the foundations of moral law, they will in fact have no authority beyond that possessed by any particular individual or group of individuals. In that case, states may do only what any individual may do to secure the mutual respect of persons, to support the discharge of obligations of beneficence, and to protect the property rights of individuals and communities. One would be able to determine the moral authority of any moral regulation by retracing it to one of the three moral principles. If the regulation failed to show such a lineage, then it may be prudent to obey the rule, but not morally obligatory.

Such questions are far from academic in health care, where state regulations dramatically influence the character of health care. For example, may a state determine what hospital charges must be for various types of admission, even if individuals and particular health insurance groups would be willing to pay more than the statutory amount for, let us say, a particular diagnostically related group? Would it be immoral to accept extra funds under the table just because there was a law against such a practice? Or what if the federal government required hospitals to condition physicians' admitting privileges on complete acceptance of assignment of in-patient Medicare patients?

Let us attempt to review the ways in which one might forward an intellectual justification for the authority of the state. I will list seven major ways in which authority for the state has been justified. This list, though somewhat arbitrary and procrustean, allows one to appreciate the major historical justifications forwarded for state authority, and the strength of their rationales.

First, one might consider the argument that the authority of the sovereign comes from God. This view has been advanced in the Christian West, often citing passages from St. Paul such as "the powers that be are ordained of God" (Romans 13:1). This account was developed by the Christian church of the Middle Ages into a doctrine of the two authorities, that of the pope and that of royal power, with the authority of royal power coming from God through the pope. One might think here of the famous arguments of Innocent III in his October 30, 1198 "Sicut universitatis conditor," where he speaks of the two luminaries in the firmament of authority, the *pontificalis auctoritas* and the *regalis potestas*.[63] This view of the standing of secular authority received an interesting articulation in the Council of Constance of July 6, 1415. Jean Petit, Master of the University of Paris, on March 3, 1408, defended the thesis that it was legitimate to kill a tyrant. The subject of this contention was the duke of Burgundy, who had killed the duke of Orleans on November 23, 1407. The council condemned as an error the claim of a right to kill tyrants.[64] This doctrine of the sovereign ruling by *jure divino* was strongly contested in the seventeenth and eighteenth centuries.[65] Indeed, the doctrine of the divine right of sovereigns is untenable in secular pluralist contexts. The premises needed to secure the notion of such a divine right depend on particular cultural and religious suppositions, which are neither agreed to by all nor open to a general rational justification.

The doctrine of the divine right of kings has often been naively replaced by a presumption regarding the (divine?) right of majorities to rule. One might think here of the maxim "Vox populi vox Dei est." However, why should a majority, in and of itself, carry authority? What authority is possessed by a righteous mob, or group, even if it constitutes a plurality, a two-thirds majority, or even a three-fourths majority of the community? What authority should laws have simply because they are endorsed by a majority? The answer is that there is no more a divine right of majorities than there is one of kings and princes. There is nothing morally magical about majorities. One will need to look elsewhere for the government's moral authority.

One might hope to establish the authority of a government by showing that it is in fact acting to achieve the morally obligatory concrete understanding of the good life. As chapters 2 and 3 have already shown, it is not only difficult but impossible to establish a particular concrete view of the moral life as morally obligatory for all. One will not be able to establish a sufficiently detailed understanding of what one is obliged morally to do so as to justify the wide range of rules and regulations imposed on citizens in general and health care practitioners in particular.

A fourth option would be to attempt to establish a justification for government authority by appeal to a hypothetical contract. One might envisage an intellectual construct somewhat similar to John Rawls's original position,[66] in which he invites us to imagine ourselves establishing general moral rules as if we were individuals ignorant of our particular advantages in society. According to Rawls, what we would rationally choose under those circumstances would count as the basic rules of just conduct in society. One could then use those fundamental rules to guide an actual constitutional convention and legislatures in developing actual laws.[67] The problem here is as before. One must impute to the hypothetical contractors a particular moral sense in order for them to rank some primary social goods (e.g., liberty) higher than others. As a consequence, the device of appealing to hypothetical contractors will not authoritatively deliver a sufficiently concrete or universal understanding of the principles of justice and of other principles of morality so as to justify the modern state and its wide range of laws and regulations regarding health care.

To derive political authority, appeal has also been made to the notion of an actual past originary agreement of all to the conventions of government in general or to a particular constitution. One might think here of the political arguments of individuals such as Jean Jacques Rousseau, Thomas Hobbes, and John Locke. Indeed, these past philosophical considerations direct many of the presuppositions of American constitutional law, which presumes that the actions of individuals between 1787 and 1790 in adopting the current American Constitution bound all Americans in the future to that constitution and to its processes for enacting, enforcing, and interpreting laws to its means for amendment.[68] Such a view is at least as metaphysical as the appeal to the divine right of sovereigns. One may agree that once all have subscribed to a particular constitution, all those who had indeed agreed were then bound. However, such was surely not the case with the American Constitution of 1789 (which provided for means of adoption in violation of the Articles of Confederacy), or for that matter any constitution written for any large-scale state. Those who object to the Constitution may presumably doubt its moral authority and be returned to the clash of asserted right with asserted right. One might think here of Blackstone's characterization of the law that binds nations, namely, the law of arms, where "the only tribunal to which the complaints can appeal is that of the God of battles."[69]

The prospect of such conflict leading to civil and intestine wars introduces the sixth possible justification for the authority of government, namely, that of prudence. Consider that one is living in a village regularly attacked by marauding groups who murder, rape, and pillage. After years of such uncontrollable, wanton carnage, the village is approached by a warlord who agrees to protect the village from the roving bands as long as he and his men are paid a tenth of the crops per year, can draft for two years' service a tenth of the women for their concubines and a tenth of the men for their army, and can establish a village health service in which all physicians must participate for a salary, while forgoing all fee-for-service practice. In addition, the warlord's men will aid in protecting against members of the village who may murder, rape, or pillage the village, other than on the orders of the warlord. If the losses of life, liberty, and property are likely to be much less under the rule of the warlord than under local independence, agreement to the authority of the warlord may be a prudent arrangement. The justification for the authority of the warlord and his men is that of prudence. In the absence of the warlord's power and the uniformity of his administration, there will be more pillage which will bring much greater costs to all. Here one might think of Hobbes's remark on the state of nature where "the life of man [is] solitary, poore, nasty, brutish, and short."[70] It is for considerations such as these that Hobbes holds that men and women fashion the mortal god, the leviathan, a government, a commonwealth, a civitas.[71]

Hobbes wishes the authority of the commonwealth to be more than one based simply on prudence. He sees the authority of a government arising out of the following explicit or implicit agreement: "I authorise and give up my Right of Governing my selfe to this Man, or to this Assembly of men, on this condition, that thou give up thy Right to him, and Authorise all his Actions in like manner."[72] He defines the essence of the commonwealth as "One Person, of whose acts a great Multitude, by mutuall Covenants one with another, have made themselves every one the Author, to the end he may use the strength and means of them all, as he shall think expedient, for their Peace and common Defence."[73]

The difficulty is that everyone has *not* in fact agreed. Not all, as Hobbes alleges, enter into "the Congregation of them that were assembled," having agreed to be bound by whatever the majority decides.[74] Many may simply respond that the commonwealth may go its way peacefully, as they will go their way peacefully. Such dissenters may include both individuals who were there as the original compact was framed, as well as children born of the original consenters. Unless one can develop a somewhat metaphysical doctrine of hereditary consent (perhaps on the model of the old doctrines regarding hereditary slavery),[75] those who are born since the covenant are not a party to it unless they, too, agree. Those who might challenge such dissenters with the maxim "Consent to the commonwealth or leave it" must be prepared for the dissenters' rejoinder, "Why shouldn't the commonwealth leave us alone? Why should we be the ones forced to leave?" There appears to be no effective retort available to the commonwealth, since it is impossible to establish a commonwealth's claim to political boundaries without exclaves. A commonwealth may surely exclude dissenters from welfare rights and the protection of civil rights. But dissenters may claim a repayment of taxes collected by coercion and proceed to hire a security force with the funds.

The dissenters can assert that they hold certain values dearer even than certain forms of personal safety, and that they will not agree to the authority of leviathan in general or in certain areas. Such dissenters, individuals who have not freely committed themselves to obey the laws and regulations of the commonwealth, when they find themselves in a commonwealth, may with moral justification refuse to participate not only in those endeavors of the commonwealth they recognize to be immoral, but also those to which they do not wish to give their energies. Thus, they need not, and ought not, aid in impeding the suicide of rational individuals by the use of state force. In fact, they would likely find themselves in opposition to the use of state force against individuals "guilty" of victimless crimes (i.e., "crimes" to which all those involved have agreed freely to participate: the sale of pornography, the conduct of prostitution, or the sale of heroin and marijuana). They would find themselves morally obliged not to participate in the use of state force against such individuals (e.g., they would find it immoral in a hard-core sense to serve as a vice officer on a police force). They would not find it immoral in a hardcore sense to run a sporting house (that is, in a sense of morality that could be generally justified by appeal to a rational argument, whose premises would be binding on all). Whether such dissenters would themselves obey or disobey such laws would turn on issues of prudence.

Such considerations of prudence could be both individually and societally directed. Consider a physician asked by a friend dying of a painful disease to kill him. If one assumes a physician has an opportunity to do so without being detected, despite the action being legally forbidden, the physician would be morally free, except for considerations of prudence, to kill his friend as long as he had not explicitly, freely, and without coercion agreed to give up that right to the state. However, he might as a prudent individual be concerned that he could be caught. He might also be concerned that if a general practice of disobeying laws were accepted, the fabric of society would begin to disintegrate, leading to the general injury of all. If he were sure that he could commit the act without being detected, he might then find himself bound out of considerations of prudence and beneficence never to mention to others that he had given aid. However, there would be no grounds to say that he had acted immorally in a generally sustainable sense if he responded to the request.

Some may find these conclusions perturbing. They indicate that the moral position of vice officers is considerably more dubious than the moral standing of whores and whore-mongers. On reflection, this should not be too surprising. As this chapter has shown, the morality of mutual respect is central to the intellectual standing of ethics itself. Insofar as whores and whoremongers can show that those involved in prostitution are engaged in it freely, the lineage of authority for action can be clearly demonstrated. Prostitutes can explain what they are doing with their clients in terms of mutual agreements. Such surely cannot be as clearly shown for vice officers. One might imagine here as well individuals who would use state force to limit access to abortion and sterilization. It is difficult, if not impossible, to establish that individuals have in fact granted to the commonwealth a right to regulate their sexual lives, or their use of mind-altering drugs. Whether the opportunity to use marijuana or heroin is more dangerous than the opportunity to join particular religions is a matter where, especially given the history of the persecution of heretics, both sides can be argued with some merit. But as long as the individuals involved agree without coercion to use particular drugs, or to be members of particular religions that forbid the use of blood products, contraceptives, or abortion, nothing has been done in violation of the morality of mutual respect.

When these reflections are taken to a more general level, one is left with this conclusion: it is prudent to obey all (most?) of the rules and regulations of one's government, but the general moral authority of governments to fashion such rules and regulations is not as strong as the moral authority of multinational corporations such as IBM, Dow Chemical, or Exxon to fashion rules for their workers, or of unions for their members, presuming that the employees and union members have joined without coercion and in agreement to such fashioning of rules and regulations. Governments are morally suspect, for they traditionally use force to coerce those in their territory to accept their authority. It is very difficult to show that individuals have agreed to the authority of the commonwealth within which they reside, absent threats of coercion. (Who reading this volume, for instance, has freely agreed that the United States Government may make it impossible for the reader to purchase heroin to control the pain of terminal cancer, should the reader need it?) What one would never tolerate from multinationals or unions is accepted as a matter of course on the part of governments. There is no evidence, for example, that Dow Chemical drafts individuals to serve in its security forces.

One is brought to the seventh and final source for the moral authority of government, namely, the actual consent of all of the citizens to the actions of the government. This condition is not as difficult to meet as one might at first suspect. Since peaceable individuals may at any time defend other innocents against the use of force, so too may governments act to protect the innocent from such crimes as murder, rape, and robbery. Since it is a morally praiseworthy act to aid individuals in the honoring of contracts to which all parties have agreed, so too it is morally permitted for governments to enforce contracts that citizens record as binding among them. All of these actions of government have undisputed authority, for all peaceable individuals involved have consented to them.[76] Beyond that, property held in common can be distributed in whatever way those who fashioned the common ownership stipulated. In this fashion, original constitutions can bind descendants who come to participate in a commonwealth to distribute such property through a democratic process. In short, within the constraints of actual consent of all those involved, one can still fashion a government with a wide range of substantial capacities and authorities. It is simply that such authority will not extend to the control of the consensual action of free individuals, including their use of their private property. The unquenchable markets for pornography, prostitution, and drugs must be tolerated because of the basic human right to the black market. Moreover, the data suggest on prudential grounds that attempts to interdict these markets lead to a level of corruption and violence whose evils are so significant that they are likely to outbalance whatever goods are naively sought from their proscription. The same might be said regarding the proposed controls of abortion or fee-for-service medicine.

These considerations suggest severe limitations on the authority of the government in regulating the practice of health care outside of governmentally owned facilities. As a moral test, one might ask oneself under what circumstances Exxon or Dow Chemical security forces may control health care with moral authority in order to disclose the moral limits of state force in the regulation of health care. Governments will be justified in protecting patients and health care workers from coercion, fraud, and breach of contract. In addition, regulations may be imposed on the use of governmental funds and properties through majority vote. But individuals will continue to possess moral rights to do with themselves and consenting others as they and those consenting others decide.

These reflections, if enacted into public policy, would lead to some rather radical changes in tax laws, in the ways in which the free consensual acts of individuals are controlled, and in the government's role in the regulation of health care. I will not explore the radical implications of these reflections at length here. It is enough to note that things would be dramatically altered. With the advent of a general, worldwide, peacekeeping authority limited by the morality of mutual respect (which is to say, with the coming of the secular millennium), one could be assured of the possibility of individuals freely joining in various associations, which need not be localized to any particular geographical area. One might think here of the ways in which individuals of different faiths may proceed to gain a divorce in Israel, on the basis of the rules of their particular religious groups. In such associations, individuals could pursue their own views of the good life. Each association could in its own way provide a level and kind of health care in accord with its guiding view of the good life. The result would likely be a world in which individuals would belong in different ways to different associations. As a consequence, individuals would have complex entitlements to health care and other support. The realization of such possibilities must at this time be but a dream, a hope, the allure of a possible utopia of free individuals in free associations.

This vision encompasses two of the major goals sought from government. First, it offers the impartial protection of citizens. The international, or if it were possible intergalactic, police force would dispassionately protect persons of whatever species from murder, robbery, and other unauthorized touchings of themselves or their property. It would protect recorded contracts and distribute to all their equal share in the revenues from the general rent on material. However, it would have no view of the good life, it would enforce no concrete sense of morality, it would provide no welfare rights such as a right to health care. For special welfare rights, the second goal of governments, one would have to appeal to particular corporate entities such as individual states, associations such as the AFL-CIO, or corporations such as IBM and Exxon. Such may hold property in common for their members and through some preestablished procedure decide how to use it and the income it produces. Finally, individuals could belong to particular, closely knit communities sharing well-articulated concrete views of the good life— communities that may not be restricted to particular geographical areas. Under such circumstances there may be the possibility for numerous objects of patriotic dedication. The polytheistic metaphor may find expression in political life.

Though these visions are fantasies, they are instructive in reminding us that states possess no special moral status. States are no more legitimate as rule makers than are multinational corporations, unions, or other large organizations. In fact, as has been noted, their legitimacy is less secure. One might observe, since there is much greater danger both to individuals and to the world at large from states claiming encompassing sovereignty than from corporations, unions, or similar voluntarily constituted bodies, the idea of the sovereign state is one whose time should pass. These visions should help to remind us of the need to inspect the claims for moral authority advanced by particular groups of rulemakers. The absence of moral legitimacy should not necessarily inspire a physician or nurse to violate the rules (including local, state, and national laws). Obeying the rules may be prudent not only for those nurses and physicians, but for their professions generally, as well as the patients under their care. Still, there is a certain moral satisfaction from knowing whether the order within which one must practice is one ordained through morality, or rather accepted out of expediency.

PRINCIPLE IV. THE PRINCIPLE OF POLITICAL AUTHORITY

Morally justified political authority is derived from the consent of the governed, not from a view of the good life, including commitments to beneficence, for the actual significance of such views or commitments must be framed by common agreement. The character of consent to an organization's authority will differ, for example, if one compares a territorial state such as Texas with a multinational corporation such as IBM.

Political or corporate entities possess authority to:

    i. Protect the innocent from unconsented-to force (e.g., against being subjects of medical experimentation without their consent, or from having their free access to consenting abortionists impeded);

    ii. Enforce contracts (e.g., the commitment to confidentiality on the part of physicians);

    iii. Develop welfare rights through the use of common resources (e.g., health care welfare rights).

A. Authority from implied consent: the notion of the peaceable community presumes acquiescence in the protection of the innocent from unconsented-to force (e.g., using patients for goals to which they have not consented).

B. Authority from explicit consent: Particular individuals, through participating in a community, can fashion a web of explicit agreements through which authority is transferred to a political entity in order to administer common endeavors and resources. In this fashion, states and corporations create specific health care rights for their members.

C. Justification of the principle: Political authority receives primary moral justification in terms of the morality of mutual respect. It receives justification as well in terms of the principle of beneficence. However, such authority must always be placed within the constraint of mutual respect, in that the principle of beneficence is specified through mutual consent.

D. Motivation for respecting political authority: To act contrary to legitimate political authority is to lose grounds for protest against punitive and defensive force. The motivation for respect is thus drawn in part from the considerations that underlie the morality of mutual respect. In addition, corporate entities provide the basis for individuals to pursue, in common, goods that would be impossible to achieve, were they to act individually. One might think here of how Plato remarks that an ample city is requisite for the luxuries of life (*Republic*, II.373). Issues of beneficence, of achieving a particular view of the good, will thus further motivate individuals to create special corporate endeavors. Finally, considerations of expedience and prudence may as well bring acquiescence in the laws and rules of government.

E. Public policy implications: The authority of governments is suspect, insofar as they

    i. Restrict the choice of free individuals without their consent (e.g., attempts to forbid the sale of human organs, the developments of contracts for surrogate mothers);

    ii. Regulate the free exchange of goods and services, beyond protecting against such evils as fraud, coercion, or violation of contracts; however

    iii. Political authority is properly exercised over commonly held land and other possessions, according to the rules established by the participants in the corporate endeavor.

F. Maxim: though respect of governmental rules and laws regarding health care is prudent, one is morally blameworthy only if one acts against legitimate moral authority. Therefore: Obey laws when one must; feel guilty about infractions when one should.

Human biological versus human personal life: some summaries

Given these reflections on the character of persons, animals, things, and states, some general classifications can be offered regarding the moral standing of such entities.

Persons strictly

Such entities are moral agents, rational, able to choose freely according to a rational plan of life, and are possessed of a notion of blameworthiness and praiseworthiness. Persons strictly are protected by the moralities of mutual respect and of beneficence. They may not be treated or experimented on without their consent (unless they have ceded that right).

FREE PERSONS. This group encompasses those who are not substantially restricted in their liberty to accept or refuse medical treatment for themselves due to agreements made explicitly or implicitly with other persons, e.g., most adult competent humans other than those serving in the armed forces.

PERSONS IN THE POSSESSION OF OTHERS. Here one would have to include not only nonemancipated minors, but also indentured servants and members of the military. Such individuals are characterized by their having given to others the right to make important choices on their behalf. The rights of parents to choose medical treatment for their adolescent children must be understood in this light.

Human biological life

Human biological life is protected by the morality of beneficence insofar as such life is capable of suffering, and insofar as such life is of significance to other persons. To the extent that such life is owned by other persons, the morality of mutual respect is also involved. One should note that concerns of beneficence toward such life will vary widely. One can have substantial concerns with beneficence toward severely mentally retarded humans. However, the opportunities to be beneficent toward a brain-dead but otherwise alive human organism vanish to the point of nonexistence.

SOCIAL PERSONS. Some instances of human life, because of their capacity to interact in social roles, are accorded some of the rights of persons strictly. Here one finds infants, very young children, the profoundly and many of the severely mentally retarded, the severely demented, including those suffering from advanced stages of senile dementia. Distinctions will need to be made among different classes of social persons: (a) infants and young children, (b) neonates prior to a commitment to full treatment, (c) the very senile who once were moral agents, and (d) the very severely and profoundly mentally retarded and demented who never were and never will be persons in the strict sense.

HUMAN LIFE ACCORDED SPECIAL LEVELS OF PROTECTION. Out of considerations of utility, one may accord a special protection to viable fetuses. Though they are not given the rights of persons, one may wish to encourage respectful treatment. As we will see in chapter 6, such treatment of fetuses ought not to include actions on the behalf of fetuses against the wishes of the women bearing them except in very specific circumstances in order to protect the future person whom that fetus is likely to become.

OTHER INSTANCES OF HUMAN BIOLOGICAL LIFE. These need not be accorded special protection, unless there are clear utilitarian arguments to support such protection, and then only when such protection does not violate the rights of persons strictly. Examples of such instances of human life would include human gametes and cells in culture. They need not be accorded any special respect. Consider, for instance, what it might mean to treat human sperm with respect.

Animal life

Animals are protected by the morality of beneficence. Since the range of the capacity for animals to suffer or achieve pleasure and fulfillment spans from that of the higher primates to that of one-cell animals, the strength of claims to beneficence will vary dramatically. The more animals can feel, suffer, and have affection for others, the more the concerns of beneficence toward them may plausibly have weight. On the other hand, concerns of beneficence with respect to roaches and amoebas are much less substantial. Still, capriciously to torment a paramecium for sport, if one were of the opinion that paramecia can be the subjects of torment, would be an act against the morality of beneficence (unless one held that a proportionate good was to be realized in or through that sport). One would need also to classify animals in terms of whether they are (1) owned by individuals or groups, or (2) unowned, in order to be clear with respect to one's duties regarding them. These considerations would place few restrictions on the use of animals in bona fide medical research.

Things

Insofar as things are rendered products or transformed by human labor, they can be owned (note: some concept of continued use will also be required). One will need therefore to distinguish between (1) owned and (2) unowned things. One will need as well to note whether, in talking about the rights of persons regarding things, one is concerned with (1) the ownership rights of private persons, (2) the ownership rights of corporate entities, or (3) the general residual ownership rights of all persons in all things.

Corporate entities

Persons can fashion corporate entities (e.g., nations) that can hold property and act as vehicles for joint action. As such, the property of these corporations belongs to the corporations, not the individual shareholders. Following corporate rules (e.g., democratic processes), corporate entities can provide for the health care of their members.

Discussions of bioethics occur against the background of this complex geography of moral distinctions. As the foregoing shows, the discussion is complex, for morality itself is complex in drawing from concerns for mutual respect and beneficence. This complexity is compounded by the real inequalities among humans (e.g., adult competent humans versus fetuses) and even among moral agents (i.e., in terms of financial resources). It is compounded as well by the special position of health care practitioners as gatekeepers of therapy roles. Health care practitioners medicalize reality in labeling problems as medical problems of a particular kind, and labeling patients as ill or disordered in a particular way. Such labels are informally tied to special social expectations, as well as to assignments of rights and duties. These may then in turn be formalized through governmental actions. What may at first appear to be purely factual judgments (i.e., X has a disease of Y kind), under closer examination can be shown to reflect hidden social and value judgments of central importance to bioethical discussions. We therefore move now to the description of reality in medical terms.

Notes

1. Kant, *Grundlegung zur Metaphysik der Sitten*, Akademie Textausgabe, vol. 4 (Berlin: Walter de Gruyter, 1968), p. 438.

148 THE FOUNDATIONS OF BIOETHICS

2. Ibid., p. 452.
3. Ibid., p. 453; *Foundations of the Metaphysics of Morals*, trans. Lewis White Beck (Indianapolis: Bobbs-Merrill, 1959), p. 72.
4. *Grundlegung zur Metaphysik der Sitten*, p. 452.
5. This point is explored at great length by Kant in his treatment of the third antinomy in the *Critique of Pure Reason*. The third antinomy presents the unavoidable contrast between the deterministic perspective and the moral perspective. This contrast or tension cannot be resolved, as Kant argues, in terms of one of the particular perspectives alone. This leads, as a consequence, to holding on the one hand that all human actions are in principle predictable (*Kritik der reinen Vernunft*, 2d ed., 1787, p. 578, B578), while on the other holding that we must think of ourselves as free, though we cannot prove that we are free.
6. Ramsey has been reluctant to allow experimentation on fetuses and children because they cannot consent. Such a line of argument presumes that fetuses can sensibly be the object of such respect. Ramsey also objects to the use of children in research not aimed at their benefit, because such would entail using that individual "without his will." However, there is no will to respect in the case of infants. Paul Ramsey, *The Patient as Person* (New Haven, Conn.: Yale University Press, 1970), p. 35.
7. Dr. Jerome Lejeune, in his testimony to the United States Senate, stated: "But now we can say, unequivocally, that the question of when life begins is no longer a question for theological or philosophical dispute. It is an established scientific fact. Theologians and philosophers may go on to debate the meaning of life or the purpose of life, but it is an established fact that all life, including human life, begins at the moment of conception." Testimony by Dr. Jerome Lejeune on the Human Life Bill: Hearings before the Subcommittee on Separation of Powers of the Committee of the Judiciary, 97th Congress (Washington, D.C.: U.S. Government Printing Office, 1982), vol. 1, p. 13.
8. St. Thomas Aquinas distinguishes between the status of the early and late fetus in *Summa Theologica* I, 118, art. 2. He also indicates in his commentary on Aristotle that Aristotle shows moral sensitivity in favoring the use of early abortion rather than infanticide or late abortion. Such early abortion was not held to be murder. *Aristoteles Stagiritae: Politicorum seu de Rebus Civilibus*, Book VII, Lectio XII, in *Opera Omnia* (Paris: Vives, 1875), vol. 26, p. 484. This issue is also discussed by St. Thomas in *Summa Theologica* II, II, 64, art. 8. See also *Commentum in Quartum Librum Sententiarium Magistri Petri Lombardi*, Distinctio XXXI, Expositio Textus, in *Opera Omnia*, vol. 11, p. 127.
9. A good overview of the history of abortion in canon law is provided by John T. Noonan, Jr., "An Almost Absolute Value in History," in John T. Noonan, Jr. (ed.), *The Morality of Abortion* (Cambridge, Mass.: Harvard University Press, 1971). The view of the Catholic church developed under a number of influences. The Septuagint translation of Exodus 21:22 suggested that there was a difference between formed and unformed embryos, between ensouled and unensouled embryos. This scriptural distinction is similar to one drawn by Aristotle, between the fetus before and after it possessed an animal soul. *De Generatione Animalium*, 2.3.736a–b and *Historia Animalium*, 7.3.583b. Theological and philosophical reflections on the bases of these and other considerations led to the development in Roman Catholic theology of the dispute between those who favored mediate animation (the soul entering some time after the conception of the body) and those favoring immediate animation (the soul entering at the time of the

conception of the body). J. Donceel, "Abortion: Mediate v. Immediate Anima-tion," *Continuum* 5 (Spring 1967): 167–71, and "Immediate Animation and Delayed Hominization," *Theological Studies* 13 (March 1970): 76–105. See also Canon Henry de Dorlodot, "A Vindication of the Mediate Animation Theory," in E. C. Messenger (ed.), *Theology and Evolution* (London: Sands, 1952), pp. 259–83. A twelfth-century canon law case entered canon law in the thirteenth century, setting a precedent that recognized the difference between the crime of murder and the act of destroying an unformed (i.e., unensouled) fetus. *Corpus Juris Canonici Emendatum et Notis Illustratum cum Glossae: decretalium d. Gregorii Papae Noni Compilatio* (Rome, 1585), *Glossa ordinaria* at bk. 5, title 12, chap. 20, p. 1713.

The change in Roman Catholic treatment of early abortion was influenced, it would appear, by the setting of the dates for celebrating the Immaculate Conception of the Blessed Virgin Mary (December 8) as nine months prior to the date for celebrating her birth (i.e., September 8).

This is not to suggest that there were not individuals who held that early abortion should be considered equivalent to acts of murder. See, for example, Pope Sextus V, *Contra procurantes, Consulentes, et Consentientes, quorunque modo Abortum Constitutio* (Florence: Georgius Marescottus, 1888). Pope Sextus for three years (1588–91) made early abortion equivalent to taking the life of a person.

10. For an excellent study of the significance of the sin of contraception and its relation to the sin of abortion, see John T. Noonan, Jr., *Contraception* (Cambridge, Mass.: Harvard University Press, 1965). See also, for a helpful treatment of current Catholic viewpoints in this matter, James J. McCartney, "Some Roman Catholic Concepts of Person and Their Implications for the Ontologial Status of the Unborn," in W. B. Bondeson et al. (eds.), *Abortion and the Status of the Fetus* (Dordrecht: Reidel, 1983), pp. 313–23.

11. Marie-Joseph Nicolas, "The Meaning of the Immaculate Conception in the Perspectives of St. Thomas," in E. D. O'Connor (ed.), *The Dogma of the Immaculate Conception* (Notre Dame, Ind.: University of Notre Dame Press, 1958), p. 333.

12. S. I. Benn, "Abortion, Infanticide, and Respect for Persons," in Joel Feinberg (ed.), *The Problem of Abortion* (Belmont, Calif.: Wadsworth, 1973), pp. 92–104.

13. The fact that many zygotes do not go to term has been appreciated for a number of years. For example, Arthur Hertig showed in 1967 that at least 28 percent if not 50 percent of all conceptions appeared to terminate in early, unnoticed, spontaneous abortions. "Human Trophoblast: Normal and Abnormal," *American Journal of Clinical Pathology* 47 (March 1967): 249–68. Such findings have recently been reviewed by John D. Biggers, "Generation of the Human Life Cycle," in Bondeson et al. (eds.), *Abortion and the Status of the Fetus,* pp. 31–53.

14. As Charles Hartshorne suggests, whales may have a higher intrinsic significance than human fetuses, since whales may be able intellectually to recognize their significance for the Deity, though human fetuses and infants cannot. This greater complexity of adult whales would then itself have a significance for the Deity in contributing more richly to the Deity's life. See, for example, Charles Hartshorne, "Scientific and Religious Aspects of Bioethics," in Earl E. Shelp (ed.), *Theology and Bioethics* (Dordrecht: Reidel, 1985), p. 42.

15. The distinction between pain and suffering is explored by George Pitcher, "Pain and Unpleasantness," pp. 181–96; David Bakan, "Pain—The Existential Symp-

tom," pp. 197–207; Bernard Tursky, "The Evaluation of Pain Responses: A Need for Improved Measures," pp. 209–19; and Jerome A. Shaffer, "Pain and Suffering," pp. 221–33, in *Philosophical Dimensions of the Neuro-Medical Sciences*, ed. S. F. Spicker and H. T. Engelhardt, Jr. (Dordrecht: Reidel, 1976).

16. Robert Nozick, *Anarchy, State, and Utopia* (New York: Basic Books, 1974), p. 39.

17. Ibid.

18. One must in fact acknowledge the wide range of ways in which Kant treats of persons, the ego, or the subject. Kant employs at least six different senses. The first is the transcendental ego, the logical form of the spontaneity of the intellect, whose functions of judgment are the categories (*Critique of Pure Reason*, B137, 140, 143). It is this transcendental ego that accompanies any and all judgments (*Critique of Pure Reason*, B406, 419). There is, second, the consciousness of the bare fact that one exists (*Critique of Pure Reason*, B156). This fact cannot be captured as true knowledge (*Critique of Pure Reason*, A346 = B404) but can be apprehended as an intellectual representation or thought (*Critique of Pure Reason*, B158). There is also, third, the empirical ego, which is the subject as it appears to itself in inner sense, but not as an object (*Critique of Pure Reason*, B278, A347 = B405, A381f.). The fourth sense, that of the ego of rational psychology, is the false hypostatization of the logical function I think (*Critique of Pure Reason*, A403f.). The fifth sense, that of the noumenal ego, is that of the person as a moral agent, through which we think our actions, but concerning which there is no knowledge, since the subject cannot be given in experience (*Critique of Pure Reason*, A538-40 = B566–68). It is this sense that is important to the reflections in this book about persons as moral agents. It is persons in this sense who exist as the constituting sources of the moral world. The last sense in which Kant treats of the subject or person is as a psychological idea read into experience through a regulative use of the idea giving a further unity to our knowledge of persons. *Critique of Pure Reason*, A665 = B693, A671–674 = B699–702, A682–684 = B710–712.

    Kant suffers from a need for a general category of subject. An account of such a category must be approached through a more expanded categorial account See H. T. Engelhardt, *Mind-Body; A Categorial Relation* (The Hague: Martinus Nijhoff, 1973). Kant's moral arguments remain useful in establishing the key position of the subject.

19. *Metaphysik der Sitten*, in *Kants Werke* (Berlin: Walter de Gruyter, 1968), vol. 6, p. 223; *Metaphysical Principles of Virtue*, trans. J. Ellington (Indianapolis: Bobbs-Merrill, 1964), p. 23.

20. Immanuel Kant, *Lectures on Ethics*, trans. Louis Infield (Indianapolis: Hackett, 1979), p. 240.

21. Ibid. Kant argues that one should keep an old dog until it dies, for "such action helps to support us in our duties towards human beings, where they are bounden duties." Ibid. However, if the man shoots his dog, according to Kant, he does not fail in his duty to the dog, "but his act is inhuman and damages in himself that humanity which it is his duty to show towards mankind." The dog owner has no duty to the dog, but a duty to humanity regarding the dog. In my arguments I have indicated that the dog owner in addition has a duty of beneficence to the dog. I agree with Kant that the purposes of humans can outweigh the considerations of beneficence to animals. "Vivisectionists, who use living animals for their experiments, certainly act cruelly, although their aim is praiseworthy, and they can justify their cruelty, since animals must be regarded as man's instruments, but

any such cruelty for sport cannot be justified." Ibid., pp. 240–1. The arguments in this book do not preclude the use of animals for purposes of sport. As an example, consider the report of a gun club using live pigeons for target practice. Olive Talley, "Gun Club Again Using Live Pigeons," *Houston Chronicle* (February 16, 1985), sec. 1, p. 32.

22. For a recent discussion of the use of animals for medical and other research, see R. G. Frey, "Vivisection, Morals and Medicine," *Journal of Medical Ethics* 9 (June 1983): 94–7; T. L. S. Sprigge, "Vivisection, Morals, Medicine: Commentary from an Antivivisectionist Philosopher," *Journal of Medical Ethics* 9 (June 1983): 98–101; Sir William Paton, "Vivisection, Morals, Medicine: commentary from a Vivisection Professor of Pharmacology," *Journal of Medical Ethics* 9 (June 1983): 102–4. For general treatments of the issue of animal rights, see M. Fox, *Returning to Eden: Animal Rights and Human Obligations* (New York: Viking Press, 1980), and Peter Singer, *Animal Liberation* (London: Jonathan Cape, 1976).

23. What I raise here is the moral equivalent of some of the arguments that have been advanced in support of tort-for-wrongful-life suits. If one initiates a pregnancy, damages the fetus, and then fails to abort the fetus over which one has authority, one can then become the author of a harm that could have been prevented had one in a timely fashion had the fetus aborted. For an overview of the issues raised by tort-for-wrongful-life cases, see Angela Holder, "Is Existence Ever an Injury?: The Wrongful Life Cases," in S. F. Spicker et al. (eds.), *The Law-Medicine Relation: A Philosophical Exploration* (Dordrecht: Reidel, 1981), pp. 225–39.

24. Richard H. Feen, "Abortion and Exposure in Ancient Greece: Assessing the Status of the Fetus and 'Newborn' from Classical Sources," in Bondeson et al. (eds.), *Abortion and the Status of the Fetus*, pp. 283–300. In Viking law the child could not be exposed once it had been given suck. P. G. Foote and D. M. Wilson, *The Viking Achievement* (London: Sidgwick & Jackson, 1980), p. 115.

25. This point is noted in *Kitzur Shulhan Arukh,* by Rabbi Solomon Ganzfried (the standard condensed version of the code of Jewish religious law, entitled *Shulhan Arukh,* compiled by Joseph Karo [1488–1575], sec. 203, par. 3): "... if an infant dies within the first 30 days of its life, or even on the 30th day of its life, and even if there has been growth of its hair and nails, you do not follow any of the observances of mourning, because it is as if there had been a miscarriage" (adapted and translated by Professor Isaac Franck).

26. Stopping treatment on defective newborns seems to have been fairly well accepted. One might think here of the suggestions by Raymond S. Duff and A. G. M. Campbell regarding the ways in which parents may be assisted in making responsible choices regarding when to refuse treatment for their severely defective newborn. "Moral and Ethical Dilemmas in the Special Care Nursery," *New England Journal of Medicine* 289 (Oct. 25 1973): 890–4. See also Anthony Shaw, "Dilemmas of Informed Consent in Children," *New England Journal of Medicine* 289 (Oct. 25 1973): 885–90.

27. The United States government has attempted to stop parents or physicians from discriminating against neonates in treatment choices on the basis of physical and mental disability. The issues raised by such interferences are discussed in chap. 6.

28. The writings of Jeremy Bentham and John Stuart Mill have had a major liberalizing influence on the laws and customs of England and indeed of other countries. One might think here, in particular, of the influence that Jeremy Bentham had through his associate, Sir Edwin Chadwick (1800–90), who served on the Royal Commission for the Reform of Poor Laws and produced the *Report*

on an Inquiry into the Sanitary Conditions of the Laboring Population of Great Britain (1842). Bentham, one might note, was also a friend and correspondent of John Quincy Adams. He also had a brief impact on South American educational systems through Simón Bolívar, and on the civil code of Guatemala through José del Valle. Mill's writings on freedom have had an enduring influence on civil libertarian thought.

29. Gary E. Jones, "Engelhardt on the Abortion and Euthanasia of Defective Infants," *Linacre Quarterly* 50 (May 1983): 172–81.
30. Alfred Schutz and Thomas Luckmann, *The Structures of the Life-World*, trans. R. M. Zaner and H. T. Engelhardt, Jr. (Evanston, Ill: Northwestern University Press, 1973), p. 47.
31. John Hughlings Jackson (1835–1902), the father of modern neurology, examined this issue in a number of his writings. See, in particular, "Evolution and Dissolution of Nervous System," in *John Hughlings Jackson: Selected Writings*, ed. James Taylor (London: Staples Press, 1958), vol. 2, pp. 45–75; reproduced from the initial publication of the Croonian lectures delivered at the Royal College of Physicians, March 1884, and published originally as "Evolution and Dissolution of the Nervous System," *British Medical Journal* 1 (1884): 591–93, 660–3; "Evolution and Dissolution of the Nervous System," *Medical Times and Gazette* 1 (1884): 411–13, 445–58, 485–7; and "Evolution and Dissolution of the Nervous System," *Lancet* 1 (1884): 555–8, 649–52, 739–44. See also H. T. Engelhardt, Jr., "John Hughlings Jackson and the Mind-Body Relation," *Bulletin of the History of Medicine* 49 (Summer 1975): 137–51.
32. Here one must recall the point made in no. 18 concerning the at least six different ways in which Kant speaks of subjects or persons. For Kant's treatment of the "synthetic unity of apperception," see *Critique of Pure Reason*, B131-144.
33. H. T. Engelhardt, Jr., *Mind-Body: A Categorial Relation* (The Hague: Martinus Nijhoff, 1973).
34. The issue of the status of the right and left cerebral hemispheres has been explored by both philosophers and scientists. See, for example, Joseph E. Bogen, "The Other Side of the Brain. I. Dysgraphia and Dyscopia Following Cerebral Commissurotomy," *Bulletin of the Los Angeles Neurological Societies* 34 (April 1969): 73–105; "The Other Side of the Brain. II. An Appositional Mind," *Bulletin of the Los Angeles Neurological Societies* 34 (July 1969): 135–62; Joseph E. Bogen and Glenda M. Bogen, "The Other Side of the Brain. III. The Corpus Callosum and Creativity," *Bulletin of the Los Angeles Neurological Societies* 34 (Oct. 1969): 191–220; T. Nagel, "Brain Bisection and the Unity of Consciousness," *Synthese* 22 (1971): 396–413; R. W. Sperry, "Forebrain Commissurotomy and Conscious Awareness," *Journal of Medicine and Philosophy* 2 (1977): 101–126.
35. A. L. Wigan, *The Duality of the Brain* (London: Longman, 1844).
36. J. Hughlings Jackson, "On the Nature of the Duality of the Brain," *Medical Press and Circular* 1 (Jan. 14, 1874): 19–21; (Jan. 21, 1874): 41–4; (Jan. 28, 1874): 63–5.
37. Derek Parfit, "Personal Identity," *Philosophical Review* 80 (1971): 3-27; Roland Puccetti, "Brain Bisection and Personal Identity," *British Journal for the Philosophy of Science* 24 (1973): 339–55; "Multiple Identity," *The Personalist* 54 (1973): 203–15; "Sperry on Consciousness: A Critical Appreciation," *Journal of Medicine and Philosophy* 2 (1977): 139–44; "The Case for Mental Duality: Evidence from Split-Brain Data and Other Considerations," *Behavioral and Brain Sciences* 4 (1981): 93-123; Jerome Shaffer, "Personal Identity: The Implications of Brain

Bisection and Brain Transplants," *The Journal of Medicine and Philosophy* 2 (1977): 147–61.

38. C. H. Thigpen and H. M. Cleckley, *The Three Faces of Eve* (New York: McGraw-Hill, 1957).

39. H. Tristram Engelhardt, Jr., "Splitting the Brain, Dividing the Soul, Being of Two Minds," *Journal of Medicine and Philosophy* 2 (1977): 89–100.

40. Roland Puccetti, *Persons* (New York: Herder & Herder, 1969).

41. One would need to imagine each hemisphere receiving special training through data being flashed on the lateral retina of each eye. See, for instance, M. S. Gazzaniga, *The Bisected Brain* (New York: Appleton-Century-Crofts, 1970).

42. Such cases would raise interesting moral problems regarding responsibilities. Imagine what would happen if John$_2$ and John$_3$ were each married during the separation of the hemispheres of John$_1$ and were then later re-fused. Would the consequent John$_4$ now be married to both women? It would seem reasonable to say that John$_4$ had inherited the debts of John$_2$ and John$_3$, and most of John$_2$'s and John$_3$'s rights and privileges. It would seem reasonable to hold that the wives had morally grounded expectations from John$_4$, though John$_4$ may be free of certain of such morally based expectations regarding "his" wives, if they consented to the fusion. However, if they had not consented ("one John is not better than two"), or had consented on the condition that morally grounded expectations remain intact, then most covenantal duties to the wives may remain. Some of the problems raised here would have analogies with the problems a wife would face if her husband underwent transsexual surgery and developed lesbian inclinations.

43. Terence Penelhum, *Survival and Disembodied Existence* (New York: Humanities Press, 1970).

44. At the moment that God created a number of exact copies of individuals who are the same in the sense of sharing equivalent structures of their brain and equivalent memory, He would have created a number of instances of the same person. As their memories diverge, they would cease to be instances of the same person, in that they would be accruing new and different moral histories. They would be similar persons.

   One must note here that the sameness of these individuals at the moment of their cocreation is quite different from the sameness of clones or of twins who would share neither the same memories nor that same exactness of brain structure that would be the substrate of those equivalent memories. Sameness here would signify not strict identity, but equivalence so that God in reading the minds of the persons created could tell no differences in their memories, or note any significant differences in the structure of their brains. They would not be identical, in that these persons would be at different places at the same time.

45. See Gazzaniga, *Bisected Brain.*

46. John Locke, *The Treatises of Government, in the Former, the False Principles and Foundation of Sir Robert Filmer, and His Followers, Are Detected and Overthrown; the Latter, Is an Essay concerning the True Original, Extent, and End, of Civil Government,* book II, chap. V, sec. 25.

47. Kant, *Metaphysik der Sitten,* Akademie Textausgabe, vol 6, pp. 245–58. For Kant, one owns external property in a state of nature in anticipation of a civil society.

48. William Blackstone, *Commentaries on the Law of England* (1765), book II, chap. 1, pp. 8–9.

49. Hegel, *The Philosophy of Right,* trans. T. M. Knox (London: Oxford University Press, 1965), 54.
50. John Locke, *The Treatises of Government,* book II, chap. V, 27.
51. Gaius, *The Institutes of Gaius,* trans. F. de Zulueta (Oxford: Clarendon Press, 1946), part I, sec. 67, p. 83.
52. Locke, *Treatises of Government,* #27.
53. Thomas Paine, *Agrarian Justice* (London: T. G. Ballard, 1798).
54. W. Ogilvie, *Essay on the Right of Property in Land* (London: J. Walter, 1781).
55. Baruch Brody, "Health Care for the Haves and Have Nots: Toward a Just Basis of Distribution," in Earl E. Shelp (ed.), *Justice and Health Care* (Dordrecht: Reidel, 1981), pp. 151–9.
56. John Locke, *Treatises of Government,* book II, chap. V, #27. This notion of the right of all to the rent on things generally does not give any person any specific right to any specific bit of land. Therefore, insofar as individuals come to work or transform particular land, they have a right not to be disturbed by others, for example, walking through their houses late at night, claiming that all land belongs to all. Such an intrusion would violate their actualized claim to that land, insofar as they have transformed it by their activities. What others have is a right to be compensated for the inconvenience of having to walk around private property and to use public parks for picnics instead of the lawns in front of private houses. The Lockean proviso is a principle of compensation for inconvenience. The person who has transformed land or properly come into possession of transformed land has a right that conflicts with the rights of those who might have wished to be able to possess that land themselves. The latter do not own that land but have a right to be compensated for the opportunities foreclosed to them.

   The answer to how much rent to charge cannot be discovered but must be created through some democratic process. This does not return us to the status quo. First, the rent may be collected only on land and raw materials. Second, the amount of the rent cannot be determined on the basis of redistributive goals. Indeed, the whole notion of the rent on the land would lead to something very close to international property tax.
57. Robert Nozick, *Anarchy, State, and Utopia.*
58. Baruch Brody, "Health Care for the Haves and Have Nots," pp. 151–9.
59. Gaius, *The Institutes of Gaius,* part II, pp. 75-80.
60. Hippocrates, "Law," trans. W. H. S. Jones (Cambridge, Mass.: Harvard University Press, 1969), vol. 2, p. 263.
61. The character of "malpractice suits" in both ancient Greece and Rome has been explored at length by Darrel Amundsen, "The Liability of the Physician in Roman Law," in H. Karplus (ed.), *International Symposium on Society Medicine and Law* (New York: Elsevier, 1973), pp. 17-30; "The Liability of the Physician in Classical Greek Legal Theory and Practice," *Journal of the History of Medicine and Allied Sciences* 32 (April 1977): 172–203; "Physician, Patient and Malpractice: An Historical Perspective", in S. F. Spicker *et al.* (eds.), *The Law-Medicine Relation,* pp. 255–58.
62. Marcia Angell, "Should Heroin be Legalized for the Treatment of Pain?" *New England Journal of Medicine* 311 (Aug. 23, 1984): 529–30; and Edward N. Brandt, Jr., "Compassionate Pain Relief: Is Heroin the Answer?" *New England Journal of Medicine* 311 (August 23, 1984): 530-2.
   From both libertarian and utilitarian perspectives, one might ask why any

access to drugs should be forbidden. Which is more dangerous to individuals, the risk of being addicted to a dangerous drug or that of being involuntarily subjected to drug-related crimes? Under current circumstances, addicts steal property to sell it at a fraction of its worth in order to buy drugs priced at many times their value. Because drugs are illegal, there is a booming illicit drug industry whose profits are in the billions. This trade is then taken to justify specially directed police forces, whose interventions succeed in maintaining the high prices of illicit drugs and therefore the continued great incentives for illegal sales.

63 Pope Innocent III, "'Sicut universitatis' ad Acerbum consulem Florentinum, 30 October 1198," in H. Denzinger (ed.), *Enchiridion Symbolorum,* 33d ed. (Rome: Herder, 1965), p. 244.

64. See "Erronea propositio de tyrannicidio," in *Enchiridion Symbolorum,* p. 326.

65. William Blackstone, *Commentaries on the Laws of England* (New York: Augustus M. Kelley, 1969), vol. 2, book I, pp. 191f.

66. John Rawls, *A Theory of Justice* (Cambridge, Mass.: Harvard University Press, 1971), pp. 62f., 136–42, 302f.

67. Ibid., pp. 195–201, 221–34.

68. One must observe that there has been a considerable dispute in the history of America regarding the significance of the original consent to the American Constitution of 1789. Though this dispute peaked during the War Between the States, its origins can be found already well articulated in the resolutions of the Kentucky legislature endorsing nullification and the general assembly of Virginia endorsing interposition during the time of John Adams's restrictions of civil liberties. See the Resolution of the Kentucky Legislature in the House of Representatives, November 14, 1799, and the General Assembly of Virginia in the House of Delegates, January 7, 1800, reprinted in *We the States* (Richmond, Va.: William Byrd Press, 1964), pp. 155–9.

69. Blackstone, *Commentaries,* book 1, p. 193.

70. Thomas Hobbes, *Leviathan, or the Matter, Forms, & Power of a Common-wealth Ecclesiastical and Civill* (London: Andrew Crooke, 1651), part 1, chap. 13, p. 62.

71. Ibid., part 2, chap. 17, p. 87.

72. Ibid.

73. Ibid., p. 88.

74. Ibid., part 2, chap. 18, p. 90.

75. One might recall here the defense of slavery given by Hugo Grotius in his *De jure belli ac pacis.* Hereditary slavery comes into existence when a person is captured in a war and not killed. In forgoing the right to kill the captive, the captive taker gains the right to the children born of the slave *ad indefinitum.* See book 3, chap. 7, esp. sec. 1–5. These morally unjustifiable considerations were in fact endorsed by theologians of the time, though Christians were held to be bound to forbear from taking Christians as slaves. See book 3, chap. 7, sec. 9.

One should note that, even if slaves were not persons before the law, the very theory of slavery still presumed that they were moral persons. This was the case even despite special rationalizations that underscored the moral and psychological infirmities or disabilities of slaves in order to justify the peculiar institution. One might note, for instance, that in both Tennessee and Texas before the War Between the States the slave was held to be in a position analogous to that of individuals in Norman villeinage, conferring upon the slave a certain standing before the law. A. E. Keir Nash, "Texas Justice in the Age of Slavery: Appeals

Concerning Blacks and the Antebellum State Supreme Court," *Houston Law Review* 8 (1971): 438-56.

76. Were this a volume focused primarily on political theory rather than bioethics, one would need to explore in detail the extent to which states might properly continue to perform the functions we now associate with them. For instance, there may be no reason to allow the state to have a monopoly on the enforcement of justice. There are, in fact, arguments to support the efficiency of the private enforcement of justice in the historical example of Iceland, where from the tenth to the thirteenth centuries the enforcement of justice was a private matter. David Friedman, "Efficient Institutions for the Private Enforcement of Law," *Journal of Legal Studies* XIII (June 1984): 379–97; "Private Creation and Enforcement of Law: A Historical Case," *The Journal of Legal Studies* VIII (March 1979): 399–415. The Icelandic experience developed out of the same general pagan Teutonic roots that gave rise to much of Anglo-Saxon law. For a study of the Icelandic legal and social system, see P. G. Foote and D. M. Wilson, *The Viking Achievement* (London: Sidgwick & Jackson, 1970). Original material concerning old Icelandic law and customs can be found in the *Njals Saga* and in the *Gragas,* the earliest compilation of Icelandic law.

One might still envisage a need for the police of the general secular pluralist peaceable society to monitor the activities of private police forces as an overseer of last resort. To this proposal there will be the reaction that the market is likely to produce a police force able to perform this function just as well or better. One may need also to consider the balance of powers between private and public police forces, as well as the arrangement of courts for the trial of public crimes. In a world where true toleration is given for the diversity of human beliefs and for the diversity of human communities likely to be formed, there will be numerous special legal systems developed as administrative laws governing rights and obligations within particular corporations, associations, and communities. One might foresee such an arrangement somewhat on the model of the relationship between civil and canon law, save for the fact that there will be numerous genres of canon law. There will be the problem of whether one may establish a single set of courts for civil law. Perhaps the general secular pluralist state could at most impose a form of arbitration upon individuals in the process of selecting a particular genre of civil courts, which arbitration process and which court would need to be in accord with the principle of autonomy. These are complex and important matters that will need to be treated elsewhere than in this volume.

5

The Languages of Medicalization

Shaping reality

Medicine medicalizes reality. It creates a world. It translates sets of problems into its own terms. Medicine molds the ways in which the world of experience takes shape; it conditions reality for us. The difficulties people have are then appreciated as illnesses, diseases, deformities, and medical abnormalities, rather than as innocent vexations, normal pains, or possession by the devil. Medical problems are clusters of phenomena seen as amenable to medical assessment, explanation, and up to a point, amelioration or cure. Here one finds clusters of difficulties often termed diseases, sicknesses, illnesses, deformities, disabilities, and disfigurements, which are beyond the immediate control of the individuals afflicted, and which are presumed to have a basis in physiological, anatomical, or psychological causal matrices. Their sense, significance, and reality are cast in terms of the social and intellectual institutions of medicine. In being seen as medical problems, they are usually characterized as circumstances that deviate from physiological or psychological ideals regarding proper levels of function, freedom from pain, and achievement of expected human form and grace. An ache or pain thus becomes a medical disorder. In addition, since medicine is a social institution, the pains, deformities, and dysfunctions are given a social valence.

Consider the transformation of experienced reality accomplished with the diagnosis of heart disease. A slight shortness of breath or the swelling of ankles after a long day of work becomes a sign of disease. Sleeping on two pillows is no longer an innocent occurrence, but a possible stigma of a deadly disease. The individual's view of life is changed by a set of expectations regarding the dangerousness of heart disease and the possibility of an early death. New relations are likely to develop with physicians and other health care personnel. New rituals are imposed with a force and character comparable to those of a religion. One must now regularly take medication and conform to a new diet in order to lower salt and cholesterol intake. What were previously innocent undertakings, such as eating, exercise, and recreation, now become serious matters of health, if not of life and death. Cigarette smoking will now clearly appear as dangerous. The individual may even worry that sexual intercourse could lead to death. The social circumstances of the individual will be transformed by the expectations of others as they learn of the diagnosis. Friends will wonder whether John can go on the ski trip, after all. Is it likely to be too much for him? Women may worry that he may die while making love with them. If he is a pilot for an airline, he may no longer be able to continue in his job. Insurance companies are likely to issue insurance now only at a markedly increased premium. In short, a major transformation of experienced reality will have taken place.

Such is not unexpected. The world in which we live is not furnitured by uninterpreted facts. We see the things around us in terms of social and theoretical expectations. We are taught early how to explain the occurrences of our world. In the West we take for granted that a set of complex, etiologic forces directs the production of illness and disease. Individuals in other cultures, or our antecedents in our own culture, untutored by our current scientific world view, do not or did not see illness as the result of infectious agents, genetic flaws, or endocrinological abnormalities. We, however, do. Our world is structured by a special set of assumptions about the rule-governed character of our experience. These scientific and metaphysical presuppositions fashion for us our everyday expectations. They give shape to our lifeworld. In addition, the particular character of our social institutions invests occurrences with social significance. The current arrangement among dentists, surgeons, physicians, and psychiatrists is the result of a set of past historical forces in great proportion peculiar to our particular culture, but which contributes to the appreciated significance of a toothache, appendicitis, heart disease, or schizophrenia.

We see the world through our social, scientific, and value expectations. The medical *facts* with which bioethics deals are not timeless truths, but data given through the distorting biases of our history and culture. Recognizing a state of affairs as heart disease, cancer, depression, homosexuality, or tuberculosis is a rich and complex process. All knowledge is historically and culturally conditioned, and the influence of history and culture is often, as we shall see, particularly marked in medicine. This is not to say that investigators do not attempt to know, timelessly unconstrained by social and cultural forces. In endeavoring to know truly, one attempts to understand the world as it would be seen from God's eye, from the viewpoint of dispassionate, scientific observers, so that the findings could be shared with other investigators, even those outside our culture—in principle, even with alien investigators on planets circling distant stars.

The goal of undistorted knowledge is a heuristic. It directs us as knowers, as scientists, toward the truth. As Charles S. Peirce (1839–1914), the founder of pragmatism, observed, "Finally, as what anything really is, is what it may finally come to be known to be in the ideal state of complete information, so that reality depends on the ultimate decision of the community; so thought is what it is, only by virtue of its addressing a future thought which is in its value as thought identical with it, though more developed."[1] Peirce is suggesting that it is impossible to speak of reality apart from possible knowers of reality. Any concept we can have of reality is that of a reality that is experienced, even if experienced by ideal observers. To speak of the nature of reality undistorted by historical and cultural context is to speak of a view that would be possessed by unbiased knowers in full possession of all information. The interest in knowing reality truly sets knowers on a journey from their unrecognized biases toward an ever more complete overcoming of those biases through a recognition of them and through endeavors to compensate for them in order to achieve a greater capacity to describe reality, unconditioned by the idiosyncrasies of one's cultural context. In pursuing the ideal of Peirce's community of perfectly advantaged scientists, one is able to distinguish between better and worse portrayals of reality by reference to an ideal, which one need not claim can actually be achieved. The ideal is ingredient in the very practice of science, in the very endeavor of science as a cultural undertaking directed toward intersubjectivity in knowledge claims secured by and regarding an external reality. As certain genre of religious undertakings turn to revealed scriptures and divine inspiration, empirical science turns to the world outside. In naming, classifying, grading, staging, and explaining diseases, we would hope to do so, as would be done by a community of ideal investigators responding to an external reality. Again, we never reach this goal.

Though there has been much recent attention to the historically and culturally conditioned character of knowledge, the roots of this appreciation are deep. Indeed, from Giambattista Vico (1168–1744) through G. W. F. Hegel (1770–1831) and Wilhelm Dilthey (1833–1911) to the present, there has been an ever-increasing appreciation of the extent to which our construals of reality exist within the embrace of cultural expectations. The recent development of these insights by Ludwik Fleck (1896–1961)[2] and Thomas Kuhn[3] has led to a better understanding of the role of historical and cultural forces in science generally and in medicine in particular. I will not address this issue here as it arises with regard to such sciences as physics and chemistry, the focus of Thomas Kuhn's interests. I will look instead at medicine. The example of medicine, it might be noted, is the one developed by Ludwik Fleck, who in fact influenced Kuhn's work, which has been so influential in the recent reassessment of the interplay between the history and the philosophy of science.[4] Medicine is a promising arena in which to explore the role of values and goals in scientific knowledge claims, for in medicine, concerns to know truly and to intervene efficiently intertwine. The role of social values is often outrageously salient.

Consider, for example, the following case history provided in Isaac Baker Brown's *On the Curability of Certain Forms of Insanity, Epilepsy, Catalepsy, and Hysteria in Females.*[5] The volume from which the case is taken is a classic in the literature that focused during the eighteenth and nineteenth centuries on the "disease" of masturbation.[6] Individuals were thought in that period to die from masturbation[7] and autopsy findings substantiated the effects of self-abuse on the spinal cord.[8] Against this background, Dr. Brown recommended that, in order to treat female masturbators, the clitoris be excised to terminate the "long continued peripheral excitement, causing frequent and increasing losses of nerve force."[9] By experience he found that the best approach was, after placing the patient "completely under the influence of chloroform, [to have] the clitoris freely excised by scissors or knife—I always prefer the scissors."[10] It is in terms of these assumptions that Dr. Brown published a number of cases to demonstrate the success of his therapeutic interventions. Consider as an example case number thirty-one of the some forty-eight cases included in his volume.

Case XXXI. Cataleptic Fits—Two Years' Illness—Operation—Cure.

M.N., aet. 17; admitted into the London Surgical Home September 4, 1861.

History.—Was perfectly well up to the age of fifteen, when she went to a boarding-school in the West of England. In the course of three or four months she became subject to all symptoms of hysteria, and from that time gradually got worse, having fits, at first mild in character and of rare occurrence, but gradually more severe and frequent, till she became a confirmed cataleptic. For several months before admission, she had been attacked with as many as four or five fits a day, and during the whole journey from the North of England to London she was unconscious and rigidly cataleptic. She was seen immediately on arrival, and there was no doubt that it was a genuine case of this disease. So sensitive was she, that if any one merely touched her bed, or walked across the room, she would immediately be thrown into the cataleptic state.

Before making any personal examination, Mr. Brown ascertained both from her mother and herself, that she had long indulged in self-excitation of the clitoris, having first been taught by a school-fellow. The commencement of her illness corresponded exactly with the origin of its cause; in fact, cause and effect were here so perfectly manifested, that it hardly wanted anything more than the history to enable one to form a correct diagnosis. All the other symptoms attending these cases were, however, well marked.

The next day after admission she was operated upon, and from that date she never had a fit. She remained in the Home for several weeks. Five weeks after operation, she walked all over Westminster Abbey, whereas for quite a year and a half before treatment, she had been incapable of the slightest exertion.[11]

The young woman was successfully diagnosed and treated.

One need not go to the nineteenth century to encounter the obvious intrusions of social values. The recent history of homosexuality has seen it develop from an instance of sociopathic personality disturbance in the first *Diagnostic and Statistical Manual of the American Psychiatric Association* (*DSM-I*),[12] to a personality disorder in *DSM-II*,[13] and, finally, to an instance of psychosocial dysfunction in *DSM-III* under the taxon, ego-dystonic homosexuality.[14] In short, it is now a mental disorder only if the individual has a persistent concern to change his or her sexual orientation. This shift in the medical understanding of homosexuality was tied to changes in ideas of sexuality, the notion of perversion, and views regarding the proper bounds of disease language.

The difficulties in becoming clear regarding what should count as a disease are not restricted to psychiatry or to sexuality. One might think of the fashionable nineteenth century disease of chlorosis, "impoverishment of the blood, constipation, dyspepsia, palpitation, and menstrual derangements and irregularities."[15] Reputable physicians from Thomas Sydenham (1624–1689) in the seventeenth century to numerous physicians in the nineteenth century described women as in fact turning green from the disease. The past is replete with views and experiences of illness at odds with our current understandings. Among such one might also include the ways in which fevers were considered diseases, not just symptoms, through the eighteenth century.[16] The more one moves to the past, the more the landscape of disease departs from the one to which we are accustomed.

In fact, the further one retreats into the past, the more difficult it is to recognize diseases with which we are familiar. Physicians then did not have the same concerns as we do. As a result, they described illnesses in somewhat different fashions. Their views of the line between what should count as noise and information were fashioned in terms of presuppositions often quite unlike ours. Consequently it is often difficult to understand what diseases they were in fact describing. Consider a case given in the Hippocratic corpus.

In Meliboea a youth took to his bed after being for a long time heated by drunkenness and sexual indulgence. He had shivering fits, nausea, sleeplessness, but no thirst.

First day. Copious, solid stool passed in abundance of fluid, and on the following days the excreta were copious, watery and of a greenish yellow. Urine thin, scanty and of no colour; respiration rare and large with long intervals; tensions, soft underneath, of the hypochondrium, extending out to either side; continual throbbing throughout of the epigastrium; urine oily.

Tenth day. Delirious but quiet, for he was orderly and silent; skin dry and tense; stools either copious and thin or bilious and greasy.

Fourteenth day. General exacerbation; delirious with much wandering talk.

Twentieth day. Wildly out of his mind; much tossing; urine suppressed; slight quantities of drink were retained.

Twenty-fourth day. Death.[17]

Though we might have a number of suppositions regarding the nature of the disease, it is difficult to advance any particular diagnosis with assurance. This is not simply because Hippocrates fails to provide us with laboratory data; he also does not provide us with the sort of physical examination we would undertake were we faced with the same case and the need to make a diagnosis in the absence of any laboratory findings. We would also provide a more complete past history, filled out in terms of our presuppositions regarding the youth's fatal illness.

We also readily recognize some constellations of findings in the descriptions of past physicians. One might think here of the famous Hippocratic description of mumps with orchitis.

Many had swellings beside one ear, or both ears, in most cases unattended with fever, so that confinement to bed was unnecessary. In some cases there was slight heat, but in all the swellings subsided without causing harm; in no case was there suppuration such as attends swellings of other origin. This was the character of them:—flabby, big, spreading, with neither inflammation nor pain; in every case they disappeared without a sign. The sufferers were youths, young men, and men in their prime, usually those who frequented the wrestling school and gymnasia. Few women were attacked. Many had dry coughs which brought up nothing when they coughed, but their voices were hoarse. Soon after though in some cases after some time, painful inflammations occurred either in one testicle or in both, sometimes accompanied with fever, in other cases not. Usually they caused much suffering. In other respects the people had no ailments requiring medical assistance.[18]

Is mumps more of a contextless, naked fact than the disease that killed the youth from Meliboea? How does one determine what is really the case in medicine? How does one protect against the errors of physicians such as Baker Brown and properly build a science of medicine on data such as the Hippocratic description of mumps?

These are practical, not just theoretical questions, because medicine's theories lead to actual interventions, as occurred with the clitoridectomies of the nineteenth century. In fact, simply regarding a phenomenon as a medical problem can alter the character of a range of societal expectations. For example, to see the process of giving birth as freighted with medical risks requiring medical interventions from episiotomies to caesarean sections is to change the meaning of giving birth and alter the socially supported rights of expectant mothers and fathers vis-à-vis physicians. As Ivan Illich has argued, the medicalization of life is ubiquitous and can be devastating.[19] Seeing an element of life as a medical problem raises more than issues of scientific medicine. The medicalization of reality raises issues of public policy and of ethics. What one classifies as a disease and how it is classified as a disease has an immediate impact on persons' lives and on society in general, in contrast with the classification of stars. In examining a Pap smear, a decision must be made regarding how many cells with deviant changes of what character must be present before the smear is read as indicating cancer. To be too liberal in classifying cells as cancerous will lead to unnecessary operations. To be too conservative in the classification will lead women to receiving treatment too late for successful cure. How one in part discovers and in part creates lines between cancerous, noncancerous, and precancerous findings is of considerable moment for individuals concerned to keep their bodies intact while avoiding cancer, and for societies interested in containing medical costs and maximizing benefits for their members.[20] How one fashions such classifications will have implications for morbidity, mortality, and financial costs.

In both strong and weak senses, medicine creates a socially accepted reality. Through denominating a problem a medical problem, expectations are created and personal destinies influenced. They are obviously strong senses of fashioning reality in the case of classifications leading to legally enforced medical viewpoints. Here one might think of the vote by the American Psychiatric Association whether to classify homosexuality as a disease.[21] The medical regard of homosexuality as a disease reinforced the legal proscription of homosexual activities. Its removal from the list of mental disorders weakened arguments for state sanctions. Somewhat less socially enforced are the particular stagings of cancer, which lead to particular levels of treatment.[22] Such systems for staging reflect decisions made by communities of physicians regarding the most appropriate and useful ways to characterize an area of reality. The acceptance of a particular staging system involves agreeing to see and react to reality in a disciplined and coordinated fashion. The difference between a stage I and a stage II cancer will be expressed in the differences between limited surgical procedures and more extensive interventions with chemotherapy and/or radiation along with a less optimal prognosis. This is a point to which we will return after an examination of the character of medical accounts of reality.

Medical reality is the result of a complex interplay of descriptive, evaluative, explanatory, and social labeling interests. The ways in which we speak of, react to, and experience medical reality are shaped and directed by these interests. These four clusters of concerns I will synoptically call the four languages of medicine. However, they are more than languages. They represent four conceptual dimensions, through which clinical problems are regarded. They are modes of medicalization. "Language," however, provides a useful metaphor by suggesting that each mode has its own grammar or rules for constructing meaning. There are four different clusters of "syntactical" and "semantical" constraints that shape the ways we speak of, understand, and experience medical reality.

The four languages of medicine

The experienced reality with which medicine deals is shaped by (1) evaluative assumptions regarding what functions, pains, and deformities are normal in the sense of proper and acceptable, (2) views of how descriptions are to be given, (3) causal explanatory models, and (4) social expectations regarding individual ills of particular forms of sickness. The more we share assumptions with physicians in the past, the easier it is to recognize the disease under study and to agree with the characterizations offered of medical reality. The more the assumptions differ, the less the descriptions will be intersubjective.

Consider the differences between current classifications of pain and those of the eighteenth century. In the twentieth century, pains are regarded, for the most part, as symptoms of diseases, rather than as diseases in their own right. Pains do not appear among the major classes of disease in the current *International Classification of Diseases*.[23] In contrast, the classification of diseases, *Genera morborum* (1763) by Carl von Linné (Carolus Linnaeus) (1707–78), listed pains as one of the eleven major classifications of disease.[24] The influential classification provided by the French physician François Boissier de Sauvages (1701–1767) also listed pains prominently as one of the ten classes of disease.[25] The differences in classification of pain turn on differences in presumptions regarding the reality of diseases. They subtly direct physicians regarding how they should take seriously the pains of their patients. Currently, for example, since pains are not considered diseases in their own right, they tend to be discounted unless they can be shown to have a pathoanatomical or pathophysiological cause. We are led to look for the pathoanatomical or pathophysiological truth value of a complaint before we acknowledge it as being fully bona fide.[26]

The interplay of descriptive, evaluative, explanatory, and social labeling languages in health care thus shapes our appreciation of a medical problem. Though the four languages inseparably intertwine, they can be distinguished. Distinguishing them can allow us to appreciate the roots of different understandings of disease in different cultural contexts. It can also aid us in seeing how hidden value and policy judgments shape the "medical facts" we accept. If the role of such value and policy judgments is not recognized, we are likely to accept uncritically what is offered to us as "the scientific facts."

What is presented as a fact, especially as a scientific fact, often has a cachet similar to the deliverances of a divine revelation to a community of believers. It may be considered a value-free timeless reality. This engenders difficulties. If homosexuality is in fact a disease, how could one vote whether it should be recognized as a mental disorder? Should not the determination of its standing be reserved for scientific investigation alone? To answer questions such as these, one will need to examine the languages of medicine in some detail.

Disease language as evaluative

To see a phenomenon as a disease, deformity, or disability is to see something wrong with it. Diseases, illnesses, and disfigurements are experienced as failures to achieve an expected state, a state held to be proper to the person afflicted. This may be a failure to achieve an expected level of freedom from pain or anxiety. It may involve a failure to achieve an expected realization of human form or grace. Or it may involve a failure to achieve what is an expected term of life. These genre of judgments characterize a circumstance as one of suffering, one of pathology, one of a problem to be solved. Such judgments may be made either by the individuals afflicted or by others regarding those individuals. In being characterized as perverted, diseased, or deformed, an adverse judgment is rendered them. This is the case even with a disfigured nose, for which the bearer seeks cosmetic surgery, or an unwanted pregnancy, for which the woman seeks an abortion.

THE SEARCH FOR VALUES IN NATURE. How does one encounter medical phenomena as problems? Is it in terms of societally conditioned values? Or are there values ingredient in natural processes that can be disclosed as guidelines for appreciating what should count as biological and psychological norms? Until recently, the answer affirmed the latter. The presumption was that nature contained ingredient goals and purposes by which dysfunctions, disfigurements, and disabilities could be objectively judged. One sees this language most fully developed in the language of sexual perversion. Consider the following statutory definition of an unnatural act and perversion.

Every person who is convicted of taking into his or her mouth the sexual organ of any other person or animal, or who shall be convicted of placing his or her sexual organ in the mouth of any other person or animal, ᴏr who shall be convicted of committing any other unnatural or perverted sexual practice with any other person or animal, shall be fined not more than one thousand dollars ($1,000.00), or be imprisoned in jail or in the house of correction or in the penitentiary for a period not exceeding ten years, or shall be both fined and imprisoned within the limits above prescribed in the discretion of the court.[27]

How does one know that such acts are unnatural? How does one discover the norm from which the activities deviate? Does one appeal to statistical frequencies regarding what individuals usually or customarily do in a particular society? If so, what moral force would such findings have? How could they disclose a biological or physiological ideal? Does the fact that the penis and vagina evolved for maximizing reproductive capacities say anything regarding the use of the anus or mouth for recreational sex? What if such recreational activities reinforce the bond between a reproducing couple, so as to maximize their interest in the successful development of their offspring? That is, what if oral and anal sex were indirectly to maximize reproductive success?

The traditional Western answer was given in terms of a view of man and of all nature as created by God and therefore designed toward the achievement of the purposes of God. To speak of perverting nature in sexual or other activities thus presupposes a divine standard ingredient in nature from creation. The Middle Ages was thus able to synthesize a set of presumptions regarding a Creator God and His designs for nature with an Aristotelian language of essences and final causes. Within the Aristotelian framework, it was presumed that one could discover the essences of things and that an examination of the essence of man would disclose ingredient purposes. These Aristotelian assumptions, when fortified by Stoic views that one's lot was maximized by following the laws of nature, made a fertile ground for the completion of the Christian synthesis in terms of which one could then discover what was natural and unnatural.

The appeal to a designing Creator God makes it plausible to presume that one will be able to discover what are truly and objectively diseases by appeal to the design of nature. One will need only to attend to *the* function of the organs in question in order to decide whether a particular condition should count as a disease. Consider color blindness, which is a disadvantage in a number of environments but which confers an advantage if one needs to recognize camouflage. In environments where spotting camouflage increased reproductive success, color blindness would confer an advantage on the individual with the trait.[28] However, in terms of the creationist view, one could still understand the trait as a defect. It is simply that in a particular deviant environment, a defect may produce an advantage. The same would be the case with respect to homosexuality, which in certain environments might confer an advantage. The creationists have as a canonical reference point the ideal nature of man adapted for the ideal environment, presumably Eden.

In terms of such presumptions regarding ideal designs, one can make moral, physio-aesthetic, and anatomico-aesthetic judgments regarding proper human form, function, and freedom from pain. Such presuppositions can support judgments such as those by St. Thomas Aquinas that, all things

THE LANGUAGES OF MEDICALIZATION

being equal, masturbation is a greater sin than a naturally performed rape, because masturbation violates the very law of nature.[29] However, once one departs from a creationist perspective, how can one appeal to a canon of normality that will provide a basis for value judgments? One cannot appeal to a creator's design or to *the* ideal environment. Nor will appealing to what is statistically normal in itself decide what ought to be the case. From the fact that most people may lie or cheat to some extent, it does not follow that such behavior is praiseworthy, proper, or ideal. The same holds for widely distributed, if not nearly universal diseases, such as caries or artherosclerosis among the elderly. This is not to deny that problems will come to be accepted if they are frequent enough. Individuals may indeed acquiesce in widely distributed diseases. However, when given the opportunity to treat them, such circumstances may be recognized as clinical problems, as illnesses, as diseases. What would be the basis for such a judgment?

DISEASE AS SPECIES ATYPICALITY, OR THE ATTEMPT TO DISCOVER DESIGN IN THE PRODUCTS OF EVOLUTION.   One might, as Christopher Boorse, attempt to discover what should count as a disease by appealing to species-typical levels of species-typical functions, which have been established through evolution. Thus, in his earlier works Boorse attempted to distinguish between a concept of illness, which is value laden, and one of diseases, which is value free. Boorse characterized illnesses as states of affairs in which one has a disease that is serious enough to be incapacitating and that is "(i) undesirable for its bearer; (ii) a title to special treatment; and (iii) a valid excuse for normally criticizable behavior."[30] In contrast, he attempted to fashion a notion of disease that is independent of desires and societal roles. Thus, he framed a concept of disease in these terms:

1. The *reference class* is a natural class of organisms of uniform functional design; specifically, an age group of a sex of a species.
2. A *normal function* of a part or process within members of the reference class is a statistically typical contribution by it to their individual survival and reproduction . . .
3. A *disease* is a type of internal state which is either an impairment of normal functional ability, i.e. a reduction of one or more functional abilities below typical efficiency, or a limitation on functional ability caused by environmental agents.
4. *Health* is the absence of disease.[31]

In this fashion, Boorse attempted to recapture the capacity to identify deviations from a norm so as to discover what ought to count as diseases. Even after the collapse of creationist presumptions, he seeks to disclose without an appeal to societal values the line between health and disease.

The difficulties with Boorse's approach are multiple. First, in placing his accent on individual reproductive fitness, he fails to accent the more generally acknowledged notion of inclusive fitness. What appears to be important in evolution is not whether a particular individual reproduces, but whether that individual maximizes the chances of his genes being spread in the gene pool. Thus, if one is a homosexual who does not marry and stays at home as a bachelor uncle, one may maximize the reproductive capacities of one's siblings with which one stays, and thus in fact maximize the chances of genes such as one's own being passed on.

It is not just that Boorse overlooks the role of inclusive fitness in evolutionary accounts of "biological design", he is unsympathetic to the fact that species may in fact be well adapted because of a balance among various contrasting traits. There may not be a single design, but rather a number of designs. When such is the case, one cannot speak straightforwardly of either species design or species typicality. In contrast, Boorse's approach reflects a somewhat Platonic view that favors a single typical way to achieve the excellence of humans. It is for this reason that Boorse is so clear that homosexuality should count as a disease.[32] In the absence of such a notion of typicality, it will not even be clear how one should determine what should count as homosexuality. Will a single homosexual encounter suffice? It is not clear whether Boorse has in mind individuals who would rate as Kinsey 5s or 6s on the Kinsey scale, which ranges from Kinsey zeros, who have never had any homosexual experience, to Kinsey 5s, whose homosexual experiences dominate their sexual lives, to Kinsey 6s, who are innocent of any heterosexual activity. What of Kinsey 4s, who although they have predominantly homosexual encounters still have heterosexual experiences, and who may reproduce at the same rate as Kinsey zeros? In short, the more one recognizes how biological and behavioral phenomena often express themselves along a continuum, the more difficult it becomes to speak of species typicality.

If one ignores this problem, one is still left with the possibility that homosexuality may be balanced with heterosexuality, because such a balance, at least at some time in the past, led to maximizing inclusive fitness.[33] A number of traits undoubtedly exist in balance, because the balance itself maximizes inclusive fitness. Here one might think of the somewhat classic case of sickle cell disease. If sickle cell disease developed, as it appears, to confer a protection for pregnant women against falciparum malaria, it is then a successful product of evolution.[34] What is to count as a species-typical blood type? A particular blood type, or a balance among types that may include sickle cell?

The problem is that it is difficult to decide what is or is not a medical problem, if one does not specify an environment and a set of goals. If one holds that it is important for all individuals to reproduce, then Kinsey 6s, in the absence of artificial insemination, will count as diseased, as maladapted. (Could gay men and lesbians cure themselves of Boorse's disease of homosexuality, if the males donated to a sperm bank to inseminate the lesbians, so that they could achieve a higher reproductive rate than heterosexuals?) One will also not be able to decide whether sickle cell disease (i.e., being homozygous for sickle cell trait) is in fact a disease, unless one knows whether one is taking a species-oriented or an individual-oriented perspective. If one is concerned about individual pain and suffering and the circumscription of life expectancy, being homozygous for sickle cell will be a disease. On the other hand, if one is concerned to maximize species survival, one will hope that sickle cell trait remains in the gene pool, in the event that through some worldwide catastrophe falciparum malaria would spread without the ability to control it through drugs (e.g., Jesuit bark). One might thus term it not a disease but an element of an evolutionarily secured advantage.

To decide what is a problem for medicine, one must make reference to a particular environment and a particular set of goals, so that one can understand whether the individual is well adapted. What will be required for the realization of particular goals will differ from environment to environment. If one is a black living in Trondheim without the availability of exogenous vitamin D, then the possession of highly pigmented skin would put one at a disadvantage with regard to survival. One will have a greater risk, for example, of developing rickets. However, if the environment were to include vitamin D-enriched milk, as is the case in modern circumstances, the individual becomes well adapted. So, too, a Norwegian with lightly pigmented skin and without adequate clothing and protection from the sun will run a markedly increased risk of developing carcinoma of the skin if transported to the tropics. The notion of successful adaptation is context specific and determined by what one wishes to achieve in a particular context.

One cannot simply turn to the results of evolution to determine what a disease is. We are the product of blind, selective forces, which, if they have been successful, have adapted us to environments in which we may no longer live. Since what is species typical may represent an adaptation to environments in which we no longer live, it may not afford us the same degree of adaptation as that provided by some species-atypical trait. Moreover, evolution is not directly concerned with the comfort and pleasure of humans or with their goals. For all these reasons, one will not be able simply to turn to biological conditions or the outcomes of evolution in order to discover what ought or ought not to be seen as a medical problem. Conditions stand out as problems because they thwart the goals of particular individuals or groups of individuals.

It might be the case that zoologists would be interested in determining what states of affairs represent species-atypical departures from species-typical levels of function. But one cannot know whether such are good or bad departures until they are seen within the context of human goals in a particular environment. Since evolution does not aim at the realization of the goals of individuals or of societies, the outcomes of evolution can fail to be in accord with individual and societal goals. Indeed, sickle cell anemia offers an example of the lack of coincidence. To speak metaphorically, the individuals who die of sickle cell disease are, from an "evolutionary perspective," sacrificed in the process of maximizing the fitness of heterozygotes. Individuals, however, will be concerned that their physicians treat them, not to maximize the survival potential of their genes or their species, but to achieve the goals of relief of suffering and avoidance of disability, which they hold to be proper. They will then join in social organizations such as medicine to relieve pain, to avoid disability, and to restore ability. Such individual or societal perspectives are alien to evolution, which as such has no perspective. Evolution is, after all, a general term for a process in which traits appear through random mutations and are selected by the blind forces of nature.

As a result, one must note yet another difficulty in appealing to the conditions of nature or the results of evolution. Such an appeal makes one's judgments regarding what ought or ought not to count as disease hostage to the past.[35] What one now finds as species-typical levels of species-typical function are the result of past selective pressures, which may have delivered biological capacities ill adapted to current circumstances. One might think, for instance, of menopause, which is most likely the result of past evolutionary forces in circumstances where few women lived to reach menopause. Consequently, the development of the phenomenon may well have conferred neither an advantage nor a disadvantage. In any event, the species-typical character of calcium metabolism for postmenopausal women is one of negative calcium balance. More calcium is absorbed than deposited, leading to the development of osteoporosis and painful debilities such as collapsing vertebrae and greater exposure to risks of fractures. Such phenomena are as species-typical as menopause itself. Yet one would not want to say that osteoporosis in postmenopausal women is not a disease. Rather, one must recognize that the blind outcomes of nature are sometimes beneficial, sometimes neutral, and sometimes undermining of our purposes and welfare. As a consequence, a physician will be unable to determine a classification of disease by simply attempting to discover what will count as species-atypical levels of species-typical functions.

In short, a project such as Boorse's must fail. A species-atypical level of a species-atypical function correlated with a decreased reproductive rate will not be a sufficient condition for acknowledging a circumstance as a disease. Even if, for example, one determined that individuals with IQs over 140 tended not to reproduce as effectively as individuals within two standard deviations from the norm, one would likely not wish to characterize high intelligence as a disease. On the other hand, as the example involving menopause suggests, having a species-atypical level of a species-atypical function is not a necessary condition for being a disease, if one can in fact identify such circumstances as osteoporosis in postmenopausal women as diseases.

The point is that Christopher Boorse has not given an adequate reconstruction or account of the ways in which patients and physicians understand diseases. One can appreciate this point if one attends to the ambiguity in terms such as normal and abnormal. As I have indicated, one can mean by natural or normal the design of the Creator. Or by normal one can mean statistically frequent. In addition, by normal or natural one may have in mind something such as Christopher Boorse's idea of species typicality. None of these concepts is central to the ways in which conditions stand out as diseases for medicine. Medicine as a secular science cannot appeal to the first notion. Second, as even Boorse will agree, statistical findings are at best suggestive, but surely not defining, of what should count as diseases for medicine. The third notion, which approximates Boorse's, is of primary interest only to biologists engaged in unapplied scientific research.[36] As a zoologist, one may have an interest in determining what levels of function characterize a particular species. One may in addition be interested in discovering the evolutionary processes that led to those circumstances. But such are not the interests of physicians or patients who have nonepistemic goals such as the relief of pain, the preservation of function, the achievement of desirable human form and grace, and the postponement of death. If Christopher Boorse has succeeded at all, he has reconstructed not clinical medicine's concept of disease, but perhaps a notion of disease that would be employed by an unapplied scientist. It is because medicine is applied to the achievement of particular individual and societal goals that Boorse's attempt fails. One must wonder, since he does not consider the notion of inclusive fitness, whether Boorse's account would be in fact adequate for a zoologist. In any event, Boorse has unwittingly done us the very important service of underscoring the special character of medicine's concerns by contrasting them with the concerns of unapplied biological science.[37]

DISEASES AND VALUE JUDGMENTS.   Problems stand out as problems for medicine because they are disvalued.[38] They are seen as pathological. They are associated with pathos or suffering, and suffering is judged, all else being equal, to have a disvalue. The very appreciation of a problem as a problem for medicine is tied to its appearing as a failure to achieve a desired state. It may be a failure to achieve a desired or expected level of freedom from pain or anxiety. It may involve a failure to achieve an expected level of function. It may involve a failure to achieve an expected realization of human form or grace. Or it may involve a failure to achieve what is an expected term of life. These genre of judgments that depend on a family of values characterize a circumstance as one of suffering, one of pathology, or of a problem to be solved. As we shall see, there is the additional presumption that the problem is of the sort that is beyond immediate willing away and is embedded in a web of causal forces of an anatomical, physiological, or psychological sort open to medical explanation and manipulation. This qualification is needed in order to distinguish these disvalued circumstances that are viewed as causally determined and that are given to medicine vis-à-vis those viewed as due to human choice and given to the charge of law. These negative judgments may be made either by the individuals afflicted or by others regarding those individuals. An adverse judgment is rendered a person characterized as diseased or deformed; this is the case whether one is concerned with tuberculosis or such circumstances as a disfigured nose for which the bearer seeks cosmetic surgery, or an unwanted pregnancy for which a woman seeks an abortion.

One encounters a wide range of problems that lie along a continuum. On one end of the continuum there are circumstances likely to be disvalued in whatever culture an individual lives, and in terms of whatever goals are possessed by individuals or societies. One need not presume transcultural values regarding the proper range of human function or form. One need only recognize that certain circumstances are likely to be impediments to the realization of goals in nearly any foreseeable environment, and in terms of any likely cluster of human purposes. Thus, on the one hand, crushing substernal pain radiating down the left arm accompanied by weakness, collapse, and a feeling of impending death is likely to make myocardial infarction a disvalued circumstance across cultures, even if there are appreciable differences in cultural values regarding human function. On the other hand, color blindness, the inability to roll up the sides of one's tongue, or the incapacity to taste phenylthiocarbamide may or may not count as genetic diseases or defects, depending on the environment in which persons live and the goals they and their cultures support.[39]

One can recognize a complex interplay among environment, cultural expectations, individual goals, and the ways in which problems stand out as diseases, while still expecting a considerable amount of cross-cultural argument regarding what should count as diseases. One will be able to acknowledge that cultures not only influence goals but also shape the environment in which the goals are achieved, while still accounting for the intersubjectivity of disease claims in terms of the many conditions that undermine goals across environments and cultures, whatever the goals might be. Since the treatment of diseases is a societal undertaking, those conditions more generally acknowledged as problems worthy of treatment will be more easily accepted as diseases. Thus, tuberculosis, schizophrenia, myocardial infarction, and osteogenic sarcoma can be straightforwardly acknowledged as diseases and need not be termed ego-dystonic tuberculosis, ego-dystonic schizophrenia, or ego-dystonic myocardial infarction. As we shall see, individuals have the right to decline treatment if they are competent and do so without direct and significant harm to others. In this sense, even the most "objective" disease categories are open to rejection.

There are, however, difficulties when conditions do not generally impede values across cultures and groups. Consider how the categorization of homosexuality as a disease or of bisexuality as a psychosocial norm would meet with greater controversy than do concepts of tuberculosis or myocardial infarction as diseases. It is not simply enough to note that one may refuse treatment if one engages in homosexual activities because there is a powerful negative judgment involved in being termed diseased, which would be protested by many homosexuals. Judgments of sexual perversity have an especially negative valence. Refusing treatment would not be enough. They would also wish to refuse the very categorization of disease for their sexual activities. Instead, one must recognize that there is a wide range of competing human understandings regarding the proper goals to be achieved through sexual function. This range makes inappropriate the use of the term *disease* with its connotations of an objective reality or a general intersubjective agreement. The term disease may function adequately for styling tuberculosis and schizophrenia, while being inappropriate for circumstances such as sexual orientation or pregnancy, which only certain persons, in certain circumstances, may see as clinical problems to be treated.

Given these reflections, one might even wish to eliminate or strongly qualify the term *disease* in situations where misunderstandings could arise. One might think of substituting the term *clinical problems* to identify those difficulties that stand out as conditions that ought to be addressed and solved by medicine.[40] Such a term would more accurately indicate the ways in which clusters of value judgments make conditions stand out as problems to be treated. It would also contribute to enlightening the long history of disputes regarding the nature of diseases. One might think here of the disputes between ontologists and physiologists of disease, between those who held diseases to be in some sense things or entities and those who held them to be artificial characterizations of physiological and anatomical phenomena.[41] If what makes a cluster of findings stand out as a disease is that it bothers individuals in a way that medicine can explain or cure, it is more accurate to consider diseases not as enduring entities, but clusters of findings collected together because of their usefulness in giving prognoses and guiding treatment. Clinical, etiological, and pathoanatomical "disease entities" serve as treatment warrants.[42] One draws a line between innocent physiological or psychological findings and pathological findings because of particular human values in a particular circumstance, not because of the discovery of an essential distinction that exists outside of particular human expectations. The more nominalist or instrumentalist views of disease are better justified in that they eschew the ontological quest to discover the essence of disease.

The term *clinical problem* underscores the fact that an attempt to give a neutralist, purely descriptive, account of disease fails. Diseases stand out for us as problems to be solved, all else being equal. Of course, attendant circumstances may make things far from equal. Having the right disease at the right time may provide one with an exemption from military service or a comfortable disability income. However, a disease is a disease because it is disvalued—in a particular way. It is a clinical problem. One may still draw a distinction, somewhat as Boorse drew, between illness and disease in order to discriminate between those physiologically, anatomically, or psychologically rooted circumstances that are in fact currently causing suffering versus those circumstances that will surely or likely lead to suffering for that individual, or those circumstances that usually lead to suffering for humans or for animals of X sort (here one will need to recall the special problem of speaking of the diseases of nonhuman animals). Such does not indicate a contextless disease reality. It acknowledges rather that an individual has a disease, a clinical problem, but is not yet, or is not now, ill. The judgment of illness will then bring with it the special negative evaluations that are associated with current suffering.

The central point is that we encounter diseases, illnesses, disabilities, sufferings through a web of important nonmoral values. The values are not those involved in holding that an individual is evil for violating the rights of others or for failing to be charitable or benevolent. The nonmoral values that structure medicine are also distinguishable from the nonmoral values employed in such judgments as "That is a beautiful sunset," "That is an ugly painting," "That is an attractive person," though they have a similarity in having aesthetic characteristics. They are values invoked in judging human function, form, and grace. They reflect ideals of freedom from pain, of human ability, and of bodily form and movement. They are aesthetic in that deformity and dysfunction are ugly. They have their special sense in depending on ideals of anatomical, physiological, and psychological achievement and realization.

To say that John is diseased, deformed, or disabled is to pass a negative value judgment. The force of such judgments will range from those that are rather mild, such as "Mary has a disfigurement," to those that are rather strong, such as "Mary is perverted." Often the values lie hidden within the disease term itself, as occurs in "George is a schizophrenic." Schizophrenia is not valued; to be judged schizophrenic is to bear a disvalue. Whether it is athlete's foot, tuberculosis, a deformed nose, or unwanted pregnancy, diseases or clinical problems are not good things to have. They are things that are good to prevent, treat, or cure. Only by appreciating this web of nonmoral value judgments that direct our bioethical judgments will one be able fully to understand the actual social transactions that occur in health care. One is not simply concerned in health care to maintain one's moral integrity or to achieve moral virtue. Health care is directed to the realization of a wide range of nonmoral values regarding bodily and mental function, form, and freedom from distress. Health care is also provided, constrained, and directed by moral values that play a role in addition to these nonmoral values.

Disease language as descriptive

Diseases do not appear simply through a web of values. They are also appreciated, understood, and seen through a set of descriptive assumptions. Language is an intersubjective undertaking and therefore requires a standardization of terms and, as a result, leads to a standardization of concepts as well. The more that precision is required, the more the standardization becomes formal. One might think here of the *Systematized Nomenclature of Pathology*, which provides three alternative ways of describing findings, so that, for instance, Wilson's disease can be described as "copper disorder," "ceruloplasmin disorder," or "hepatolenticular degeneration."[43] One can provide descriptive terms that are etiological, anatomical, or clinical, depending on one's context. The choice is not an innocent one, for it already skews the ways in which one comes to appreciate the matter at hand. One might think here of the criticism by Alvan Feinstein of *The Standard Nomenclature of Diseases and Operations and of the International Classification of Diseases*.[44] As he argues, such classifications may press a clinician to be more specific than the data justify. For this reason Feinstein defends the clinical category of stroke against the more precise terms *cerebral arteriosclerosis* or *encephalopathy*.[45]

Describing reality is always infected by expectations. Those expectations usually include both evaluative and explanatory expectations. One sees in terms of the interpretations one has in mind. It is for this reason that medicine provides excellent examples of missteps in the psychology of discovery. The fact that one sees reality already in terms of one's expectations has been well explored in science generally.[46] But in medicine it has recurring practical importance, as Henrik Wulff has argued with regard to the impact of diagnostic interpretations. The very description of medical findings casts them in terms of explanations, often importing unnoticed infections by values and theories. Such diagnostic data transformations occur when one sees a shadow in a lung as pneumonia. But they also occur when one terms someone's heavy breathing "dyspnea" or "shortness of breath." Even to put matters in medical terms is already to appreciate the findings not as innocent rapid breathing, but as a likely difficulty in need of further diagnostic intervention and possible treatment.[47]

Consider the case of Koplik's spots, which are pathognomonic of measles. Whenever one sees Koplik's spots, one can make the diagnosis of measles with a 100 percent probability of being correct. This is the case because Koplik's spots are by definition an element of the beginning of measles. A diagnostic data transformation takes place, however, when one sees small irregular bright red spots on the buccal and lingual mucosa *as* Koplik's spots. One may see some irregular bright red spots with bluish-white specks in the center and yet not be sure that they are Koplik's spots. What one will see will turn in part on one's expectations under the circumstances.

One may attempt to describe medical findings as innocently as possible of values and theories, as has been suggested by Lawrence Weed.[48] But even to see problems as medical problems is to put them in a context rich with expectations and presumptions. Descriptions require standardizations of terms. Such standardizations will be fashioned through quasi-political or societal discussions and against background assumptions about what will be useful in achieving particular goals and purposes. Those assumptions are themselves structured by explanatory views.

Disease language as explanatory

The language of medicine is structured around its explanatory assumptions. Problems are seen as medical problems because they are presumed to be embedded in a pathophysiological, pathoanatomical, or pathopsychological nexus because the problems are not experienced as removable at the immediate will of the sufferer. As such, they are not legal problems or religious problems, but problems to be resolved through the manipulation of the elements of a special causal web. How one understands this web has major implications. What one accepts as underlying causal forces will influence one's views of how to frame descriptions and regarding what one should judge to be good or bad prognostic signs. Explanatory models bring coherence, as we have already seen, to the multiplicity of events we encounter in medicine. They give a sense to the stories we tell about illness and disease. As we noted in exploring the clinical accounts offered by Hippocrates, such stories differ in terms of what the storyteller takes to be relevant to a coherent account. Explanatory models structure the very sense of what we see and experience.

One must note before even proceeding that the very nature of explanation is a puzzle for philosophers. Here it will be enough to distinguish between the issues raised by the structure of explanation, and the issues raised by its goals. Explanation provides, to use a Hegelian idiom, a structure for reflection. It relates different sorts of elements: appearances and laws, observations and regularities. They are related so as to weave being together in terms of correlatives. Thus, one comes to understand the fevers, pains, rashes, sweatings, diarrhea, and so forth of a patient in terms of underlying laws, intelligible patterns, anatomical understandings, or physiological mechanisms. The laws and regularities acquire their sense through that to which they give regularity and coherence. The hidden pathological forces and disease mechanisms have content in their expressions. The various expressions of disease gain meaning and coherence through the mechanisms they are seen to presuppose and express.

The cardinal example in medicine of this intertwining of findings and understandings is the relation between the data of clinicians and the data of pathoanatomists and pathophysiologists, which is provided by the laws of pathoanatomy and pathophysiology. Two worlds of observations are related. The findings of the clinician are related to the observations of the pathoanatomists and pathophysiologists and take on a new significance through these anatomical and pathological observations. The observations of the pathoanatomist and pathophysiologist take on clinical significance through being related to the world of the clinician. This exchange of meanings is effected through a web of mechanisms, laws, and regularities. Explanation affords a coherence among groups of observations and findings.[49] The development of clinical-pathological and pathological-clinical correlations offers an expansion, as we will see, of the explanatory powers of medicine through allowing two different domains of observation to be correlated and reinterpreted through wide-ranging organizational schemes (e.g., through laws in pathology and anatomy). New explanations of diseases can then be tested in different ways by observations within the domains of both clinicians and basic scientists.

This correlation of observations, one with the other, through mechanisms, laws, and regularities, is undertaken in medicine not just to give insight. It is undertaken primarily in order to manipulate reality, that is, to treat diseases, pains, deformities, disabilities, and so forth, as well as to predict the course of diseases, that is, to provide prognoses. Science is in general concerned to provide explanations and predictions and to allow for the manipulation of nature. However, in health care the concerns with predictions and manipulations have a salient nonepistemic character. One is not predicting primarily in order to know or manipulating primarily in order better to understand. Rather one is framing explanations in order to come to terms with the human

pains, anxieties, disabilities, and deformities associated with clinical problems. These goals of explanation, as we will see, direct applied sciences such
as medicine to mold the character of explanation in order to facilitate the
achievement of these nonepistemic goals. One will highlight those explanations most useful in curing disease, ameliorating pain, and giving the kinds of
prognostic information with which patients are usually concerned.[50]

Medical findings are seen within prevailing etiological, pathological, and
psychopathological theories. The contribution made by theories to the ways
in which we experience medical reality can be appreciated if one compares
how the description of medical problems changes with changes in accepted
explanatory accounts. For instance, the various problems associated with
tuberculosis, which were once separated within different taxa of traditional
nosologies, can now be gathered together under one rubric, given our current
etiological model. We see consumption, King's evil, and Pott's disease as all
manifestations of *one* disease. On the other hand, we can now clearly
distinguish between typhoid and typhus, which were once seen as one
disease. There is a dialectical interplay between the descriptions of diseases
and the explanatory models used in accounting for them. As a consequence,
if one were to enter the world of an eighteenth-century clinician, one would
not find the same understanding we possess today of the significance of
tuberculosis, typhus, gonorrhea, or syphilis. The findings we associate with
these diseases today were in the past gathered under different rubrics.

Consider the description given by Thomas Sydenham of venereal diseases.
In his description, he mixes in a way we no longer would the signs and
symptoms of both syphilis and gonorrhea. They were for him one disease.

This disease proceeds in the following manner. The patient, sooner or later,
(according as the woman with whom he has lain was more or less infected, and
according as his constitution renders him more or less disposed to receive the
infection) is first seized with an uncommon pain in the parts of generation, and a kind
of rotation of the testicles; and afterwards, unless the patient be circumcised, a spot,
resembling the measles in size and colour, seizes some part of *glans*, soon after which,
a fluid like *semen* flows gently from it; which differing every day therefrom, both in
colour and consistency, does at length turn yellow, but not so deep as the yolk of an
egg . . .[51]

We are likely to experience similar changes in classification when we develop
better etiological accounts for that cluster of diseases we term cancer. We are
likely to discover that what we took to be a particular form of cancer may in
fact be caused by more than one cluster of etiological factors, leading us in
the future to rearrange our descriptions in accord with our explanatory
assumptions. Explanatory assumptions frame how medicine is experienced
by both patients and practitioners.

Consider one of the better-known classifications of disease, or nosologies, of the eighteenth century, that of François Boissier de Sauvages. Sauvages's final classification was presented in a work entitled *Nosologia methodica sistens morborum classes juxta Sydenhami mentem et botanicorum ordinem.*[52] As the title indicates, it is a systematic classification of diseases that follows the suggestions of Thomas Sydenham and that is placed in a botanical order. Thomas Sydenham was himself highly influenced both by the works of Sir Francis Bacon (1561–1626) and by the successes of botany in the seventeenth century. The influence of Bacon and Sydenham remained strong in medicine throughout the eighteenth century, having not only an impact on Sauvages, but on William Cullen (1710–90), among others. In addition, botany continued to offer a paradigmatic example of a successful classification of reality. One sees the influence of botany on medicine in a number of ways, including the fact that Linnaeus, the well-known naturalist and botanist, also provided a classification of diseases.[53] In addition, Sauvages and Linnaeus maintained a correspondence regarding classifications.[54]

The result was a view of diseases and of the reality of illnesses that is strikingly different from ours. Consider the ten major classes under which Sauvages united forty-two orders, some three hundred fifteen genera, and two thousand four hundred species of diseases (depending on which edition one consults).[55]

I.	Vitia	Defects, blemishes and symptoms treatable by the mechanisms of surgery (this class includes everything from vitiligo and exophthalmos to fractures and herpes)
II.	Febres	Fevers
III.	Phlegmasiae	Inflammations
IV.	Spasmi	Spasms
V.	Anhelationes	Difficulties in breathing
VI.	Debilitates	Weaknesses
VII.	Dolores	Pains
VIII.	Vesaniae	Insanities
IX.	Fluxus	Fluxes
X.	Cachexiae	Constitutional disorders and deformities in volume, symmetry, weight, and color (the class includes such "deprivations" as depigmentation and "deformities" as pregnancy)

For Sauvages and for others of his time, fevers and pains were diseases in their own right, as the classification shows. Moreover, phenomena were brought together in a way that may appear strange to many of our contemporaries. For instance, under fluxes were included both bloody discharges and diarrhea. The classification was clinical, rather than etiological or anatomical, though Sauvages also provided such classifications.

Sauvages developed his classification for reasons very similar to those that influenced the American Psychiatric Association in the development of its *Diagnostic and Statistical Manual of Mental Disorders* (*DSM-III*): the provision of a theory-neutral description of diseases.[56] Medicine in general was at the time of Sauvages as ignorant of the causes of diseases, and as overwhelmed by conflicting theories, as psychiatry is today. Sauvages, and those who fashioned similar classifications, pursued as unbiased a description of reality as was possible. In this they followed Sydenham, who with Bacon presumed that (1) the world had a general rational structure that (2) could be disclosed by careful examination, were one only (3) to free oneself from distorting prejudices. Sydenham shared with Bacon a view regarding the intrinsic rationality of reality and the capacity of the human mind to know that structure. Consider, for example, Sydenham's injunction in the preface to the third edition of his 1676 *Observationes medicae*:

In writing, therefore, a history of diseases, every philosophical hypothesis which hath prepossess'd the writer in its favour, ought to be totally laid aside, and then the manifest and natural phenomena of diseases, however minute, must be noted with the utmost accuracy; imitating in this the great exactness of painters, who, in their pictures, copy the smallest spots or moles in the originals. For 'tis difficult to give a detail of the numerous errors that spring from hypotheses, whilst writers, misled by false appearances, assign such phenomena for diseases, as never existed, but in their own brains . . .[57]

Sauvages and the other writers of the eighteenth century who were influenced by Sydenham inherited these presuppositions along with Sydenham's influential commitment to the task of understanding the natural histories of diseases. From Sydenham they inherited as well the assumption that descriptions of the reality of disease would disclose species of disease.

What must be underscored is the special, almost paradoxical, distrust in theory and faith in empirically inquiring reason that guided Sydenham, Sauvages, Linnaeus, Cullen, and others. They had no sense that their very attempt to see the world free of theory was itself rich in theoretical assumptions concerning the nature of knowledge and of reality. To have a sense of this, consider one of the explanatory footnotes provided with Sydenham's *Observations*.

Hypotheses owe their origin to ostentatious vanity and idle curiosity; whence 'tis easy to conceive how much they must needs obstruct the improvement of physick, which is a science that depends chiefly upon well-conducted experiments and close and faithful observation; whereas hypotheses are always built in great part upon feign'd, precarious, and often very obscure principles.[58]

The endeavors of Sydenham, Sauvages, and Cullen, and the nosologies they produced, which appear to us as highly elaborated products of a theory imposed upon reality, were to their authors attempts to free the mind from the burdensome theorizing that characterized much of medicine in the seventeenth and eighteenth centuries.

Endeavors similar to those of Sydenham and Sauvages remain in areas of medicine where theory has had little success in effectively explaining phenomena. As indicated, a good example is the nosology developed by the American Psychiatric Association and reframed under the direction of Robert Spitzer and the Task Force on Nomenclature and Statistics. Robert Spitzer in his introduction observed:

For most of the DSM-III disorders, however, the etiology is unknown. A variety of theories have been advanced, buttressed by evidence—not always convincing—to explain how these disorders come about. The approach taken in DSM-III is atheoretical with regard to etiology or pathophysiological process except for those disorders for which this is well established and therefore included in the definition of the disorder.[59]

We can see, though the classification is atheoretical with respect to certain theories, that it is surely not innocent of theoretical assumptions, any more than were the classifications of Sauvages and Linnaeus. There is rather an attempt to frame a classification with very little dependence on etiological and pathogenic assumptions.

Through the success of anatomy and physiology in providing etiologic and pathogenetic accounts of medical phenomena, the ways in which diseases were experienced by patients and physicians were refashioned as medicine entered the nineteenth century. Though there were anticipations of the role of pathoanatomical correlations with clinical findings in the *Sepulchretum* (1689) of Theophile Bonet (1620–1689)[60] and in the *De sedibus et causis morborum per anatomen indagatis* (1761) of Morgagni, (1682–1771)[61] it was with the beginning of the nineteenth century that the clinical world was radically restructured in terms of work done in the laboratory and the anatomical dissection room. The world of illness that was open to experience by the patient and the clinician alike became correlated with, and reinterpreted in terms of, the findings of the pathoanatomist and the physiologist. Foucault makes this shift central to his work, *The Birth of the Clinic*.[62] As he documents, the gaze turned inward as a result of the work of Xavier Bichat (1771–1802) and François-Joseph-Victor Broussais (1772–1838), among others. The true disease is no longer that which is experienced by the clinician or the patient; the real disease becomes the lesion. As Broussais put it, "... true medical observation is that of the organs and their modifiers, it is in fact an observation of the body itself..."[63] In the nineteenth century, diseases become, as Rudolf Virchow (1821–1902) put it, "altered vital state[s] of larger or smaller numbers of cells or cell-territories."[64]

One must appreciate what a major shift this involved. The whole language of disease changed. Fevers were no longer diseases in their own right, but became merely symptoms. Jaundice was now a symptom of the disease hepatitis. This required a major recasting of medical reality and a retreat from taken-for-granted clinical nosologies, such as those of Sauvages. Consider, for example, how this shift was experienced by Bichat.

It is well known into how many errors we have fallen, so long as we had confined ourselves to the simple observation of symptoms. Let us take for example consumption. It has been considered as an *essential malady*, before we had recourse to post-mortem examination; since, it has been shown that marasmus was only a consecutive symptomatic malady of the affection of an organ. Jaundice has been for a long time considered by practitioners as an *essential malady*; post-mortem examination has also proved that this affection, though primitive, was in reality only consecutive to diverse alterations of the liver, of which it is always the symptom. The same has happened with respect to dropsies, which although for a long time considered as essential affections, have never been other than the result of some organic disease. It is, then, ignorance of organic affections, resulting from a total neglect of post-mortem examination, which is the cause that has misled the ancient practitioners on most diseases; thus, *Cullen* and *Sauvages* have erred in their classifications.[65]

What had been considered to be diseases became symptoms; the reality of diseases is now to be found in changes in organs. A few remnants of the language of eighteenth-century classifications remained. For instance, the term *essential hypertension* recalls when clusters of symptoms, with an unknown causal basis, were held to be a disease in their own right.

The shift offered the possibility of explaining under one rubric phenomena that had once been scattered across the nosological frameworks of the eighteenth century. In short, it made it possible to unify observations through a new explanatory model. The shift offered insights into the mechanisms of disease that had not previously been available. But most important, it offered a research program through which the bewildering findings of medicine could now be examined, criticized, and organized in terms of emerging understandings of anatomy and physiology. It redirected the energies of medicine in a way that led to major advances in medical understanding during the first part of the nineteenth century and to major advances in therapeutics in the last part of the nineteenth and during the twentieth century.

What one finds in the 1800s is the correlation of two domains of medical description. The first is the traditional domain of clinical findings, which had been the focus of Sydenham, Sauvages, and Cullen. The second is a relatively new domain of descriptions provided by anatomists, physiologists, pathologists, and microbiologists. The two domains were brought together by new accounts of disease that allowed the descriptions to interact. Clinical findings, as well as laboratory findings, could falsify theoretical assumptions. The result was a set of complex opportunities for studying the nature of medical reality. Clinical findings invited the fashioning of theoretical models through which laboratory findings were sought in order to account for those clinical findings, which were then redescribed, now in terms of the emerging basic scientific models. On the other hand, laboratory findings invited the clinician to look for phenomena that could be predicted in terms of the basic scientific models.

A dialectic interaction was established. Clinical findings were redescribed in terms of theoretical models. The redescribed reality could itself then lead to puzzles that would engender further changes in the theoretical models and so on, ad indefinitum. The laboratory findings had their real sense as being part of the mechanisms used in explaining the clinical findings. Anatomical findings became lesions because they were the underpinnings for clinical problems. On the other hand, the clinical findings had their sense colored by the theoretical models and the laboratory findings employed in explaining them. There was a dynamic interaction between the explanans and the explanandum, between that which explained and that which was to be explained, each conferring on the other part of its own significance.

Past ways of understanding medicine had come to appear implausible. Consider Broussais's reflections on past medical investigations.

One has filled the nosographical framework with groups of most arbitrarily formed symptoms ... which do not represent the affections of different organs, that is, the real diseases. These groups of symptoms are derived from entities or abstract beings, which are most completely artificial ουτοι; these entities are false, and the resulting treatise is ontological.[66]

However, both Broussais and in fact Foucault failed to appreciate the full significance of this shift. They understood that the world of symptoms had been recast in terms of the presuppositions of a new and powerful research problem. They failed to appreciate that this restructuring carried with it an ideology that discounted the significance of patient complaints. Patient problems came to be understood as bona fide problems only if they had a pathoanatomical or pathophysiological truth value. Absent a lesion or a physiological disturbance to account readily for the complaint, the complaint was likely to be regarded as male fide. This requirement was credible because the laboratory sciences had become the basic medical sciences in an important ontological sense. They were seen as disclosing the reality underlying clinical findings. On the other hand, clinical observations, which for Syden-ham and Sauvages had been integral to the basic medical science, clinical medicine, now became secondary. Clinical medicine became a manifestation of a deeper reality. This was in a very restricted sense correct with regard to the development of explanatory models. Accounts of disease were now formulated in terms of underlying pathophysiological and pathoanatomical mechanisms. The error lay in failing also to accent the goals and purposes of medicine. As an applied science, medicine remains focused on caring for human suffering. Clinical medicine begins from and returns to the problems of patients. However, the changes in explanatory assumptions, and the development of the basic sciences, led to certain unfortunate changes in the ideology of symptoms.

To appreciate this, one must note that the clinical nosologies accented the problems the patients experienced. Pains constituted, as has been noted, one of the ten classes of disease in the nosology of Sauvages. They were the fourth (dolorosi) of Linnaeus's eleven classes.[67] Consider, for instance, Sauvages's category, "dolores vagi, qui nomen a side fixa non habent" (wandering pains that do not have a name from a fixed site), the first of his five orders of pains.[68] Sauvages's classification allowed him to take patient anxieties and distress as serious problems in their own right. His classification highlighted these symptoms through considering them diseases.

By legitimating such complaints, Sauvages legitimated the social role of those who complained of a wide range of pains and sufferings. As we will see, the explanatory and descriptive assumptions of medicine tie into major social views regarding the assignment of social status. By deciding whether a symptom is bona fide or male fide, medicine authenticates an individual's claim to particular forms of treatment. Medicine's concern with evaluative, descriptive, and explanatory endeavors is thus also intimately tied to the performative role of language, through which social reality is shaped.

Disease language as shaping social reality

In addition to describing and evaluating problems as medical and explaining them, physicians and other health care workers place these problems within social practices. Such individuals are gatekeepers of therapy roles, or to use Talcott Parsons's more restrictive term, sick roles.[69] To characterize a patient as sick is not only to say that he or she has a problem that ought to be solved and that the problem can be explained in medical terms. It is also to cast that individual in social roles where certain societal responses are expected. If the individual is placed in a full-fledged sick role, he or she is usually held to be not responsible for being in that role, is excused from social duties that the illness impairs, and is enjoined to seek treatment from a set of individuals socially recognized as appropriate therapists.[70] A therapeutic imperative is established. In determining that someone is sick one accepts a prima facie claim regarding ways in which the person ought to be treated, in that sickness is a state that, ceteris paribus, is not valued. Sickness is a state in which, all else being equal, people do not want to be. There is thus a defeasible presumption that sick people want to be treated. In addition, a diseased individual may lose particular social rights and prerogatives. Determinations such as insanity will relieve a patient of particular social prerogatives. On the other hand, if the individual is held to be partially or totally disabled, the individual may be able to receive welfare payments.

Medical language thus has a performative character. Just as a sheriff changes legal reality, not simply describes it, when saying to a lawbreaker, "You are under arrest," a physician changes reality when saying to a patient, "You have cancer"; "You have syphilis"; "You are fifty percent disabled"; or "You have a terminal disease." The patient is placed in a social context with a set of taken-for-granted social expectations. These routinized expectations stabilize the social world through a web of stereotyped roles.[71] It is because medicine focuses primarily on "caused" rather than chosen phenomena that such roles tend to remove blame for *being* in a state of illness (though blame still may be assigned for becoming ill or remaining ill, insofar as this can be influenced by personal choice). It is because states of affairs become clinical problems against the background of health care institutions that offer hope of cure or care that certain individuals (e.g., physicians, dentists, etc.) stand out as persons appropriate to address such problems.

The set of expectations that typically defines being sick differs, given different diagnoses. Consider the different ways in which there will be typical, formally or informally established, social responses to a diagnosis of heart disease, cancer, venereal disease, or acne. There will be different responses on the part of insurance companies, employers, welfare agencies, friends, and lovers. Diagnosis is a complex means of social labeling, as is the process of arresting a criminal. Such labeling shapes social reality toward the achievement of therapeutic goals.

The social construction of medical reality and the challenge of clinical judgment

The values presumed in seeing particular circumstances as diseases or clinical problems are conditioned by societies, their views of the good life, and the social roles they support. So, too, common endeavors to describe reality presuppo.p: informal, if not formal, agreements with regard to canonical, descriptive terms. Finally, as the history of medicine has shown, medicine's explanatory goals are pursued by particular groups of scientists with particular understandings of what should count as the proper rules of evidence and inference, which may conflict with lay understandings of disease and treatment or with the understandings of other investigators. To resolve such controversies, those involved will need to make clear what rules of evidence ought to be accepted and why. This question may be confronted by a single scientist when raising the question whether his or her explanation should be accepted as *the* explanation, even in the absence of a particular controversy. Explanation is thus always potentially communal, in that one advances knowledge claims with the presupposition that they ought to be accepted by other investigators. Knowledge claims presume their intersubjectivity—that they should be able to be justified generally, even if they are articulated by particular men and women within particular communities and cultures.[72]

There is thus a tension between the universal aspirations of knowers and the particular context in which real individuals actually know and frame explanations. From past experience and on the basis of what one ought to anticipate, given the limitations of human reason, one should expect that not all such controversies will allow of resolution by an appeal to sound arguments alone. One will not always be able decisively to determine what is the correct set of rules of evidence and inference, or the proper set of conclusions. As a result, one will need to appeal even in science to rules of fairness in debate and in the resolution of scientific controversies. One will need to establish fair procedures, which may often involve committees and votes. A set of nonepistemic considerations will need to be employed in order to bind knowers peaceably in their task of knowing truly.

Science as a social endeavor must mediate the particular passions, jealousies, and controversies of scientists in order to pursue goals that transcend time, culture, and idiosyncratic controversy. Much of the mediation is informal. Scientists come to see certain classes of problems as more interesting than others. Common terminologies are fashioned, and incentives such as the approbation of members of the Royal Society direct the inquiries of investigators even in the most abstract of undertakings. The very presence of the Nobel Prize, for instance, motivates scientists across national boundaries and contributes to the cohesiveness of scientific endeavors. The same can be said of funding agencies, which are more likely to support "orthodox" investigations and to shy away from undertakings that appear eccentric.

Such informal constraints are supplemented by formal modes of standardization the more a science is applied. In medicine, this is expressed in the phrase "the usual and customary standards of medical practice." Though these may not have a fully formal articulation, they come to be the object of public discussion and court testimony. In addition, in order for physicians to evaluate the efficacy of different therapies, collective endeavors such as the American Joint Committee on Cancer are organized to fashion rules for the use of descriptive terms in diagnostic categories. In such circumstances the social reality of the applied sciences is settled by votes within committees.

The decisions in such circumstances are made not simply in terms of the character of reality as it is taken really to be, but also in terms of which modes of classification will be most useful in organizing treatment and care.

Here one might think in particular of the ways in which cancers are staged.[73] The classification and stagings of cancer are fashioned to

allow the physician to determine treatment for the patient more appropriately, to evaluate results of management more reliably, and to compare statistics reported from various institutions on a local, regional, and national basis more confidently.[74]

As already indicated, such classifications and stagings of cancer are the result of particular social organizations balancing the interests, albeit scientific and therapeutic, of various groups. One has, for instance, the results of a group organized January 9, 1959, as the American Joint Committee for Cancer Staging and End-Results Reporting:

Each of the sponsoring organizations designates three members to the Committee. The American College of Surgeons serves as administrative sponsor. Subcommittees, called "task forces," have been appointed to consider malignant neoplasms of selected anatomic sites in order to develop classifications. Each task force is composed of committee members and other professional appointees whose special interests and skills are appropriate to the site under consideration.[75]

As a point of history, there has been a problem in coordinating these classifications of the American Joint Committee on Cancer with the recommendations of the TNM Committee, originally known as the Committee on Clinical Stage Classification and Applied Statistics of the Union Internationale Contre le Cancer. This has involved compromises. "In a few instances, arbitrary changes have been made to make the recommendations of the AJCC consistent with those of the TNM Committee of the International Union Against Cancer. Consistency at all anatomic sites has not as yet been achieved."[76] The picture is that of the social construction of reality through various formal processes that fashion agreements for common endeavors.

It should be obvious that the ways in which one decides to describe phenomena such as cancer are not of interest to physicians alone. The interests of patients are also involved. The classification of cancer is not like the classification of stars. The choice among different ways of classifying cancers sets the conditions for the ways in which physicians will choose therapeutic interventions. The number of stages selected (why, for instance, use three, four, or five stages for any particular carcinoma) presupposes cost–benefit calculations and understandings of prudent actions that have direct implications for the ways in which patients are treated. They involve more than purely scientific judgments; they concern as well the proper balancing of benefits and harms in the organization of therapeutic choices around a particular number of stages of cancer. The choice to subdivide stages (e.g., stages IA and B) will reflect the decision that a more complex assessment of therapeutic options is appropriate. There are limitations to the number of subdivisions one can make and still have them remain useful. Human physicians can only remember and easily organize data in terms of a limited number of classifications. Since the treatment of patients and the assessment of the treatment of patients are a collective endeavor, there must be a choice among the competing possibilities for division, subdivision, and classification. It must be emphasized that there are no unique natural lines in reality to which the classifications correspond. Rather, the categories are as much created as discovered through endowing certain findings with significance.

After one has decided on classifications and systems for staging diseases and clinical problems, one will need to come to terms with the fact that the decisions one will make will at times be wrong. This involves a complex set of moral and prudential concerns that have been gathered under the rubric of clinical judgment and medical decision making.[77] In deciding whether an individual has a disease or a clinical problem of a certain sort, one will need to assess the consequences that will follow from being wrong and then take account of that likelihood in establishing the threshold of certainty required to make the diagnosis. One will need, in short, to ask what the costs are of holding a particular diagnosis to be true. For example, if one operates to remove a breast on ambiguous data that indicate the presence of a cancer, one may have imposed major costs upon the woman so treated. On the other hand, if one delays the treatment of certain diseases in order to acquire better data, the condition of the patient may worsen. Even the acquisition of diagnostic data is associated with costs. These costs are not only financial but often include risks of morbidity and mortality. Here one might think of the risks of liver biopsy, heart catheterization, and other invasive diagnostic tests. Before one acquires information, one must first judge that the knowledge will likely make a sufficient difference in the treatment of the patient to merit the risks and costs to which the patient will be exposed. In medicine, acquiring knowledge and making knowledge claims have direct implications for the ways in which patients are treated.

Because of the difficulty of deciding what is a proper balance between the risks of over- and undertreating patients, it will often be very difficult to determine whether particular therapeutic interventions are warranted. One will not be able *simply* to discover whether physicians are performing unnecessary hysterectomies, or unnecessary tonsillectomies. One will not be able simply to discover, by appeal to factual issues alone, what treatments are indicated, what treatments are appropriate, what treatments are ordinary, or what treatments are extraordinary. Integral to such judgments will be appeals to particular hierarchies of values and to peaceable processes for resolving disputes in these matters. Such judgments will not be purely epistemic. Judgments in such matters depend on deciding how important it is to avoid the problems solved by surgery versus how important it is to avoid the problems that may be caused by surgery (including transfer of funds to surgeons). Because surgical interventions are often predicated on the availability of funds through third-party payers, the definition of necessary versus unnecessary interventions becomes an issue of importance to all who participate in a particular insurance plan (including government welfare policies). One needs to find mechanisms for fairly choosing particular criteria. Since a community of individuals is involved, problems of fairness and democratic procedure become salient.

Most of the crucial terms in bioethical debates share in a complexity of this sort. Determinations of death are made against the background of judgments regarding how sure one must be that one can avoid significant numbers of false positive and false negative determinations of death. What will count as a *significant* number is again not a purely factual question. As we will see, what one will mean by a viable fetus in the abortion debate will also not be a purely factual matter. In scientific debates with a heavy ethical and political overlay or in ethical debates with a heavy scientific focus, one will find concerns with values and facts intertwined. By this I do not mean to suggest that the fact–value distinction is not appropriate in abstract contexts. Rather, the factual and evaluational components, which are distinguishable, occur inseparably bound in actual debates.

Seeing a problem as a medical, rather than as a legal, religious, or educational problem

The world of medical findings is only one of a number of finite provinces of meaning controlled by major social institutions. The ability of physicians to create social roles ("You are diseased"; "You are perverted") must be contrasted with the socially established capacities of priests to declare individuals clean or unclean, or of judges to declare persons guilty or innocent. Health care professionals are gatekeepers within one of a number of major social institutions. As a result, it is not simply a question of how circumstances ought to be construed within medicine, but whether they should be construed within medicine at all, rather than within a collateral and competing institution, such as the law or religion. Each of the major social institutions identifies problems for its care in terms of sets of values that make the problems stand out as suboptimal, as failing to meet a standard, as a difficulty to be set aside. The institutions of education, religion, morality, law, and medicine in this fashion variously characterize circumstances as those of ignorance, ritual uncleanliness, sinfulness, blameworthiness, criminality, civil liability, or disease. To see a circumstance as one of sinfulness, criminality, or disease is to place it within the province of one of the major social institutions with its peculiar models of explanation and with its own special directing goals.

The facts available within the spheres of religion, law, morality, and medicine are seen as problems of a particular kind in terms of particular webs of values, descriptive conventions, explanatory models, and social roles. Religious accounts of reality are likely to involve supernatural causal models dependent on views regarding the final destiny of individuals and the universe. It is in this fashion that religions give ultimate meaning to life, suffering, and death. Legal accounts will incorporate particular systems of evidence and proof, which determine which findings can be assessed in what ways in order to achieve the goals of particular practices of blaming and praising. One might think here of Hart and Honoré's classic account of causation and the law.[78] As they point out, when flowers in a garden wither due to a gardener's failure to tend them, the gardener is held as having caused the flowers to die, though from a more neutral perspective, the failure of passersby to water the flowers and the absence of sufficient rainfall are equally causes. It is the social presumptions regarding the duties of gardeners that make these other circumstances assume the role of background conditions and underscore the gardener's failure to water the flowers as *the* cause of their dying. A set of social relevances is employed to establish a particular account of causation, so as to highlight certain causes because of their role in a social practice.

Medicine similarly accents some causes over others because of the usefulness of this practice. Consider how diseases are characterized as genetic, infectious, or environmental diseases, though the particular disease may be influenced by all three factors. Tuberculosis, for example, is "due" to genetic, infectious, and environmental influences. One usually speaks of it as an infectious disease because of the general usefulness of that designation. Seeing it as an "infectious" disease focuses our attention and directs treatment to the causal factor that is usually most useful to address. Medicine accents those causal factors most amenable to medical intervention.

One must note, even if only in passing, the complexity of the notion of cause. The term *cause* can be used to identify conditions that are sufficient to produce effects, necessary to produce effects, or that contribute to the likelihood of an effect's occurring. In medicine, where the data are often statistical, causal factors will often be identified in the last sense. In all of these senses of cause, factors are identified that are part of experiencing reality coherently and of explaining how events take place according to rules. In applied sciences, one is not interested simply in giving a coherent account, but in selecting among the possible coherent accounts those accounts that are more useful in achieving certain goals and purposes. In many circumstances, it will not be worthwhile to attend to all of the factors involved in giving a complete causal account. One turns one's attention instead to those factors, which are most easily manipulable, and highlights them in the account offered. Medicine, like the law, tends to underscore those causes that can be prevented or usefully manipulated.[79] Each such major institution underscores certain elements of a neutral, encompassing, scientific account of reality, because of the importance of some elements for the particular social institution, such as assigning sinfulness, criminal or civil liability, or directing treatment in a useful manner.

As already indicated, the major social institutions also differ in the character of the adverse judgments they give in characterizing undesirable circumstances. Consider how antisocial behavior can be understood alternatively as a sin, as a crime, as a moral fault, or as a disease (i.e., as a mental disorder). In seeking to characterize a circumstance as a disease rather than a sin, a moral fault, or a crime, one is not simply attempting to place such behavior in a social institution more able to resolve the problem. One is also choosing among values to be assigned to the phenomenon. Again, terming a circumstance a disease is not a value-free finding. If a circumstance is seen as one of disease, deformity, disability, or dysfunction, it is found to have fallen short of a physiological or psychological norm. So, too, when a circumstance is seen as a crime or a sin. It is disvalued in terms of a special set of value judgments. To decide between seeing a circumstance as a disease, a crime, or a sin is to choose from among competing value frameworks in terms of which to understand a state of affairs.

It is therefore important to decide where a problem falls. In deciding where to place a problem, one changes the frame of reference for interventions. In medicalizing a set of problems, one may relieve afflicted individuals of one set of disvaluations and encumber them with another. Consider the shift from holding drug addicts to be immoral to holding them to be diseased. Or consider alcoholism, which can be characterized as a sin, a moral fault, a crime, or a disease. One will need to decide where the accent should fall, in that shifting the accent from one major social institution to another changes the character of the responsibility one expects from individuals alternatively viewed as sinful, sick, diseased, or criminal. Past debates regarding whether homosexuality should be viewed as a crime, a sin, a disease, or a particular lifestyle are another good example.

Major difficulties have occurred through overmedicalizing problems. One might think here in particular of controversies regarding the use of the insanity plea as a means of determining that an individual's problem is one that justifies treatment, rather than punishment.[80] Or consider the use of psychiatric hospitalization in the Soviet Union to control political dissidence.

Such political problems are medicalized, undoubtedly in part, because they offer an efficacious way of controlling free expression.[81] They may also represent a sincere misuse of the social institution of medicine. It is a matter of considerable importance when to regard behavior not as freely chosen but as causally determined and open to medical cure. Such choices are made regularly when puzzling over disruptive children and adult criminals. They are choices with major moral presuppositions and consequences. They have their past instructive analogues, such as the special diseases assigned to slaves in the American South before the War Between the States, for example, drapetomania and dysaesthesia aethiopis, through which runaway or laggard slaves were seen as diseased.[82]

The problem is not simply to decide on the correct sick role or the correct staging or characterization of a disease, but whether to see a problem as a disease at all. The major social institutions offer competing construals of reality with competing costs and benefits. There are advantages and disadvantages in seeing disruptive behavior as a crime, a sin, a moral fault, or a disease. In some circumstances it is more important, useful, and plausible to see individuals as responsible for their actions. In others it is more useful and plausible to see behavior as determined and open to technological manipulation. The general moral is to understand that these choices are often not clear-cut. One must make them as best one can in terms of the plausibility of the account and its usefulness. In many circumstances, anything but a medical account will be highly implausible. Samuel Butler and *Erewhon* notwithstanding, it will be highly implausible to hold individuals responsible for developing appendicitis. In other circumstances, as for instance in drug addiction, the argument may plausibly go more than one way. In some circumstances, it may not make sense to choose between accounts; instead, it will be more plausible and useful to employ two or more accounts. It may make perfect sense to treat alcoholism as a disease, while at the same time regarding it as a moral problem. The proper choice may be one of both . . . and, rather than either . . . or.

The choice of how to view a circumstance will not simply be an epistemic or knowledge-based determination. It will be a determination based on a set of value considerations. The choices may not simply be right or wrong. They are often best understood as chosen in fair or unfair fashions. The very characterization of reality can thus become a moral issue. Reality as approached within the social institutions of medicine and the law will need to be understood in terms of the two major social practices of attempting to know truly and to treat fairly.

In this volume, we have looked in some detail at the conceptual constraints that structure ethics. In doing so, we have found that the rules that we can lay out generally and atemporally will be formal and will possess only a minimal content. The same is the case with science. Particular scientific communities at particular times embrace particular facts, findings, and rules of evidence and inference that we later find to be idiosyncratic, just as particular moral communities involve the acceptance of particular moral rules and views of the good life. Actual scientific controversies depend on conflicts between individuals united in a general commitment to science as an endeavor of intersubjectively establishing claims regarding the nature of the world, but divided due to different particular understandings of rules of evidence and inference. The same applies, mutatis mutandis, to moral debates. When the debates involve scientific issues with heavy ethical and political overlays, the conflicts become, as one would expect, complex. The individuals involved in such controversies will be participants in different moral and scientific communities and, as a result, will be in conflict with regard to different particular understandings of knowing truly and deciding fairly. They will be united in certain presuppositions of the very endeavors of morality and of science.

Such differences in understandings regarding what it means to know truly and decide fairly are often at the root of conflicts regarding the proper characterization of medical facts, or regarding whether a problem should be understood as a medical, legal, or moral problem. Concerns with evaluation and explanation thus intertwine in health care in decisions about whether problems are medical problems, and about how medical problems ought to be understood and classified. The very naming and characterization of a problem can thus raise the question of what values ought to be invoked, and of how they ought to be ordered. It will raise as well the question of who should participate in framing the classifications, and whose hierarchies of costs and benefits are involved. This issue must be answered in part, as has been indicated, through the practice of free and informed consent. It must also be answered through public knowledge of, and influence on, the ways in which problems are classified as medical, legal, religious, and so on. The answers must in part be created. Since the fashioning of such characterizations depends not just on knowing reality truly, but on deciding in a fair manner among various ways of classifying reality, problems of individual rights and democratic prerogatives become salient. If classifications are natural, no one is at fault for describing reality as it is. One may not like the way reality is, but the scientist has not taken away anyone's rights by describing things the way they are. However, if one is fashioning a classification in order to pursue particular goals, the choice of the particular goals is open to negotiation among those involved.

The democratization of medical reality: some conclusions

How should one choose in a fair fashion among competing descriptions of reality? As this chapter shows, there are choices to be made among alternative accounts of medical reality. Since these choices are not simply determined on epistemic grounds, we become accountable for the ways in which we fashion that reality. The portrayal of reality is a cultural product. Though there are constraints placed upon us as knowers by the given character of the object, the object appears to us through our concepts and in terms of the conditions of our experience. In the case of the unapplied sciences, where one's choice among different construals of reality is dictated by the ideal of a fully intersubjective account free of idiosyncratic values and purposes, there is a commitment to avoid imposing the values and perceptions of one particular group of knowers. Within an unapplied science one attempts to know anonymously and impersonally. As we have seen, the matter is different in applied sciences such as medicine. The goals to which we may apply medicine are varied and dependent on the visions of particular individuals and communities. We have seen this illustrated by the staging of cancer and by questions regarding medical decision making. Different ways of staging cancer and different balancing between over- and undertreatment depend in part upon different understandings of the values involved.

The question is, who gets to choose? The issue of who decides is thus moved from the area of individual free and informed consent to a communal area of negotiations regarding construals of reality. This is not a plea that staging systems for cancer be decided by referendum. But one must recognize that the choice among different understandings of reality within the applied sciences is a matter of communal interest. Communities must begin with a recognition of the constructed character of medical reality. This recognition underscores our choices and indicates our responsibilities as individuals who not only know reality but also know it in order to manipulate it. One must also recognize that these manipulations tend to be communal. Systematic programs for treatment and for the assessment of treatment, or communal insurance policies, are in principle not the undertakings of isolated individuals. As a result, communities of physicians, insurers, and the general public will need to negotiate regarding the characterization of medical reality where the interests of these three groups do not coincide. Such negotiations may take on either a formal or an informal character. In either case, they represent a democratization of reality. One comes to construe reality as the outcome of the choices of various communities of individuals, insofar as they are conducted openly and are under public control. Because of the principle of autonomy, individuals have rights to participate freely in such negotiations. The more one recognizes and respects these conditions, the more the medicalization of reality will enhance human goals and not constrain individual choices. It can be the thoughtful expression of our understanding of ourselves.

Notes

1. Charles S. Peirce, *Collected Papers of Charles Sanders Peirce*, ed. Charles Hartshorne and Paul Weiss (Cambridge, Mass.: Belknap Press, 1965), 5.316.
   The view I am defending here has, as did Peirce's view, a substantial indebtedness both to Kant and to Hegel. This is a point already acknowledged in chapter 2 but worth repeating and enlarging here. First, Kant's arguments are essentially correct (at least when given an Hegelian accent): we know reality only through our concepts. We never know reality uninterpreted by our understandings. To use the Kantian idiom, we do not know things as they are in themselves, as they are totally apart from our categories, but only as they are given to us through our categories of understanding. "What the things-in-themselves may be I do not know, nor do I need to know, since a thing can never come before me except in appearance." Kant, *The Critique of Pure Reason*, trans. Norman Kemp Smith (London: Macmillan, 1964), p. 286, A277 = B333. We cannot make out an account of reality apart from our understandings of reality. From Hegel one can derive the suggestion that one might as well cease speaking of an inaccessible reality in itself. Even as a limit on experience, as a direction toward the object, a mere "something = x" (*Critique of Pure Reason*, A250), to which one turns in empirical investigation, the thing-in-itself is itself a product of thought (G. W. F. Hegel, *The Encyclopedia of the Philosophical Sciences* [1830], sec. 44). If one never encounters the purely other, the object as it is in itself, one can then regard the struggle to know reality as one of overcoming otherness and incompleteness in ever more coherent accounts of reality. The element of otherness directs us to seek accounts that can set that otherness aside.
   This undertaking is a cultural endeavor. Consider Hegel's reflections on this task. "By thinking things, we transform them into something universal; things are singularities however, and the lion in general does not exist. We make them into something subjective, produced by us, belonging to us, and of course peculiar to us as men; for the things of nature do not think, and are neither representations nor thought." *Hegel's Philosophy of Nature*, trans. M. J. Petry (London: Allen & Unwin, 1970), p. 198, sec. 246 Zusatz. Our aim is to grasp and comprehend nature, to make it ours, so that it is not something beyond and alien to us. As a result, in our attempt to know nature, we do not simply see nature. We come, as Hegel observes, to see ourselves, "to find in this externality only the mirror of ourselves." Ibid., vol. 3, p. 213, sec. 376 Zusatz.
   Hegel recognized, as Kant did not, that categories of knowledge are historical. The ways in which we see nature, the concepts through which appearance is given to us, if those concepts are specified in any detail, will develop through time. Revolutions occur in science when the basic categories change. "All cultural change reduces itself to a difference of categories. All revolutions, whether in the sciences or world history, occur merely because spirit has changed its categories in order to understand and examine what belongs to it, in order to possess and grasp itself in a truer, deeper, more intimate and unified manner." Ibid., vol. 1, p. 202, sec. 246 Zusatz. The quote from Peirce underscores both the direction for

investigation, namely, the attempt to find ever more articulated understandings of nature, and the realization that science is a historical process.

For an introduction to the philosophical issues involved in Hegel's notions of knowledge as negation, versus knowledge as an encounter with an object in its otherness, see Werner Flach, *Negation und Andersheit* (Munich: Ernst Reinhardt, 1959).

2. Ludwik Fleck, *Entstehung und Entwicklung einer wissenschaftlichen Tatsache: Einfuehrung in die Lehre vom Denkstil und Denkkollektiv* (Basel: Benno Schwabe, 1935); English version, *Genesis and Development of a Scientific Fact*, ed. T. J. Trenn and R. K. Merton, trans. F. Bradley and T. J. Trenn (Chicago: University of Chicago Press, 1979).

3. Thomas Kuhn, *The Structure of Scientific Revolutions* (Chicago: University of Chicago Press, 1962; 2d ed., enlarged, 1970).

4. For other discussions of the contextual character of scientific thought, see Peter Achinstein, *Law and Explanation* (Oxford: Oxford University Press, 1971), and *The Nature of Explanation* (New York: Oxford University Press, 1983). Imre Lakatos and Alan Musgrave (eds.), *Criticism and the Growth of Knowledge* (Cambridge: Cambridge University Press, 1970). Larry Laudan, *Progress and Its Problems* (Berkeley: University of California Press, 1977).

5. Isaac Baker Brown, *On the Curability of Certain Forms of Insanity, Epilepsy, Catalepsy, and Hysteria in Females* (London: Robert Hardwicke, 1866).

6. H. Tristram Engelhardt, Jr., "The Disease of Masturbation: Values and the Concept of Disease," *Bulletin of the History of Medicine* 48 (Summer 1974): 234–48.

7. For the reports of death due to masturbation, see, for example, *Report of the Board of Administrators of the Charity Hospital to the General Assembly of Louisiana* (for 1872) (New Orleans: The Republican Office, 1873), p. 30; and *Report of the Board of Administrators of the Charity Hospital to the General Assembly of Louisiana* (for 1887) (New Orleans: A. W. Hyatt, 1888), p. 53.

8. A published autopsy report from Birmingham, England, concerning a dead masturbator showed that masturbation "seems to have acted upon the cord in the same manner as repeated small haemorrhages affect the brain, slowly sapping its energies, until it succumbed soon after the last application of the exhausting influence, probably through the instrumentality of an atrophic process previously induced, as evidenced by the diseased state of the minute vessels." James Russell, "Cases Illustrating the Influence of Exhaustion of the Spinal Cord in Inducing Paraplegia," *Medical Times and Gazette, London* 2 (1863): 456.

9. Baker Brown, *On the Curability of Certain Forms . . .*, p. 11.

10. Ibid., p. 17.

11. Ibid., pp. 51–2.

12. American Psychiatric Association, *Diagnostic and Statistical Manual of Mental Disorders* (Washington, D.C.: American Psychiatric Association, 1952), pp. 38–9.

13. American Psychiatric Association, *Diagnostic and Statistical Manual of Mental Disorders*, 2d ed. (Washington, D.C.: American Psychiatric Association, 1968), p. 44.

14. American Psychiatric Association, *Diagnostic and Statistical Manual of Mental Disorders*, 3d ed. (Washington, D.C.: American Psychiatric Association, 1980), p. 281.

15. T. Gaillard Thomas, *A Practical Treatise on the Diseases of Women* (Philadelphia: Henry C. Lea's Son, 1880), p. 778.

THE LANGUAGES OF MEDICALIZATION 197

16. William Cullen, *Synopsis nosologiae methodicae* (Edinburgh: William Creech, 1769).
17. Hippocrates, *Epidemics* III, case 16, in *Hippocrates*, trans. W. H. S. Jones (Cambridge, Mass.: Harvard University Press, 1962), Vol. I, pp. 285, 287.
18. Hippocrates, *Epidemics* I.1, Vol. I, pp. 147, 149.
19. Ivan Illich, *Medical Nemesis* (New York: Pantheon Books, 1976).
20. Lee B. Lusted, *Introduction to Medical Decision Making* (Springfield, Ill.: Thomas, 1968), pp. 98–140.
21. Ronald Bayer, *Homosexuality and American Psychiatry* (New York: Basic Books, 1981).
22. American Joint Committee on Cancer, *Manual for Staging of Cancer* (Philadelphia: Lippincott, 1983).
23. U.S. Department of Health, Education, and Welfare, *Eighth Revision International Classification of Diseases*, 2 vols. (Washington, D.C.: U.S. Government Printing Office, 1968).
24. Carolus Linnaeus, *Genera morborum, in auditorum usum* (Upsalae: Steinert, 1763).
25. François Boissier de Sauvages de la Croix, *Nosologia methodica sistens morborum classes juxta Sydenhami mentem et botanicorum ordinem*, 5 vols. (Amsterdam: Fratrum de Tournes, 1763); 2d ed., 2 vols. (Amsterdam: Fratrum de Tournes, 1768), vol. 2, pp. 1–149.
26. Horacio Fabrega, Jr., "Disease Viewed as a Symbolic Category," in H. T. Engelhardt, Jr., and S. F. Spicker (eds.), *Mental Health: Philosophical Perspectives* (Dordrecht: Reidel, 1977), pp. 79–106.
27. Maryland Annotated Code (1979 Cumulative Supplement), art. 27, sec. 554. One might note that the punishment for unnatural acts was once more severe in America. Consider Benjamin Goad, who was hung and his mare executed in his sight after he had been discovered in 1673 committing the "unnatural & horrid act of Bestillitie on a mare in the highway or field." *Records of the Court of Assistants of the Colony of the Massachusetts Bay 1630–1682* (1901), vol. 1, pp. 10–11.
28. Richard H. Post, "Population Differences in Red and Green Color Vision Deficiency: A Review, and a Query on Selection Relaxation," *Eugenics Quarterly* 9 (March 1962): 131–46.
29. St. Thomas Aquinas, *Summa Theologica* II-II, pp. 153–4.
30. Christopher Boorse, "On the Distinction Between Disease and Illness," *Philosophy and Public Affairs* 5 (Fall 1975): 61.
31. Christopher Boorse, "Health as a Theoretical Concept," *Philosophy of Science* 44 (1977): 562, 567.
32. Christopher Boorse, "On the Distinction between Disease and Illness," *Philosophy and Public Affairs* 5 (Fall 1975): 63.
33. Robert Trivers, "Parent-Offspring Conflict," *American Zoologist* 14 (1974): 259–64.
34. F. B. Livingstone, "The Distributions of the Abnormal Hemoglobin Genes and Their Significance for Human Evolution," *Evolution* 18 (1964): 685. Christopher Boorse acknowledges the existence of polymorphic traits and intraspecific variations. He does not come to terms with the way various balances among traits maximize fitness, often at the price of individual suffering. Christopher Boorse, "Health as a Theoretical Concept," *Philosophy of Science* 44 (1977): 542–71; see especially pp. 546–7, 558, and 563.

35. William K. Goosens, "Values, Health, and Medicine," *Philosophy of Science* 47 (March 1980): 100–115.
36. A helpful distinction among the different senses of normality and a discussion of the difference between a biologist's taxonomic interest in normality and that of a physician are provided by Marjorie Grene, "Individuals and Their Kind: Aristotelian Foundations of Biology," in Stuart Spicker (ed.), *Organism, Medicine, and Metaphysics* (Dordrecht: Reidel, 1978), pp. 121–136.
37. For a neo-Aristotelian attempt to discover the boundaries between health and disease, see Georg Henrik von Wright, *The Varieties of Goodness* (New York: Humanities Press, 1963).
38. There is a considerable literature supporting what could be termed a weak normativist account of disease, that is, a view that concepts of disease, though in part based on empirical determinations, have an essential evaluative component. These views contrast with the neutralist views of individuals such as Christopher Boorse who hold that concepts of disease are descriptive and explanatory, but not evaluative. For a classic article supporting the weak normativist view, see Lester King, "What is Disease?" *Philosophy of Science* 21 (July 1954): 193–203. One should note that the normativist view suggests that concepts of diseases for animals and plants depend on human understandings of the purposes of animals and plants. Therefore, the paradigm examples of diseases in animals and plants are those that afflict pets, or animals and plants grown for food, and so on. It is difficult to speak of feral animals and plants as being diseased (or at least diseased in a clinical sense) except by analogy. One would also be able to develop a Boorsian, neutralist notion of the diseases of wild animals and plants in terms of species-atypical levels of species-typical functions. But such would not focus on the sufferings of animals. The concept of disease held by veterinarians or agricultural scientists is, in contrast, dependent on what humans hold to be the proper functions, levels of pain, and characters of grace and form for particular groups of living entities. "Diseases" universal to a particular species of animals and plants could be recognized as diseases only if the animal or plant is being raised as a pet or for profit, and the "disease" impedes such goals. See, for example, Peter Sedgwick, "Illness—Mental and Otherwise," *Hastings Center Studies* 1 (1973): 19–40, and H. T. Engelhardt, Jr., "Is There a Philosophy of Medicine?" in F. Suppe and P. D. Asquith (eds.), *PSA 1976*, vol. 2 (East Lansing, Mich.: Philosophy of Science Association, 1977), pp. 94–108.
39. For a development of this point, see Joseph Margolis, "The Concept of Disease," *Journal of Medicine and Philosophy* 1 (Sept. 1976): 238–55; H. T. Engelhardt, Jr., "Ideology and Etiology," *Journal of Medicine and Philosophy* 1 (Sept. 1976): 256–8.
40. One should note that attempts such as those by Clouser, Culver, and Gert to introduce a term such as malady will not provide what is needed here. K. Danner Clouser, Charles M. Culver, and Bernard Gert, "Malady: A New Treatment of Disease," *Hastings Center Report* 11 (June 1981): 29–37. They offer the following definition of malady: "A person has a malady if and only if he or she has a condition, other than a rational belief or desire, such that he or she is suffering, or at increased risk of suffering, an evil (death, pain, disability, loss of freedom or oportunity, or loss of pleasure) in the absence of a distinct sustaining cause" (p. 36). Medicine, however, treats a number of "maladies" with distinct sustaining causes as, for instance, infertility by providing artificial insemination from a donor. Such a "malady" is not a malady under the rubrics of Clouser et al., since

there is a distinct sustaining cause, that of the husband's infertility. Hence, a more general term is required. I have proposed the term *clinical problem*. Engelhardt, "Clinical Problems and the Concept of Disease," in L. Nordenfelt and B. I. B. Lindahl (eds.), *Health, Disease, and Causal Explanations in Medicine* (Dordrecht: Reidel, 1984), pp. 27–41.

41. For a review of the conflicts between so-called ontological accounts of disease (those that portray diseases as entities, as in some sense things) and physiological or functional accounts of disease (those that articulate nominalists in their views of the reality of diseases and portray disease taxa as artificial designations), see A. L. Caplan, H. T. Engelhardt, Jr., and J. J. McCartney (eds.), *Concepts of Health and Disease* (Reading, Mass.: Addison-Wesley, 1981), esp. pp. 143–263.

42. John L. Gedye, "Simulating Clinical Judgment," in H. T. Engelhardt, Jr., S. F. Spicker, and B. Towers (eds.), *Clinical Judgment: A Critical Appraisal* (Dordrecht: Reidel, 1979), pp. 93–113.

43. Committee on Nomenclature and Classification of Disease, *Systematized Nomenclature of Pathology* (Chicago: College of American Pathologists, 1969), p. xvii.

44. *Eighth Revision International Classification of Diseases*, 2 vols. (Washington, D.C.: U.S. Government Printing Office, 1968).

45. Alvan R. Feinstein, *Clinical Judgment* (Huntington, N.Y.: Kreiger, 1974), p. 968.

46. Norwood R. Hanson, *Patterns of Discovery* (Cambridge: Cambridge University Press, 1961); *Perception and Discovery* (San Francisco: Freeman, Cooper, 1969).

47. Henrik Wulff, *Rational Diagnosis and Treatment*, 2d ed. (London: Blackwell Scientific, 1981), pp. 30–41.

48. One might think here of Lawrence Weed's problem-oriented medical record, which includes an injunction to describe patient problems at least in part in terms of how they are experienced by the patient. See *Medical Records, Medical Education, and Patient Care* (Chicago: Year Book Medical Publications, 1970).

49. These points are explored by Hegel in the second book of *The Logic*, "Wesen" (Essence), and in the second section of the first part of the *Encylopedia*, "Die Lehre vom Wesen" (The Doctrine of Essence). These points are developed as well in Hegel's *Phenomenology of Mind*, his *Phaenomenologie des Geistes*, in his study of sense certainty, perception, and force and understanding. Hegel provides a detailed analysis of the ways in which the meaning of appearance and the laws that are held to lie behind appearance presuppose each other in the very structure of explanation.

50. For an introduction to some of the issues raised by the roles of prediction and manipulation in the fashioning of scientific explanations, see R. G. Collingwood, *The Idea of Nature* (New York: Oxford University Press, 1960). See also Stephen Toulmin, *Foresight and Understanding* (New York: Harper & Row, 1961), and *The Philosophy of Science* (New York: Harper & Row, 1953).

51. Thomas Sydenham, "Answer to Henry Paman, M.D. Fellow of St. John's College in Cambridge, publick Orator of that University; and Professor of Physic in Grethan College; containing the History and Treatment of the Venereal Disease," in *The Entire Works of Dr. Thomas Sydenham*, ed. and trans. John Swan, 3d ed. (London: E. Cave, 1753), p. 339.

52. See n. 25, this chapter.

53. See n. 24, this chapter.

54. Fredrik Berg, "Linné et Sauvages: Les rapports entre leurs systèmes nosologiques," *Lynchonos* (1956): 36.

55. Sauvages, *Nosologia Methodica* (1768), vol. 1. pp. 92–5.
    The reader must note that it is difficult to convey the significance of the major classes in Sauvages' clinically oriented nosology. The classification brings diseases and problems together in unaccustomed ways. For example, under class X, *cachexiae: coloris, figurae, molis in corporis habitu depravatio* (constitutional disorders: distortion of the body's condition in color, figure, and shape) [vol. 1, p. 95] is the order *tumores, corporis generalis intumescentia, seu adauctum volumen* (swellings: general tumescence of the body or increase of volume), which includes the *genus graviditas*, or pregnancy. It might appear peculiar to list pregnancy within a classification of diseases. That peculiarity is in part dispelled if one recognizes that the classification is one of clinical problems and that pregnancy can occasion clinical difficulties. The difficulty lies in seeing pregnancy under the classification of swellings and then regarding swelling as a form of constitutional disorder. The sense of inappropriateness is tied to our contemporary accepted views of how one should classify clinical phenomena. It is tied as well to the difficulty of giving *cachexiae* (wastings, consumptions, bad conditions of the body) enough breadth of meaning.
    In addition to his clinically oriented classification of diseases, Sauvages provided some eighty pages devoted to an etiological classification (*Classes morborum aetiologicae*) and an anatomical classification (*Methodus anatomica morborum*). In short, Sauvages developed three alternative classifications from which one could select, depending on the circumstances.
    For an overview of the accomplishments of Sauvages, see Lester S. King, "Boissier de Sauvages and 18th Century Nosology," *Bulletin of the History of Medicine* 60 (Spring 1966): 43–51.
56. American Psychiatric Association, *DSM-III*.
57. Sydenham, in *The Entire Works*, (E. Cave, 1753) sec. 9, pp. iv–v.
58. Ibid., p. v.
59. *DSM-III*, pp. 6–7.
60. Theophile Bonet, *Sepulchretum sive anatomia practica ex cadaveribus morbo denatis* (Geneva: L. Chouet, 1679).
61. Giovanni Morgagni, *De sedibus et causis morborum per anatomen indagatis* (Venice: Ex Typographis Remondiniana, 1761).
62. Michel Foucault, *Naissance de la Clinique* (Paris: Presses Universitaires de France, 1963). *The Birth of the Clinic: An Archaeology of Medical Perception*, trans. A. M. Sheridan Smith (New York: Random House, 1973).
63. F.-J.-V. Broussais, *On Irritation and Insanity*, trans. Thomas Cooper (Columbia, S.C.: S. J. McMorris, 1831), p. ix. *De L'irritation et de la Folie* (Paris: Delaunay, 1828).
64. Rudolf Virchow, "One Hundred Years of General Pathology (1895)," in *Disease, Life, and Man*, trans. L. J. Rather (Stanford, Calif.: Stanford University Press, 1958), p. 214.
65. Xavier Bichat, "Preliminary Discourse," in Bichat, *Pathological Anatomy* (Philadelphia: John Grigg, 1827); reprinted in A. Caplan, et al., *Concepts of Health and Disease*, pp. 167–8.
66. F.-J.-V. Broussais. *Examen des Doctrines Medicales et des Systems de Nosologie* (Paris: Meguignon-Marvis, 1821), vol. 2, p. 646.
67. Carolus Linnaeus, *Genera morborum in auditorum usum* (Hamburg: Buchenroeder & Ritter, 1773[?]), pp. 16–17.
68. Sauvages, *Nosologia* (1768), vol. 2, pp. 1–42f.

69. Talcott Parsons developed this point in a number of works. See, in particular, *The Social System* (New York: Free Press, 1951); and "Definitions of Health and Illness in the Light of American Values and Social Structure," in E. G. Jaco (ed.), *Patients, Physicians and Illness* (Glencoe, Ill.: Free Press, 1958), pp. 165–187.

70. M. Siegler and H. Osmond, "The 'Sick Role' Revisited," *Hastings Center Studies* 1 (1973): 41–58.

71. Alfred Schutz and Thomas Luckmann, *The Structures of the Life-World*, trans. R. N. Zaner and H. T. Engelhardt, Jr. (Evanston, Ill.: Northwestern University Press, 1973).

72. For discussion of the social construction of medical reality, see P. Wright and A. Treacher (eds.), *The Problem of Medical Knowledge* (Edinburgh: Edinburgh University Press, 1982).

73. Consider as an example the following staging scheme for cancer of the bladder offered in a handbook of surgery used by residents and others.

Stage 0: Papillary tumor not invading the lamina propria
Stage A: Invasion of the lamina propria but not the muscle
Stage B: Superficial (B_1) or deep (B_2) invasion of the bladder muscle
Stage C: Tumor extending outside the bladder wall to perivesical fat or overlying peritoneum
Stage D: Distant metastases

Theodore R. Schrock (ed.), *Handbook of Surgery*, 7th ed. (Greenbrae, Calif.: Jones Medical Publications, 1982), p. 374.

74. American Joint Committee on Cancer, *Manual for Staging of Cancer*, 2d ed. (Philadelphia: Lippincott, 1983), p. vii.

75. Ibid., p. viii.

76. Ibid., p. xi.

77. See A. S. Elstein, L. S. Shulman, and S. A. Sprafka (eds.), *Medical Problem Solving* (Cambridge, Mass.: Harvard University Press, 1978): Alvan R. Feinstein, *Clinical Judgment* (Huntington, N.Y.: Krieger, 1967); Edmond A. Murphy, *The Logic of Medicine* (Baltimore: John Hopkins University Press, 1976); and Wulff, *Rational Diagnosis and Treatment*.

78. H. L. A. Hart and A. M. Honoré, *Causation in the Law* (Oxford: Clarendon Press, 1959); see esp. pp. 35–6.

79. For an exploration of the notions of causality and causation in medicine, see Kenneth F. Schaffner, "Causation and Responsibility: Medicine, Science and the Law," pp. 95–122, and H. T. Engelhardt, Jr., "Relevant Causes: Their Designation in Medicine and Law," pp. 123–7, in S. F. Spicker et al. (eds.), *The Law-Medicine Relation: A Philosophical Exploration* (Dordrecht: Reidel, 1981).

80. B. Brody and H. T. Engelhardt, Jr. (eds.), *Mental Illness: Law and Public Policy* (Dordrecht: Reidel, 1980).

81. A. Koryagin, "Unwilling Patients," *Lancet* 1 (1981): 821–4.

82. S. A. Cartwright, "Report on the Diseases and Physical Peculiarities of the Negro Race," *New Orleans Medical and Surgical Journal* 7 (May 1851): 691–715.

6

The Endings and Beginnings of Persons: Death, Abortion, and Infanticide

Persons are central to the very idea and undertaking of morality. Only persons have moral problems and moral obligations. The very world of morality is sustained by persons. The problem is that not all humans are persons. At least, they are not persons in the strict sense of being moral agents. Infants are not persons. The severely senile and the very severely or profoundly mentally retarded are not persons in this very important and central way. Nor are those who are severely brain damaged. But as chapter 4 discussed, there is more than one sense of person. Medicine is concerned with persons in the strict sense of moral agents, which includes patients who discuss their problems with their physicians and come to agreements about treatment. Medicine is concerned as well with numerous humans to whom a portion of the rights and prerogatives of persons is imputed. Infants and the senile are regarded in many ways as if they were persons. *Person* is used to refer to both competent adults and the profoundly mentally retarded. This potential ambiguity is significant because definitions of death may appear to focus on the death of persons in the strict sense, while in fact their focus is upon the death of persons in other senses as well. So, too, at the beginning of life, one might think that the arguments regarding abortion and infanticide focus on the point at which persons in the strict sense come into being. But, of course, this cannot be the case, since humans do not become persons in the strict sense of moral agents until years after their birth.

These philosophical issues have already been explored in chapter 4. Here we turn to their further elaboration and application. Physicians, after all, must apply abstract concepts of being alive or being dead to actual situations. Physicians declare individuals dead. The determination of when fetuses are viable is made by physicians as well. As the last chapter has shown, such determinations are not merely factual, if for no other reason than that such findings can usually not be made without exposure to the possibility of false positive and false negative. Deciding on which side one ought to err requires a balancing of costs and benefits. Moreover, as we shall see in the case of the notion of viability, one is establishing a criterion for interventions that has a major bearing on the rights of women to determine their reproductive destinies.

The question is how ought one to approach the world, once it is clear that the entities to whom we have the strongest obligations, persons in the strict sense, come into being only some time, likely years, after birth, and likely cease to exist sometime before the death of the organism. One must recall here the distinction in chapter 4 between human biological and human personal life. Mere human biological life precedes the emergence of the life of persons in the strict sense, and it usually continues for a while after their death. Because of this circumstance, because of the concerns that persons have to raise children, and because of the interests that persons have to nurture sentiments of sympathy and care, a social sense of person is often imputed to nonpersonal, human biological life. Thus, infants are treated as if they were persons. So, too, the severely senile are regarded as persons, though they are not such in the strict sense.

The definition of death

The controversies concerning definitions of death spring in great part from unclarities regarding the kind of life that is being declared at an end. One can have a sense of this from the different wordings in American statutes defining death. The first two statutes in the United States, that of Kansas, which was enacted in 1970,[1] and that of Maryland, enacted in 1972,[2] speak to the determination of the death of a person. However, after the *Roe* v. *Wade* decision in 1973, legislatures began to shy away from the term person because it had taken on a political significance for the abortion debate. Notions of when persons end have implications for understanding when persons begin. Even contrasting human personal life with human biological life suggests that fetuses are not persons just because they are living humans. The contrast itself favors one side of the abortion debate. Against this background one finds, for example, the statutes in Montana, Oklahoma, Tennessee, and Wyoming speaking of the death of a human body[3] and that in Colorado referring to the death of an individual.[4] The statutes of other states such as Connecticut, Florida, and Illinois simply speak of death.[5]

These may appear to be innocent variations. However, the distinction between human biological and personal life shows that they are in fact central to the debate. It is one thing to be interested in when human biological life ceases and another to be interested in when persons cease to exist. To speak of the death of a human body suggests an organismic focus on human biological life. The development from a whole-body-oriented definition of death to a whole-brain-oriented definition of death can be interpreted as a move away from a definition focused on human biological life to one focused on the life of a person. The recent statutes that eschew reference to the death of a person can then be seen as a reaction against the conceptual developments that underlie the brain-oriented definition of death.

Indeed, the history of the debates concerning the definition of death can be seen to hinge on this point, as well as on two others. First, what is the kind of life, the death of which one is to determine? Here the controversy focuses on the contrast between human biological and personal life and can come to involve the various senses of person discussed in chapter 4. Second, how and where is that life embodied? The issue at stake is whether the brain or some other part of the brain is the unique locus, embodiment, or sponsor of the kind of life whose death one seeks to determine. Third, how many false positive and false negative determinations of death ought one to tolerate or find acceptable?

Bodies, minds, and persons

The first issue concerns the development of a distinction between the life of a human organism and the life of a person. Those two concepts were tied more closely together when the human body was seen to be enlivened by a rational soul. The soul was understood not only to be the source of moral agency, but also to include animal and vegetative functions, which enlivened the body. Thus, St. Thomas argued that all of the soul was in every part of the body: "tota in toto" and "tota in qualibet parte." One must recall that St. Thomas distinguished among nutritive, sensitive, and intellectual souls,[6] though the intellectual soul included the reality of the other souls in its embodied life. This led to the soul being seen as a kind of catalyst for organic processes. Such views gave special significance to the work of Friedrich Woehler (1800–82), who in 1828 first synthesized urea in vitro. Such was considered impossible by many vitalists, who held that organic compounds required life for their synthesis.

The development of the life sciences has contributed to our knowledge of the ways in which biological functions can be understood without an appeal to a vital principle. It has contributed as well to our mastery of the ways in which those processes can be substituted for by technological surrogates. Life as a biological process has ceased to be a mystery requiring special soul-like catalysts. The systematic integration of the body can be understood without invoking the presence of either the soul or a moral agent. On the other hand, moral agency requires the presence of self-consciousness. Self-consciousness has a sense and meaning that contrast with mechanical, chemical, and biological structures. The life of minds, if it is to be understood adequately, must be captured, at least in part, in introspective psychological terms.[7]

It is for this reason that the principles of biological life contrast with the principles of mental life, and here in particular, the life of persons.[8] The biology that has been marked by successes such as Woehler's helps us to come to terms with various biological functions, including the systematic integration of the body, though it does not suffice for understanding the lived experiences of minds. This is the case, even if one might foresee the artificial synthesis of organisms that would have a mental life and perhaps even be persons, as was HAL in the novel and movie *2001*.[9] To make a judgment about the moral standing of entities, one will need to decide about their capacities for consciousness and self-consciousness and their abilities to conceive of moral goods and to have a rational plan of life. The more an entity is self-conscious, able to choose on the basis of reason and able to make moral claims, the more it must be recognized as a moral agent. However, entities that fall short of this status but that can suffer and have pleasure will still be worthy of our moral attention. As chapter 4 has shown, one must distinguish between entities that have mental lives but are not persons, and those that are persons. We ought to have moral regard for entities with a mental life because they suffer and have pleasure. We ought to show respect for those entities which are persons because they (and that respect) sustain the practice of morality.

This should be plain when one considers the contrast between a human body in which all of the brain except for the lower brain stem has been destroyed, and an adult human body with a fully functioning brain. To understand the first, one need only appeal to the principles of biological life. To understand the second, one will need to appeal to the principles of mental entities, including here that of persons. It is not mere biological life that is of central moral interest. A human body that can only function biologically, without an inward mental life, does not sustain a moral agent. It need not be regarded with the special moral concern that one ought to show for a living, intact opossum or raccoon, which can exquisitely feel pain and know fear and suffering. The death of a mere animal marks the passing of a mental life that can suffer and have pleasure. The death of a person marks the passing of an entity that can make promises and fashion strong moral claims. To underscore this point with regard to definitions of death: a body with whole-brain death, or with death of the whole brain except for the brain stem, does not support a mental life, much less the life of a person.

To look at things in this way requires a momentous conceptual step. It requires recognizing that mere human biological life is of little moral value in and of itself. It requires acknowledging that it is the life of human persons in the strict sense that is central to moral concerns. It also means confronting a whole set of new puzzles. One must decide how to regard those levels of human mental life that are not yet the life of a person. In particular, one must decide how to regard the standing of young children, the severely demented, and those who are brain injured. The focus shifts to determining when a particular level of human mental life has ceased.

Embodiments

When the determination of when the death of a human person has occurred involves ascertaining whether human mental life has ceased, problems of the embodiment of human life have taken on their modern character. If one asks simply about the embodiment of human life, one can come to an answer somewhat similar to St. Thomas's: human life is in all of the parts of the human body. One might think here of the classic definition of death given in the fourth edition of *Black's Law Dictionary* as "the cessation of life; the ceasing to exist; defined by physicians as a total stoppage of the circulation of the blood, and a cessation of the animal and vital functions consequent thereon, such as respiration, pulsation, etc."[10] Once one's interest is not in the preservation of mere biological life, but in the continuance of a mental life, the focus is on the brain as the sponsor of sentience and consciousness. It is the brain that sustains mental life. The body, in contrast, comes to be seen as a complex, integrated mechanism that sustains the life of the brain, which sponsors the life of a person. One can replace various parts of the body with transplanted organs or prostheses and the person remains the same person. But if one successfully transplanted a brain, one would successfully transplant a person from an old body to a new body. As Roland Puccetti has phrased it, where the brain goes, there goes the person.[11]

This leads to distinguishing among the various embodiments of various mental functions. One may recall the historical antecedents of this debate in the nineteenth-century disputes regarding these issues. Much of our modern ways of understanding cerebral localization are deeply indebted to the phrenologists, Franz Josef Gall (1758–1828)[12] and Johann Spurzheim, (1776–1832)[13] who argued for the strict localization of mental functions. Though they were attacked by such latter-day Cartesians as M. J. P. Flourens (1794–1867), who in 1845 dedicated one of his books to Descartes in defense of a view that the mind acted as a unity upon the cerebral hemispheres,[14] Gall and Spurzheim influenced in a complex and important fashion the development of the notion that mental functions can, however nonstrictly, be mapped upon various parts of the brain.[15] They also influenced, although indirectly, the work of John Hughlings Jackson (1835–1911), who created the modern idiom of neurology and of cerebral localization.[16] It is from this debate and through this idiom that we come to distinguish among various levels of mental life. Mental life could be seen as admitting of various levels with different embodiments.

Living and dying with less than absolute certainty

Understanding (1) the criteria for being a person or an entity with a mental life, and (2) what parts of the brain sponsor the life of persons or other levels of mental life will not suffice for fashioning acceptable tests for death. Even after one has achieved sufficient conceptual clarification regarding what it means to be alive as a mind or as a person, and a sufficient understanding of the embodiment presupposed by that life, one will still need to find ways to test safely for when that life's embodiment has gone. Even if one is clear conceptually regarding what it means to be alive in this world, one will still need to fashion reliable operational tests to determine when that life has ceased.

As the President's Commission report on defining death shows, there have been periods of obsessive fear about avoiding false positive tests even with whole-body-oriented definitions of death. For example, affluent individuals in the eighteenth and nineteenth centuries were occasionally interred with complex mechanisms to allow them to signal others if they revived in their coffins.[17] Such coffins were supplied as well with special provisions for ventilation. So, too, whole-brain definitions of death have raised the issue of what tests are reliable indicators that the brain has died. One might think here of contemporary concerns regarding how often one need repeat tests for reflexes or for EKG activity in order to declare an individual dead. However, one may not need to be as concerned with false positives as one might think, when one considers that a possible survivor with severe brain damage may not have a life worth living. On the other hand, one may be properly concerned with false negative tests. If one falsely finds an individual to be alive who is really dead, one may see oneself committed to discharging costly moral obligations of care and treatment.

Such concerns are only indirectly focused on what it means to be alive or on the embodiment presupposed by such life. They are rather primarily focused on ways of determining the end of that life or the destruction of that embodiment with as few false positives as possible. This may lead to an important ambiguity. One may select a whole-body- or whole-brain-oriented test for death, not because one holds that the life of persons is sponsored by the body or the brain as a whole, but because one fears false positive determinations of death that may result from employing a neocortical definition. Or to take a more colorful example, just because one does not wish to be declared dead until one is odoriferous in the Texas sun does not necessarily imply that one believes one will be alive up until that very point— the point employed for determining death.

To avoid some of these potential ambiguities, I will use the term *concept of death*, and such variants as *whole-brain-oriented concept of death* and *neocortically oriented concept of death*, to identify conceptual understandings regarding the significance of mental life or of the life of a person and/or the embodiment of that life, such as would lead one to hold that persons are embodied in the brain as a whole or in the neocortex. In contrast, I will use the term *test for* or *determination of death* to identify particular operations used to ascertain whether death according to a particular concept of death has occurred. I will use the term *definition of death* to encompass both concepts of death and tests for death.

The development of a whole-brain definition of death

To a great extent, all of the conceptual distinctions were well in hand at the end of the nineteenth century for a whole-brain-oriented, if not a higher-brain-centers-oriented, definition of death. It was clear that the brain was the sponsor of consciousness and that in fact the cerebrum was the necessary condition for consciousness.[18] The major problems would have been operational, not conceptual. The difficulty would have been in establishing a whole-brain- or a neocortically oriented test for death that would not have involved an unacceptable number of false positive determinations. The twentieth century contributed not simply more information, but a practical need to develop whole-brain-oriented, if not neocortically oriented, tests for death.

This need sprang from the development in the 1950s of intensive care units and of respirators able to sustain brain-dead but otherwise alive human bodies for a number of hours if not days. This technological advance engendered new financial and psychological costs, due to the false negative determinations delivered by whole-body-oriented definitions of death under contexts of high technology. In the 1950s the development of kidney transplant techniques and in 1967 of heart transplantation further underscored the need to develop a whole-brain definition. If one waited for the individual to be dead on the basis of whole-body tests, one ran the risk of severe damage to the kidneys and profound damage to the heart, which one hoped to transplant. Technological advances, rising costs, and an interest in transplantation pressed the question of whether one could not hold brain-dead but otherwise living human bodies to no longer be the bodies of a living person.

The first hesitant step toward a whole-brain-oriented definition of death was made in 1968 by the Ad Hoc Committee of the Harvard Medical School, chaired by Henry Beecher. It is important to note that the committee did not forward a definition of death *in sensu stricto*, but rather concluded that individuals with irreversible coma could be declared dead. The committee did not clearly equate destruction of the entire brain with death of the person.[19] Despite these limitations, this proposal had immediate and substantial impact on the understanding of what was to be meant by death. Shortly after the committee's publication of its criteria, the Twenty-Second Congress of the World Medical Association in its "Declaration of Sydney" acknow-ledged the possible usefulness of encephalographic determinations in declar-ing death.[20] In the next year, 1969, the Ad Hoc Committee of the American Electroencephalographic Society on EEG Criteria for Determination of Cerebral Death published criteria that equated death with brain death. Though the title suggests a cerebrally oriented definition of death, the committee in fact supported only a whole-brain-oriented definition.[21]

These developments led to changes in the law by statute, beginning in 1970. Whole-brain-oriented definitions of death became well established over the next decade. The initial and potentially pernicious confusion between when a person is dead and when one is no longer obliged to sustain a person's life was in the main dispelled. It was generally acknowledged that when the whole brain was destroyed, it was not simply that one was no longer obliged to sustain that individual, but rather that that individual was dead, no longer existing in this world. This was a painful and difficult step. Brain-dead but otherwise alive human bodies are warm to the touch and are respiring, albeit with mechanical assistance. They appear to be alive because they are in fact alive. It is because human biological life continues unabated that transplant surgeons are interested in such bodies as an ideal source for harvesting organs. There is no reason why a brain-dead but otherwise alive male could not function as a sperm donor. In addition, neocortically dead but otherwise alive pregnant women have been sustained until parturition.[22] Such bodies meet one of the significant criteria for biological liveliness, namely, repro-ductive capacity.

It is because brain-dead but otherwise alive human bodies are biologically alive that it was so difficult for the general public to accept whole-brain-oriented definitions of the death of persons. An example of this difficulty is provided by a 1952 Kentucky case, *Grey et al.* v. *Sawyer et al.*, in which it was important for purposes of inheritance to determine which of two individuals

died first. One individual, who was decapitated in the accident, had continued to spurt blood from her carotids after her companion no longer
demonstrated a pulse. As the court record indicates, she was found "decapitated, her head lying about ten feet from her body, which was actively
bleeding 'from near her neck and blood was gushing from her body in
spurts...'" However, physicians testified to the court that "a body is not
dead so long as there is a heartbeat and that may be evidenced by the gushing
of blood in spurts."[23] For us, the determination of the court is ludicrous, in
that we accept a whole-brain-oriented standard. When we read this case, we
understand that the head of the decapitated woman began to suffer from
anoxia at least at the same time as the brain of her companion. We have gone
through a major paradigm shift in our understanding of what it means to be
alive and embodied in this world.

Being there

These philosophical reflections concerning the life of persons and the
meaning of embodiment can be put in terms of a rather straightforward
fantasy. Imagine that one consults one's neurologist and is diagnosed as
suffering from a serious neurological disease. The bad news is that it will
destroy one's whole brain. The good news is that due to the advances in
medicine a normal life expectancy can still be assured. If one's reaction to this
information is not simply that such a life would be of no use to oneself, but
that one would *not be there* for the life to be either useful or useless, one has
embraced a whole-brain-oriented concept of death.

The step toward a neocortically oriented (or more precisely, a higher-
brain-centers-oriented) definition of death is taken when the physician
returns the next day, stating that the bad news is not that bad. Though the
patient will lose the entire cerebrum, the lower brain stem, pons, and
cerebellum will be able to be preserved. The patient will be able to continue
normal breathing unsustained by a respirator. However, there will be no
sentience, no experience of the world; the patient will be permanently
comatose. If one still concludes that one would not be there, not just that
such life would be useless, one has taken the further step toward a higher-
brain-centers-oriented concept of death. One has concluded that whatever it
means to be in the world as a person requires at a minimum some level of
sentience and consciousness. The mere persistence of biological functions is
not sufficient. One recognizes the higher brain centers as a necessary
condition for the life of persons because they are required for even a
minimum of conscious awareness. When there is no cerebrum, there is no
person. One also recognizes that the mere existence of a brain stem, pons,
and cerebellum is insufficient for the life of a person (or even the life of a

mind). A functioning and intact brain stem, pons, and cerebellum do not of themselves secure the existence of a person, because they are not sufficient for consciousness. In short, if the cerebrum is dead, the person is dead.

For reasons of caution, one may still wish not to employ higher-brain-centers-oriented tests for determining death, even though one accepts as an intellectual point a higher-brain-center-oriented concept of death. The basis may be a fear of an inordinate number of false positive determinations of death. Such a position would lead one to decide that avoiding such risks is worth the costs of false negative determinations. There is also the problem of the emotional and social costs of disposing of a body whose higher brain centers are dead but that is still spontaneously breathing. As a result, one may judge that individuals such as Karen Quinlan are long dead, though one may not wish to establish a policy of declaring such individuals dead because of its adverse consequences.

Despite these hesitations, we appear to be moving to higher-brain-centers-oriented definitions in much the same way we moved toward whole-brain-oriented definitions of death. Though the law does not allow such individuals to be declared dead, it is becoming acceptable to stop all treatment for such individuals if their relatives agree. The President's Commission for the Study of Ethical Problems in Medicine and Biomedical and Behavioral Research made the following recommendation in its March 21, 1983, report:

The decisions of patient's families should determine what sort of medical care permanently unconscious patients receive. Other than requiring appropriate decision-making procedures for these patients, the law does not and should not require any particular therapies to be applied or continued, with the exception of basic nursing care that is needed to ensure dignified and respectful treatment of the patient.[24]

The meaning of "basic nursing care" has been resolved in at least one jurisdiction through the case of *The People* v. *Barber*, in which the Court of Appeals of the Second Appellate District of California held that stopping all treatment, including the provision of intravenous hydration and nourishment, on a permanently comatose individual at the behest of his family, and in the absence of a contrary opinion expressed by the patient while competent, did not constitute murder.[25]

Permanently unconscious individuals currently fall into a limbo between those individuals recognized to be persons alive and in the world, and those unambiguously recognized as dead. That it is licit to stop all treatment, including intravenous hydration and nutrition, seems only reasonable in that there is no one home in the body to suffer from the dehydration and starvation or to derive pleasure from hydration and nutrition.[26] On the other hand, would it be justifiable for patients or their families to demand treatment under such circumstances? Should one convict an individual of murder who killed such a body? The arguments to this point suggest an answer in the negative on all these points. To demand to keep such bodies alive, other than for purposes such as research, would appear to be unreasonable in that one would not be sustaining someone's life. There would be no general grounds to require such an expenditure of money and energy. One would not be obliged to honor such a request unless prior special guarantees had been made. Such bodies, since they are recognized no longer to be the embodiment of persons or even of a mind, cannot even be the object of beneficence. If others wish to sustain a corpse, that should be their prerogative, if they have private funds. Also, an individual who killed such a body may very well be guilty of a moral offense, as is the desecrator of a corpse, but the offense would not be that of murder. There would be no one there in the body to kill. Malpractice awards could not be made to sustain the lives of such entities.

The problem is where to draw the line. One may not be clear how much consciousness is required for there to be the life of a person. Again, it is for such reasons that one may err on the conservative side. Thus, one may require the lack of all electroencephalographic activity, in the absence of hypothermia or central nervous system depressants, to declare death, even though the presence of some EEG activity will surely be insufficient to establish the presence of a person. Such an approach may be acceptable because it is clear that the capacity for EEG activity is a necessary condition for the embodiment of human persons, although it is far from clear how much EEG activity, and of what kind, is *sufficient* for the life of a person. One may be willing to accept the absence of all sentience and consciousness as a criterion for the death of a person, though the presence of minimal sentience and consciousness will not be sufficient for the presence of a person. Even a higher-brain-centers-oriented definition of death, which required destruction of the *entire* neocortex, would be conservative.

An illustration of the problem of such borderline cases is provided by In re Claire C. Conroy, which involved a petition to discontinue naso-gastric feeding on an eighty-four-year-old woman, who suffered from organic brain syndrome. A chancery court initially ruled that the patient's guardian had a right to remove the nasogastric tube,[27] the Superior Court held to the contrary,[28] and the Supreme Court of New Jersey reversed. It held that all treatment, including artificial feeding, may be discontinued, even when there was no instruction from the patient, as long as (1) there was no instruction to the contrary, and (2) the harms of continued existence, especially pain, outweighed the benefits to the patient. The ruling was limited to nursing home patients and special conditions were set.[29] Though Conroy suffered from severe organic brain syndrome, as the Superior Court noted, she was neither comatose nor in a vegetative state. She was still able to move her hands voluntarily and smile when her hair was combed, although she was unable to communicate and was severely demented. One's view of cases such as Conroy's will depend on (1) how much of a mental life one judges to be sufficient for the life of a person, and (2) the protection one holds is due to entities that are the successors of persons. The facts of the Conroy case appear to make the claim implausible that she was still a moral agent. However, we may have concerns for those states of mental life dimly illuminated by reason that may succeed the persons we were, should we become severely demented.

This is an ontological problem: how ought we to regard the imperfectly unified mental life of the severely senile? It is too easy simply to say that they should be regarded only on a par with other animals that possess similar levels of mental life. They surely possess at least the rights of such animals. These human entities also once *were* persons. One knows who they were. Such entities have a moral status quite different from that of children and the profoundly mentally retarded, who are not yet, or who will never become, persons in the strict sense. One does not know in these cases who they will be. Here one may have moral obligations to those former persons with respect to their bodies as one has obligations to honor the testamentary wishes of the dead. Indeed, in such borderline cases one will have duties to such entities (1) because of the persons they were, (2) because of the actual persons to whom they belong (i.e., their family), (3) because of one's unclarity regarding the extent to which such former persons live on in a successor entity (i.e., a mental life which is no longer that of a moral agent), and (4) because of the adverse social consequences for practices of giving sympathy and aid to those in need that may follow from removing protections from such entities, which are still minimally sentient.

The first and second points by themselves would only support respectful treatment of the body as one now treats corpses. These points would perhaps justify basic nursing care, as long as the body of a former person dies. It is the last consideration, along with a modified version of the third point, which has the greatest force. They already support the practice of imputing many of the rights of persons strictly to young children and the very severely mentally retarded. By making permanent loss of consciousness the point at which humans are declared dead, one would be able to establish a practice that would provide uniformity for the declaration of death for infants, the retarded, adults, and the senile. One would also resolve in a conservative fashion the issue of the treatment of entities with a mental life that may succeed the life of a human person. This approach would also require not imputing a social sense of person to anencephalic infants or other infants born with similar profound neurological defects. Individuals such as Claire Conroy will be treated as alive and individuals such as Karen Quinlan declared dead.

Toward a higher-brain-centers definition of death

We have been brought to the conclusion that a whole-brain-oriented concept
of death is insufficient. Whatever we mean by persons requires at least the
presence of that sentience that is lost forever to the permanently comatose.
Whole-brain-oriented definitions of death focus on structures that are
insufficient for the embodiment of persons. This error, implicit in whole-
brain definitions generally, was made even worse by the Uniform Determination of Death Act proposed by the President's Commission for the Study
of Ethical Problems in Medicine and Biomedical and Behavioral Research in
its July 9, 1981, report, *Defining Death*. That act retreated from proposals
that clearly accented the brain as the embodiment of the life of persons.
Consider here the sparse clarity of the American Bar Association's 1975
model statute: "For all legal purposes, a human body with irreversible
cessation of total brain function, according to usual and customary standards of medical practice, shall be considered dead."[30] In contrast, the
President's Commission underscored the importance of brain stem function
for the life of individuals. It also explicitly incorporated a circulatory and
respiratory test for death.

An individual who has sustained either (1) irreversible cessation of circulatory and
respiratory functions, or (2) irreversible cessation of all functions of the entire brain,
including the brain stem, is dead. A determination of death must be made in
accordance with accepted medical standards.[31]

The proposed act is a conceptual step backward.

First, there is no need explicitly to incorporate a circulatory and respiratory test for death. If circulatory and respiratory functions fail for only a
short period of time, the brain will die. Failure of circulatory and respiratory
function can be used in most circumstances as a test for brain death in accord
with "the usual and customary standards of medical practice". One need
only explicitly focus on a determination of brain function when circulatory
and respiratory function continues after possible brain death. Second, and
even more disturbing, is the commission's attempt to construe the importance of the brain, not as the sponsor of consciousness, but rather as either the
primary organ for integrating the functions of the major organ systems, or as
a hallmark for bodily integration.[32] The commission's report represents an
endeavor to reconstrue the whole-brain definition of death in organismic and
vitalistic terms, rather than to acknowledge its implications for a correct
understanding of the special significance of the embodiment of persons in
their brains. To put it somewhat bluntly, the commission has attempted to
turn the whole-body definition of death into a special test for whole-body
death. For the commission, the death of the brain was seen to be important in

signaling the death of the body as an integrated whole. This approach serves as well to impede the development of a higher-brain-centers definition of death. This last point advances a barrier in principle to adopting a higher-brain-centers-oriented definition of death in suggesting that a body with a living brain stem, but without a living cerebrum, is still a person.

Given the circumstance that human bodies whose higher brain centers are dead have no mental life (and, as I have argued, are therefore not moral subjects, much less persons), the only general, secular grounds for hesitation with respect to the adoption of higher-brain-centers-oriented definitions of death (in the absence of special, e.g., religious, agreements) will be consequence-oriented ones (issues in part recognized by the commission). First, one may be concerned whether higher-brain-centers-oriented tests for death will not involve the risk of a significant number of false positive determinations. Such is a technological problem that is likely superable. The enduring moral issues will turn on the psychological costs involved in discontinuing treatment as a matter of course on permanently comatose individuals. For example, the commission finds it difficult to declare cerebrally dead but otherwise alive bodies to be no longer the embodiments of persons.[33] Will generally allowing such individuals to die of dehydration and starvation have an adverse impact on important moral virtues and practices? Would active steps to effect death have significant adverse effects? The reflections of the President's Commission appear to be in the negative on the first point (the commission presumably would be positive on the second point). Societies would need to investigate carefully the costs of the second. Likely, in time, as people came to understand that such interventions to expedite death are not against any person (no one is at home in the body), such actions would cease to carry the danger of undermining the virtues of character that protect persons. Also, given concerns about state abuse of power, and because of the limits of state authority, authority to expedite the death of such entities should probably be in private hands.

Certain communities because of their beliefs will not be able to accept a higher-brain-centers-oriented definition, as many currently cannot accept a whole-brain-oriented definition of death. One might think here of the Orthodox Jewish position that an individual is dead only when the last breath is drawn.[34] There would never be grounds to use force to prevent individuals of communities from using private resources to sustain the biological life of a body with whole-brain or higher-brain-centers death. One might even in such cases agree to allow wills to become operative for such communities only when the testators' criteria for whole-body or whole-brain tests for death had been met. The use of state power to enforce such wills might not be too costly. On the other hand, it would be improper for the state to punish as murder actions taken by others to terminate the lives of such entities (human bodies without living neocortices). Murder is the taking of life of a person, and there are no generally available arguments to establish that such entities have a mental life, much less that they are persons. From a general secular point of view, such killings would need to be regarded as lesser crimes than murder, such as the violation of a corpse. The crime would need to be understood as a violation of the wishes of the family of the dead individual whose body it had been.

Abortion, harm to fetuses, and infanticide

The previous section of this chapter focused on the endings of human life. Because the deaths of persons are not always coincident with the cessation of the biological lives of their bodies, we faced a number of puzzles. Here we encounter reciprocal puzzles. The start of human biological life is not quickly followed by the beginning of the life of a person. Rather, in human ontogeny months of biological life transpire before there is good evidence of the life of a mind, and years go by before there is evidence of the life of a person. As a result, the moral status of zygotes, embryos, fetuses, and even infants is problematic.

As we saw in chapter 4, it is not plausible to hold that fetuses are persons in in the strict sense. In fact, there is not even evidence to hold that infants are persons in the strict sense. Whatever sort of mental life might exist for fetuses and infants, it is minimal, so that the moral standing of adult mammals, ceteris paribus, would be higher than that of human fetuses or infants. Despite this state of affairs, many established practices in Western culture discourage the killing of human fetuses and newborns, more so than killing adult great apes. From the vantage point of arguments sustainable in general secular terms, these practices can at best be understood as imputing, because of its usefulness, certain rights of persons to these forms of human biological life. As argued in chapter 4, these practices involve treating instances of human biological life within a social sense of person. These practices have similarities with the ways in which we treat the very senile and severely demented adults. There is a difference in that one does not yet know the persons that the fetuses or newborns may with luck become, as one knows who the very senile once were.

In the case of death, we saw the recognized line between personhood and nonpersonhood move from whole-body death to whole-brain death to a proposal to employ higher-brain-centers death. This movement constitutes a retreat from imputing the status of persons to a set of individuals who are not persons strictly, but who were once treated as persons in the social sense. A superficial symmetry had existed between the use of whole-body definitions of death and life as the lines of demarcation for the imputing of personhood.

One withdrew the status of being a person when the last breath was drawn; one gave the status of personhood when the first breath was drawn. With the introduction of a whole-brain definition of death one might in error seek a new symmetry. This search might falsely suggest that the criterion of the absence of EEG activity, which had been adopted as a test for death, might in reverse serve as a test for the beginning of the life of a person. One would then in error decide that when EEG activity begins, a person begins. In the declaration of death the presence of EEG activity is used as a test for a necessary, not a sufficient, condition for the presence of a person. The presence of EEG activity does not show the presence of a person. There is no evidence at all that fetuses are moral agents.

The symmetry, lost when one moved to a whole-brain definition of death, will not be regained with a higher-brain-centers definition. At the end of life one is trying to mark when consciousness ceases. When, with the partial death of the higher brain centers consciousness becomes greatly obtunded, it may still not be certain that the life of the person has ended. On the other hand, when only the first most meager indications of consciousness begin, one can be sure that there is not yet a person in the strict sense. The presence of some neocortical activity is not sufficient for the presence of a moral agent. This asymmetry stems from the fact that with dying persons one knows who is dying and one may have special duties to them to protect their interests, even in a twilight zone of nonpersonal mental life. In the case of fetuses and newborns, one does not yet know who they will be. There are no special duties to persons who are not yet extant. In contrast, one can have made special promises to dead persons regarding the care of their corpses. Also, in the case of death, one has a concern to avoid practices that may expose oneself to the risks of false positive or premature determinations of death. In the case of fetuses and newborn children, there is no such risk; there is no evidence that they are in some clandestine fashion moral agents. At most one has a duty not to malevolently injure the future persons the fetuses may become.

The status of zygotes, embryos, and fetuses

To understand the moral status of the beginning of human biological life, one will need to examine how that life is important for persons. Since that life is not the life of a person strictly, the persons involved will not be embodied in that life. If a human fetus has more than the moral status of an animal with a similar level of development, it will be because of the significance of that life for the woman who has conceived it, for others around her who may be interested in it, and for the future person it may become.

Considered simply in and of itself, a zygote, an embryo, or a fetus can make a claim on us as would an animal with a similar level of development and capacity for pain and suffering. Given the minimal development of such human life, the moral claim is minimal as well. It would require a sort of moral fineness (if not wrongheadedness) to choose a less optimal abortion procedure in order to minimize the risk of pain and suffering to the fetus. If one assigned such a substantial significance to the pain of fetuses, one would be forced as well to take very seriously the pain of organisms with a similar level of mental capacity. That seems implausible. Organisms of the general development of fetuses do not show the capacity for suffering possessed by adult cats, dogs, or monkeys. It is enough if one offers a sincere, nonmalevolent reason to justify such pain. Imposing pain on a human fetus might thus be justified because a particular abortion procedure minimizes the health risks to the woman, is more convenient for the woman, or more effectively ensures the death of the fetus. (See chapter 4 for an analysis of the claims of animals.)

Such choices are not only within the rights of women since they, not fetuses, are persons, but those choices are innocent of a disproportionate harm to the fetuses as instances of animal life. It is highly unlikely that fetuses with their underdeveloped and underconnected frontal lobes are able to experience suffering, even if they are able to experience pain. Suffering requires an appreciation of pain as threatening, as negative, as something to be avoided. Suffering requires more than simply a noxious quale. It requires an appreciation of that quale, that sensation, as something improper, harmful, and hurtful. It is questionable whether early-gestation fetuses even experience pain. Withdrawal reflexes occasioned by noxious stimuli do not demonstrate an experience of that stimulus as a negative sensation. A fetus's pain has no significance for that fetus, because giving significance to pain is beyond its scope; such would require a reflective capacity, which even neonates do not possess.

For this reason, one turns to those to whom fetuses belong in order to determine their worth. The fetus of a woman who wants a child takes on considerable significance. It gains value from her interests and love, and that of others around her. The would-be mother, father, grandmothers, grandfathers, uncles, and aunts can vest a wanted embryo or fetus with great value. The opposite can obtain as well. Because of the circumstances of the conception, the probable circumstances of the birth, or because the fetus is defective or deformed, a negative worth may be given. The fetus may be seen as something that is threatening, harmful, disvalued, or even hated.

Those who are most closely involved have the first claim on determining the value of the fetus. This is usually the father and mother who conceived it, expecially the woman because she is bearing it. They produced it, they made it, it is theirs. The fetus can be seen as a special form of very dear property:

the biological lineage of a family, a couple's attempt to fashion another person on whom to bestow their love and give their care and concern. Others may become involved with the procreators through special agreements. One might think of surrogate motherhood or of the insertion in a woman of an embryo, conceived with another woman's ovum and an anonymous third party's sperm. The procreators can contractually transfer their rights, as is the case if an embryo were donated, or maintain them if the woman serves only as a temporary host. But the point remains the same. It is persons who endow zygotes, embryos, or fetuses with value. Those who made or pro-created the zygote, embryo, or fetus have first claim on making the definitive determination of value. Privately produced embryos and fetuses are private property.

Societal groups through various communal choices may support some pregnancies but not others. They may provide or hold back funds that would increase or hinder reproduction. There may be a choice to fund a program that either will decrease miscarriages in a third-world country with unchecked population growth or preserve the country's wild life. One might decide that the country is already overpopulated with humans. On the other hand, many species of mammals are in danger of extinction. It would be quite reasonable to invest money in wildlife refuges rather than in a program to decrease miscarriages in a country with an unchecked population increase. In fact, if there were two diseases, one causing an increased rate of miscarriages among humans in such a country and another among an endangered species of nonhuman mammals, one might properly see investing in research to save the nonhuman mammals as having a higher priority. Once such a country solves its demographic and economic problems, it can always turn to address the diseases that increase the rate of miscarriages.

Though society may offer incentives for reproductive actions or omissions of various sorts, the limited authority of the state and the status of the fetus as private property make it improper to use unconsented-to force to determine the abortion choices of women. Unless the procreators have transferred their rights to others (e.g., by donating the embryo to another woman or couple), they have a right to abort the fetus, even if others would gladly adopt the child it could become. The parents, and especially the woman, have produced the fetus. Next to one's own body, the sperm, ova, zygotes, and fetuses one produces are most primordially one's own. They are the extension of and fruit of one's own body. They are one's own to dispose of until they take possession of themselves as conscious entities, until one gives them a special standing in a community, or until one transfers one's rights in them to another. As a result, it is within the rights of parents to decide whether that extension of themselves should fall into others' hands. They have a right to decide that they do not wish to be parents even in the limited sense of having produced a child for adoption. The sense of right here draws attention to the lack of authority of others to impose their will on such private choices.

One might imagine courts being invited to resolve conflicts between prospective fathers and mothers with respect to conflicting wishes regarding whether to procure an abortion. Since it will be quite difficult to determine who promised whom what, and out of respect for the privacy of the family as a social unit, it would appear prudent to follow the example of the United States Supreme Court in not intervening with state force to resolve such issues.[35] Since the woman is investing the major energies in developing the fetus, and in that it would be her body that would be the subject of control, it would be appropriate to allow her the legally protected choice. Arrangements with the father would need to be worked out privately as an understanding within the family. On the other hand, a prospective father's offer to pay the costs of an abortion should prevent a suit for child support if the father is not the husband of the mother. A woman who proceeds with a pregnancy under such circumstances (i.e., without a prior explicit or implicit commitment by the father to help raise the child) does so for her own reasons and at her own risk, not that of the father. The same protection against costs of child care should be available to men who renounce all interests in having a child as a part of a prenuptial or similar agreement.

State force could with moral probity be used to prevent a surrogate mother from seeking to abort a fetus she has contracted to bring to term. The state may choose to enforce contracts of various sorts. But, though there is a moral right to use such force, there is no duty to do so if greater harm would come from enforcing such contracts. In the absence of special contracts, abortion choices should be made without the threat of force or coercion. Others may lament what I do with that which is mine. But in that it is mine, it falls to me to make the final choice regarding its disposition, including the disposition of zygotes, embryos, and fetuses.

Wrongful life

There is an important limitation. If one decides not to abort a fetus, if one decides not to kill it, one must take care not to injure the future person it may become. Injuring the fetus, unlike killing it, sets into motion a causal chain that may injure the future person the fetus will become. This moral obligation to refrain from actions that will injure a fetus likely in the future to become a person has been explored in the law under the rubric of tort for wrongful life. Tort-for-wrongful-life suits must be contrasted with tort-for-wrongful-conception and tort-for-wrongful-birth suits, in which individuals have sued because they have been harmed by the failure of a contraceptive or of a sterilization process.[36] In tort-for-wrongful-life suits, the child has sued for being born under circumstances connected with injury or harm.

What is interesting about such suits is that the plaintiff is complaining of a harm that could have been avoided only by not conceiving that individual or by having aborted that individual. The history of these suits has been somewhat colorful. They have included an action by an illegitimate son against his father, arguing that to be born a bastard in Illinois was a harm (unlike some other states where it is a qualification for being elected to political office), for which the child should be able to collect financial damages.[37] That suit was unsuccessful, as were others such as one brought by a girl conceived when her mother was raped by a fellow mental-hospital inmate in the state of New York.[38]

New ground was broken by a California appellate court in *Curlender* v. *Bio-Science Laboratories*.[39] The court not only awarded damages for a tort-for-wrongful-life claim to the couple and to the child of the couple, who had been misinformed that they were not carriers of Tay-Sachs disease, but also added in a dictum that had the information been properly transmitted by the laboratory and by the physician, the parents could have been sued by their child. The court argued that there was a parental duty to avoid the birth of defective children. Knowing procreation of a defective child was held to be a negligent act, actionable under tort law.[40] As a moral issue, this view appears implausible if the future life of the child is such that harms do not outweigh benefits. One will on balance not have harmed *that* future person. If it is reasonable for the parents to assume that there will be a favorable balance of goods over harms to the child, procreation would be morally justified as long as the child did not constitute an unagreed-upon burden on communal resources.

An interesting scholastic question is raised because the analysis of this issue requires distinguishing between foreseen and intended harms. Are there circumstances under which it is allowable to reproduce, foreseeing, but not intending, harms to one's child?[41] Perhaps one can imagine the case of a king in a constitutional monarchy who must reproduce in order to pass on his line and where in the absence of an heir a repressive government would be established, but where the heir would inherit a very painful disease. The issue is whether procreating a person under circumstances in which the conception is unavoidably tied to future harms should count as an unconsented-to injury to that future person. If existence is tied to the injury itself, and the injury is not intended but only foreseen, has one violated another's autonomy?

This question must be answered in part by an understanding of what it means to produce a child. One need not produce a child for that child's sake. A great number of the children born are probably not directly intended or explicitly planned. They are rather the result of habit and accident. Even those planned may not be procreated for their sake alone. In fact, such is likely rarely the case. People conceive children because of the need for agricultural laborers and for support in old age. They do so as well because of a deep human desire to have children, to have the companionship and love of others, but not simply to do good to those others by giving them existence. There are as well traditional goals such as the continuation of families and traditions that require fashioning another generation. Such can make procreation a fairly selfless and dedicated act, even if not directed primarily to the child. In any event, children are produced for goals that are not theirs, but that may become theirs, and to which they have not consented. The gift of life is given along with burdens.

Given the opacity of the future, which includes our ignorance of the preferences of future individuals, if one acts in a nonmalevolent way toward those future individuals, one has not violated the very notion of a peaceable community. This is so even if in the future those individuals who are conceived do not celebrate the consequences of that procreation. Bear in mind, there will not be specific duties of beneficence to future individuals. One will not be required (in general secular terms) to provide them with any special legacy of goods (though providing a legacy would surely be praise-worthy). Without appealing to a particular moral community and its vision of the good life, perhaps the most one would be required to provide as a legacy would be a state of life no worse than that available to humans prior to the development of any particular culture or technology—a sort of status quo prior to any transformation of the world in terms of visions of the good life. To require more than that is to appeal to a particular vision of the good life, and to impose it on actual persons. But such impositions on future persons are unavoidable and not improper, since such persons do not exist and therefore do not have a particular understanding of the good life. Choosing for them does not violate the principle of beneficence. Nor does it violate the principle of autonomy since future individuals cannot disagree or refuse such actions. There is a problem of giving content to the principle of autonomy when the persons are not yet actual.

The notion of the peaceable community will preclude certain acts against future persons. If the bomb setter mentioned in chapter 4 sets a bomb to explode years in the future so as to kill future individuals, it seems plausible to hold that the bomb setter has not only acted in a nonbeneficent fashion, but has violated the autonomy rights of those future individuals. The bomb setter would have acted in a way that can reasonably be presumed to be against the wishes of those future persons. Such an action against future persons must be done under the assumption that one will not only be harming those injured, but harming them against their will. But where the wishes of future persons are far from certain, the most one can say with surety is that one should not directly act to affect those persons in ways that are very likely to be against their wishes. One is allowed a great deal of leeway in acting on one's own view of the good life when it comes to possible future persons, because of the difficulty in showing that one is acting against the general notion of a peaceable and beneficent community of persons. To live in the future is to be at the mercy of past visions of the good life and to be forced to receive their benefits and their banes. Parents frequently must make such choices. They choose in nonmalevolent fashions futures their children may or may not find pleasant. They cannot secure their infants' permission. They cannot even know with certainty that their infants will become persons to be benefited or hurt by their plans. At most, they are forbidden to reproduce when it appears likely that harms to the child will outweigh benefits. In such circumstances, the presumption must be that the child would not consent to such circumstances.

These reflections apply to our puzzles about conceiving or allowing a pregnancy to go to term when one recognizes that the child will face severe pain and hardship as a consequence of a genetic disease or defect. As long as (1) there is no malevolent intent, and (2) likely benefits to the future child outweigh likely harms (so as not to create a circumstance in which life would not be worth living), and, one might add, (3) there is no coercive force against children when in the future they wish to emancipate themselves, even through suicide, once they appreciate and understand the nature of their circumstances, then there is no violation of either the principle of autonomy or that of beneficence. Within particular moral communities there may be special moral principles, including special principles of beneficence, to forbid such reproduction. The first point acknowledges that the achievement of goods is rarely unmixed with harms. One cannot ask that all harms be avoided, only that they not be intended. If they are intended, the action becomes one against the principle of beneficence, even if the individual consents. The second point addresses the problem of the consent of future persons by forbidding actions that would clearly be against their wishes. The last point also underscores the obligation consequent upon the principle of autonomy not to do injury to a third party without that individual's permission. Once the child can understand and appreciate the circumstances in which it lives, it must be able to free itself from an unbearable state.[42] With respect to the moral issues raised by tort-for-wrongful-life suits, we can conclude that, within certain constraints, it is not morally forbidden to conceive a pregnancy and allow it to go to term, knowing that it carries with it genetic or other congenital harms.

Interventions on behalf of the fetus: cesarean sections,
fetal surgery, and civil commitment

These reflections apply not only to decisions to reproduce, knowing that the child will carry a genetic defect. They apply as well to the putative right of the state to force a woman to submit to surgical and medical interventions to prevent damage to her fetus or to cure fetal diseases or defects. This issue has been joined in a number of recent cases in which women have been compelled to submit to cesarean sections to preserve the life and/or health of the fetus. One of these, *Jessie Mae Jefferson* v. *Griffin Spalding County Hospital Authority*, was decided by the Supreme Court of Georgia, which ordered a cesarean delivery, though a vaginal one in fact occurred.[43] The case concerned a woman with a placenta previa in her thirty-ninth week of pregnancy. As a member of the Shiloh Sanctified Holiness Baptist Church of Butts County, Georgia, her religious scruples brought her to refuse a cesarean section. A vaginal delivery would have led to profuse bleeding from the placenta, which could be avoided only by a cesarean section. The court was given evidence that the fetus stood a 99 percent chance of dying and the woman a 50 percent chance of dying if a cesarean were not approved. Given this information, Justice Hill observed, "We weighed the right of the mother to practice her religion and to refuse surgery on herself, against her unborn child's right to live. We found in favor of her child's right to live."[44]

This court ruling raises a number of puzzles. Why should it be wrong for someone to refuse lifesaving treatment for herself and for her fetus? The court in *Jessie Mae Jefferson* found grounds for intruding on the basis of the fetus's viability. Thus, it raised the issue of whether some of the rights of persons should be imputed to fetuses, or at least viable fetuses. As we saw in chapter 4, infants become persons through having most of the rights of persons in a strict sense imputed to them. This is currently not the case with fetuses, for even viable fetuses may be aborted to save the life or health of the mother. In this case the court also intruded because by declining a cesarean section the woman risked her life as well. However, we have already seen that competent individuals have a prima facie right to commit suicide, a point to which we will return in the next chapter. But there is the additional issue that if the fetus does not die, it may be harmed. This returns us to the issue joined in the last section, the duty of parents to avoid harming the future individuals their fetuses may become. There we concluded that it was allowable for the parents to engage in reproductive activities they could foresee would bring harm to the child to be born, as long as the parents did not intend that harm, as long as they could reasonably hold that benefits to the child would outweigh harms, and as long as the children in the future could commit suicide if they came to a contrary conclusion. In order to understand the duties of women to submit to cesarean sections, fetal surgery, or other interventions to preserve the health of their fetuses, we will need to address the issue of injuries that take place during gestation.

The similarity of these issues to general issues of parenting must be stressed. Children are set at risk when their parents choose dangerous areas to live, work, or vacation. The choice to live in an inner-city area rather than a small town frequently entails risks not only to the parents but to the children as well. Similarly, individuals in the last century who migrated to the American West often made a choice that exposed themselves and their children to danger. So, too, individuals who maintain certain traditional ways of life, such as the BaMbuti discussed previously, may expose their children to a much higher infant mortality than would be the case were they to live otherwise. Parents usually make such choices in order to secure a favorable balance of benefits for the family. Such choices are made because of the availability of jobs or social support, because of the virtues of a traditional way of life, or because the promises of a new frontier make the risks worthwhile. They are usually understood as proper choices in terms of a particular understanding of the good life to which the parents subscribe.

Parents also expose their children to risks as a part of their lifestyle, and without a justification in terms of their vision of the good parent. Parents often smoke, drink, or ski, not because they believe such actions help fashion a moral community that will benefit their children, but simply because they enjoy them. Are such actions illicit? Again, an answer will depend on the extent to which a foreseeable but nonintended risk to a future child is incompatible with the notion of the peaceable, beneficent community. If it were to violate the notion of the peaceable community, it would be forbidden under the principle of autonomy. If it were to violate the notion of the beneficent community, it would be forbidden under the principle of beneficence.

How is one to test whether actions violate the principle of autonomy when the individuals involved are merely possible future persons? My proposal so far has been that malevolent actions against such persons are incompatible with the notion of a peaceable community. But what about irresponsible actions? What of those individuals who recognize that their actions are not beneficent, but who deny that the actions are malevolent? Let us consider here the case of a woman who smokes or drinks, recognizing that this may pose a hazard to her fetus. She does not smoke or drink in order to injure her fetus; in fact, she wishes the fetus well. She is simply of the opinion that the claims of the fetus on her are not strong enough to force her to change such habits. She may claim that the future person who that fetus may become should be happy that it has the gift of life and that it should not protest about possible detriments due to her habits. If the child is not satisfied with the gift it receives, it will surely be free to liberate itself from the burdens through suicide.

As has been argued in the last section, more is required here. If one harms a fetus so that it is likely that the future person will not find life worth living, providing the option of suicide will not be sufficient to defend one against the charge of having acted contrary to the principles of autonomy and benefi-cence. One will have acted to produce a future person, knowing that the individual will have to live with an unfavorable balance of benefits to harms. Under such circumstances one cannot presume that the individual would consent to be procreated. In other circumstances one can plausibly say, "Look, if I hadn't allowed you to go to term and develop into a person, you would not have the balance of benefits over harms that you possess." But when it appears that banes will outweigh benefits, one must presume that one will injure an unconsenting future person. Where it is plausible that benefits will outbalance harms, consent can be presumed. If one is in error in the latter case, at the very least one will be obliged to respect the choice of suicide. Out of considerations of beneficence, one may be constrained as well to aid and abet that suicide.

We are brought to conclude that force may not be used to compel cesarean sections, fetal surgery, or other invasions of a woman's body or to constrain her freedom so as to protect the future health of a possible future person, as long as (1) the woman's harmful omissions or commissions are not malevo-lent, and (2) the anticipated state of the future possible person is not so disadvantageous as to make life not worth living. In addition, then (3) the woman must protect the opportunities of that future person to commit suicide, should the calculations be wrong. A violation of any one of these three conditions will justify force to protect an innocent future person. However, a qualification must be added to the second condition. The mere residence of a fetus in a woman's womb cannot be enough to establish duties to the person the fetus may become that are strong enough to oblige the woman to submit to serious risks to health of life. The omission or commission on the part of the woman that leads to a negative balance of harms over benefits cannot justify state intrusion if the omission or commis-sion is a part of her strategy to protect herself against serious threats to her life and health, which threats she could not have reasonably anticipated and avoided without serious burdens. The woman must have had an opportunity to avoid duties to the future person who may develop from the fetus before she can be responsible for injuries to that future person whose body is developing without consent as a trespasser in her body. For example, a woman who is raped and not provided with funds for an abortion has a defense against state interventions on behalf of the fetus. However, if she refuses an abortion when it is offered, in the absence of strong moral beliefs forbidding abortion, she must then take steps to ensure that the person the fetus may become will likely have a life worth living.

But why may a woman not choose a late abortion or infanticide to prevent harm to the person the fetus could become? If the woman is faced with the need for a cesarean section or fetal surgery to protect the future health of the child, may she agree to infanticide to preclude any possibility of injuring the person the child will become? If that option were available, there would be no risk to the future person. We will need to turn next to the issue of infanticide before we can fully answer our puzzles concerning the duties of women to their fetuses.

Before we turn to these more controversial issues, it is worth noting that our reflections in this section do not leave us with radical conclusions. They restore us to the traditional understandings of the duties of women to their fetuses. Until recently, there was no serious threat of women being forced to forgo the use of major tranquilizers to control their psychoses and to be committed instead to a mental hospital in order to avoid possible risks to their fetuses, or to submit to cesareans against their will.[45] The arguments in this section would secure things more or less as they traditionally have been: women would not need to fear being forced to submit to caesarean sections or fetal surgery without their consent, except in circumstances where the outcome for the possible future person would be worse than no life at all, and then only when the woman, if pregnant with an unavoidable pregnancy, had had a reasonable opportunity to abort the fetus (in the absence of moral impedimenta) rather than face such rigors. There would be grounds for intervening, but the tests would be very stringent.

The conclusions of this and the last section are not meant to undermine the ideal of responsible reproduction. The use of genetic counseling, prenatal diagnosis, and abortion where necessary in order to avoid the birth of a defective child can reflect an exemplary commitment of beneficence to the children one wishes to have. In those circumstances where the birth would cause unavoidable costs to society, which costs society does not wish to accept, there can be a morally enforceable obligation to use such modalities. As knowledge regarding the genetic basis of diseases increases and the capacity to make prenatal diagnoses develops, there will be even greater opportunities to intervene so as to avoid harms to one's children. It will be morally improper to hinder the access of men and women to the knowledge and services required in order to take advantage of these opportunities. It will be good to take advantage of such opportunities. However, these sections have shown the limits of legitimate state authority in requiring that one use such opportunities.

Infanticide

An examination of infanticide must begin with the observation that it has been widely practiced throughout the world as a means not only of disposing of deformed newborns, but of controlling population. It is difficult to argue that there is a close connection between the practice of infanticide and the general civility of a population. In the Middle Ages, when infanticide was officially condemned, there was persecution of heretics and Jews alike. Twentieth-century Germany, which forbade infanticide, produced the tyranny of Hitler. The same may be observed with respect to the vast slaughter of the innocents perpetrated by the Soviet Union, which was also free of any official tolerance of infanticide.

Though one might associate infanticide with primitive cultures or non-European traditions, it has deep roots in Western cultural foundations. There was a wide acceptance of infanticide in the Greco-Roman world. Plato endorsed the practice of infanticide (*Republic*, V.460c). Infanticide was also recommended by Aristotle in his *Politics*: "Let there be a law that no *deformed* child shall live..."[46] One should note that the toleration of infanticide among the Athenians goes back at least to the great law-giver Solon, one of the seven wise men of Greece. Sextus Empiricus states that Solon by law legalized infanticide, though in fact he seems only to have tolerated infanticide through exposure, a practice generally accepted by the Greeks: "Solon gave the Athenians the law 'concerning things immune,' by which he allowed each man to slay his own child..."[47] Rome through the Twelve Tables did provide for explicit parental rights to commit infanticide. There even appears to have been a duty to kill deformed children. Cicero remarks in his *de Legibus*, "A dreadfully deformed child ought to be killed quickly, as the Twelve Tables ordain" (*de Legibus* III, 8, 19).

These views were incorporated in medical practice. In the oldest extant textbook of gynecology, Soranus (A.D. 98–138) included a section on how to determine whether a newborn child is worth rearing. As Soranus put it, the midwife

should also consider whether it is worth rearing or not. And the infant which is suited by nature for rearing will be distinguished by the fact that its mother has spent the period of pregnancy in good health, for conditions which require medical care, especially those of the body, also harm the fetus and enfeeble the foundations of its life. Second, by the fact that it has been born at the due time, best at the end of nine months, and if it so happens, later; but also after only seven months. Furthermore by the fact that when put on the earth it immediately cries with proper vigor; for one that lives for some length of time without crying, or cries but weakly, is suspected of behaving so on account of some unfavorable condition. Also by the fact that it is perfect in all its parts, members and senses; that its ducts, namely of the ears, nose, pharynx, urethra, anus are free from obstruction; that the natural functions of every [member] are neither sluggish nor weak; that the joints bend and stretch; that it has due size and shape and is properly sensitive in every respect. This we may recognize from pressing the fingers against the surface of the body, for it is natural to suffer pain from everything that pricks or squeezes. And by conditions contrary to those mentioned, the infant not worth rearing is recognized.[48]

This passage gives a sense of what it meant to act upon Cicero's injunction to follow the fourth Table. It provides a reasonable sketch by an intelligent physician of how to take into account factors that are predictive of futility and cost of treatment, and of quality of life.

As this history shows, the moral fabric does not appear to depend on condemning infanticide. The fabric seems to be quite able to sustain a highly advanced and intricate culture with notions of generosity and magnanimity, while not condemning the killing of newborns in general or deformed neonates in particular. As a result, it is difficult to mount a plausible, nonculturally biased, strong argument against infanticide. The best that can be produced is a speculative, circumstantial argument. It may very well be that societies will sustain with greater success virtues of sympathy and care for the defenseless, if they do not permit active or passive infanticide, except in very special cases. In addition, the availability of effective contraception, sterilization, prenatal diagnosis, and safe abortion procedures relieves many of the traditional ethical, social, and public policy pressures that favor infanticide.

A suggestive argument can be made that, in order to protect the general practice of parenting, one should forbid active or passive infanticide in the absence of special justifying circumstances. Such a proscription would need to be established on the basis of its consequences and could not be a proscription in principle, since infants are not persons in the strict sense. One could contend that it would be good to protect and sustain a moral concern for newborns by, inter alia, generally forbidding infanticide because of the good consequences such a proscription may have for the care and rearing of children and the development of important moral attitudes. Even if one endorses the establishment of such a general prohibition of infanticide, one will need to stress that infanticide is not forbidden on principle but because of its adverse social and moral consequences. As a result, exceptional circumstances will override the rule and justify infanticide (1) when the consequences of not breaking the rule are more costly than adhering to the rule, and (2) when the reasonableness of such exceptions is sufficiently apparent as not to undermine the rule itself.

Such an understanding of exceptional circumstances lies in the background of recent reflections regarding when it is appropriate to discontinue treatment for severely defective newborns. A 1973 review by Anthony B. Shaw of cases in which stopping treatment so as not to extend life might be employed suggests approval only when there are serious questions regarding the ultimate quality of life of the child and substantial costs likely to be borne by the family or society if the child is treated.[49] In fact, a review in 1973 by Raymond S. Duff and A. G. M. Campbell showed that of 299 deaths that occurred in a special-care nursery, 43 (14 percent) were related to a choice to withhold treatment. Of this group 15 newborns had multiple abnormalities; 8, trisomies (i.e., as occurs in Down's syndrome, when there are three of one chromosome, rather than a pair); 8, cardiopulmonary disease; 7, meningemyelocele (a herniation of part of the spinal cord and its covering through a defect in the vertebral column); 3, other central nervous system disorders; and 2, short bowel syndrome (insufficient small intestine).[50] The authors concluded that it was proper for parents to withhold treatment when the prognosis for "meaningful life" for the newborn was poor or hopeless.

This approach endorses the general rule of protecting and caring for newborns. It allows exceptions when the quality of outcome is low and costs are high. It is under such circumstances that we generally acknowledge that duties of beneficence are defeated. The less likely it is that a beneficent act will succeed, the less claim the duty has on us. Moreover, the greater the difficulties in discharging a duty, the easier it is to show that the duty has been defeated. Though I may generally have a duty to come to the aid of a friend dying of thirst, that duty can be defeated if the friend is at the top of a high mountain, accessible only at great risk. In addition, the less likely it is that the friend would find his quality of life acceptable if saved, the weaker the duty: the friend would likely forward a less strong claim. Also, if the friend is injured and is likely to die soon even if saved, the duty weakens as the amount of life to be secured decreases. Further, in the case of the infant, it is not yet a person to make a claim. It is not a person in the strict sense. One may properly wish to avoid persons in the strict sense coming into existence with severe handicaps, who could make major claims upon duties of beneficence. In addition, one may wish to expend major resources in order to bring persons into existence, only if that existence will be of sufficient quality and quantity. The concept of quality of outcome is itself complex, for it must include both quality of life as it is likely to be judged by those associated with that life and quality of life as it is likely to be perceived by the individual living it. The principle of beneficence can justify both interpretations. We derive both benefits and harms from our perceptions of the quality of the lives of others. As a result, all things considered, there will be circumstances when it will be proper to let the infant die, and for the couple to attempt again to produce a child who will grow to be a person without serious handicaps.

These considerations, with certain qualifications, can be expressed in an algorithm:

$$\text{Strength of the duty of beneficence} = \frac{\text{Chance of success} \times \text{Quality of life} \times \text{Length of life}}{\text{Costs}}$$

The duty to preserve the life of a newborn is defeated as the chance for success diminishes, as the quality and/or quantity of life for the newborn decreases, and as the costs of securing that quality of life increase. Appealing to such an algorithm to justify selective nontreatment pays tribute to the general prohibition of infanticide. It recognizes that exceptions should be allowed only with good justification.

Though this general approach would seem reasonable, it is difficult to establish the authority of the state to impose such a rule by force, as long as parents do not employ communal resources. The rule requires a particular ordering of harms and benefits that can be justified only with great difficulty, if at all. This is a very unpleasant conclusion but still a strong consideration in support of the proposition that the Athenian and Roman noninterference with the practices of infanticide was morally justifiable in many circumstances in terms of considerations of respecting the autonomy of the parents. To prohibit infanticide on the basis of considerations of beneficence (e.g., in order to realize a particular view of good parenting) would require establishing authority for overriding parental autonomy. It should be clear from these considerations why the onus will be on those who intervene, since the difficulty is in showing authority to impose a particular view of how to protect societies from risks and harms. Those who will defend infanticide will see the virtue of that privilege outweighing the goods that will accrue from prohibition. Because of the principle of autonomy, the burden of proof will lie on the shoulders of the interveners to show that the parents' actions are morally incorrect, rather than for the parents to show that they are acting correctly.

One can approach this problem with confidence that one can forbid at least the killing or exposure of older children who are persons in the strict sense. Also, when commitments of care have been made, implicitly or explicitly, infants can be protected by state force. Perhaps it is possible to prohibit infanticide, insofar as parents *freely* accept societal and communal support for health care and social welfare, and to endow the status of being a social person with strong protections. For the acceptance to be free, there would likely need to be sufficient acknowledgment of the rights to decline treatment under circumstances such as those outlined earlier. It is implausible to hold that most individuals would accept a general prohibition of infanticide in return for additional benefits (i.e., in addition to their payment on the basis of the general rent on the land; see chapter 4) without provision for such exceptions. Finally, states would need to acknowledge the rights of individuals to form special moral exclaves. One might think here of the Yanomamo of Brazil and Venezuela who routinely practice infanticide. Their independent life as a self-supporting social group should be sufficient to exempt them morally from Brazilian laws that stand to the contrary.[51] I will presume that, given these exceptions, and within these constraints, infanticide can in fact be prohibited. This position is an important compromise between (1) the view of those who would hold that the sanctity of life requires the preservation to the extent it is possible of the lives of all newborns, and (2) the respect of the rights of parents fully to effect their reproductive and parenting decisions.

This compromise makes it very difficult to establish viability as an upper level for abortions on request. The prohibition of infanticide involves an organism external to the mother's body. Controls on abortion involve living material that is internal to the woman's body. Even if one can envisage circumstances in which particular women have actually agreed to compromise their general liberties regarding abortion, there will likely remain a number of exceptions or restrictions. First, the generally acknowledged right of women to secure an abortion at any time on the basis of considerations of danger to life or health would likely not be ceded. Second, viability is unlikely to be accepted as a bar to an abortion when information develops late in pregnancy that the fetus is deformed or in some fashion defective.[52] And third, the concept of viability must not be understood simply as a biological phenomenon that will move ever earlier in gestation as medical technology advances, but rather as a point at which near-term infants will survive without the technological provision of what is tantamount to a surrogate womb and who therefore should be protected because of their similarity with newborn infants. Otherwise, the progress of technology would indirectly undermine the rights of women.

This progress of technology gives the issue of infanticide its modern cast through the questions it raises regarding the rights of parents to forgo the use of such technology. These new technologies have advanced our capacities to preserve the lives of newborns who are born with major physical handicaps and promise of mental handicaps, who would not have been able to survive in the past. We have the ability now not only to salvage premature infants who would have died in the past, but to salvage them at times with dim prospect of a normal life and a significant likelihood that they will suffer from severe mental deficiency, cerebral palsy, convulsions, and even hydrocephalus. The question has been when to respect parents' choices to stop treatment and to allow a child to die who would have died in the very recent past prior to current technological advances.

Recent controversies were precipitated by a case that developed from the birth on April 9, 1982, of a child with Down's syndrome complicated by esophageal atresia (i.e., no passage from the mouth to the stomach) and tracheal esophageal fistula (i.e., an anomalous connection between the windpipe and the gullet). The case of Infant Doe of Bloomington came to an informal hearing before the Indiana Supreme Court, which upheld the parents' right to refuse treatment.[53] The analyses in this volume support that court in its decision, in that significant costs are involved in raising a child with physical and mental handicaps that can defeat the usual duties of beneficence to an entity not yet a person in the strict sense. In response to this case, the federal government first imposed and then, after a judicial reversal, proposed regulations on March 7 and July 5, 1983.[54] These were contested on a number of procedural and other grounds.[55] On January 12, 1984, the government imposed the following rules on all hospitals receiving federal funds:

(i) Withholding of medical beneficial surgery to correct an intestinal obstruction in an infant with Down's Syndrome when the withholding is based upon the anticipated future mental retardation of the infant and there are no medical contraindications to the surgery that would otherwise justify withholding the surgery would constitute a discriminatory act, violative of section 504.

(ii) Withholding of treatment for medically correctable physical anomalies in children born with spina bifida when such denial is based on anticipated mental impairment, paralysis or incontinence of the infant, rather than on reasonable medical judgments that treatment would be futile, too unlikely to success given complications in the particular case, or otherwise not of medical benefit to the infant, would constitute a discriminatory act, violative of section 504.

(iii) Withholding of medical treatment for an infant born with anencephaly, who will inevitably die within a short period of time, would not constitute a discriminatory act because the treatment would be futile and do no more than temporarily prolong the act of dying.

(iv) Withholding of certain potential treatments from a severely premature and low birth weight infant on the grounds of reasonable medical judgments concerning the improbability of success or risks of potential harm to the infant would not violate section 504.[56]

The government was joined in this view by the American Academy of Pediatrics, which stated that:

When medical care is clearly beneficial, it should always be provided. When appropriate medical care is not available, arrangements should be made to transfer the infant to an appropriate medical facility. Considerations such as anticipated or actual limited potential of an individual and present or future lack of available community resources are irrelevant and must not determine the decisions concerning medical care. The individual's medical condition should be the sole focus of the decision. These are very strict standards.[57]

These rules and this viewpoint clearly reject reliance on quality-of-life considerations in decisions to withhold lifesaving treatment.

In late 1984 the rules by the Department of Health and Human Services regarding nondiscrimination on the basis of handicaps continued to be the focus of considerable controversy. One of the judicial challenges sprang from the case of Baby Jane Doe, whose parents initially attempted to choose a conservative over a surgical approach for the treatment of their child born with multiple birth defects, including spina bifida manifesta (exposure of the spinal cord and membrane).[58] Because of the questions raised in the courts regarding the authority to implement such regulations on the basis of section 504 of the Rehabilitation Act of 1973, Congress passed amendments to the Child Abuse Prevention and Treatment Act authorizing such regulations.[59] This has led to yet further proposed rules[60] and to final regulations.[61] As the matter stands, the 1984 law provides that withholding medically indicated treatment will constitute child abuse when it involves

the failure to respond to the infant's life-threatening conditions by providing treatment (including appropriate nutrition, hydration, and medication) which, in the treating physician's or physicians' reasonable medical judgments, will be most likely to be effective in ameliorating or correcting all such conditions, except that the term does not include the failure to provide treatment (other than appropriate nutrition, hydration, or medication) to an infant when, in the treating physician's or physicians' reasonable medical judgment, (A) the infant is chronically and irreversibly comatose; (B) the provision of such treatment would (i) merely prolong dying, (ii) not be effective in ameliorating or correcting all of the infant's life-threatening conditions, or (iii) otherwise be futile in terms of the survival of the infant; or (C) the provision of such treatment would be virtually futile in terms of the survival of the infant and the treatment itself under such circumstances would be inhumane.[62]

Again, no provision is made for quality-of-life judgments; in fact, such judgments are forbidden, save with respect to chronically and irreversibly comatose existence. It should be clear, given our analyses of the principles of autonomy and beneficence, that both the federal government and the American Academy of Pediatrics are mistaken. Quality-of-life judgments and issues of cost are central to proper moral decision making in these areas, as we have argued. One may dispute the level of deformity or the amount of cost that justifies selective nontreatment. The fact that the child, which is not yet a person in the strict sense, falls within the authority of the parents as their possession sets limits to the authority of the state to intervene. In addition, the use of force to impose a particular federal understanding on unwilling parents should oblige the government, at the very least, to sustain the costs entailed in the care of the child imposed against the wishes of the parents.

This approach is not that radical. The American Medical Association quite clearly states that "quality of life is a factor to be considered in determining what is best for the individual."[63] Moreover, it endorses the role of parents in making such quality-of-life decisions.

In desperate situations involving newborns, the advice and judgment of the physician should be readily available, but the decision whether to exert maximal efforts to sustain life should be the choice of the parents. The parents should be told the options, expected benefits, risks and limits of any proposed care; how the potential for human relationships is affected by the infant's condition; and relevant information and answers to their questions. The presumption is that the love which parents usually have for their children will be dominant in the decisions which they make in determining what is in the best interest of their children. It is to be expected the parents will act unselfishly, particularly where life itself is at stake. Unless there is convincing evidence to the contrary, parental authority should be respected.[64]

Although the AMA does not characterize the burden to the family or society involved in treating severely defective newborns as a primary consideration, it also does not exclude it.[65]

Western societies have generally allowed infants to die when the costs of treatment have been significant and the likelihood of success restricted.[66] It is rather that such omissions have not been described as infanticide, given moral scruples against directly intending the death of the child, though its death was often a foreseen consequence of discontinuing treatment. One should note that the traditional Christian doctrine of extraordinary treatment gives a basis for discriminating against newborns who will likely be encumbered by serious physical or mental handicaps. One was generally excused from providing treatment if that treatment constituted a serious burden on oneself or on society. As Pope Pius XII phrased it,

normally one is held to use only ordinary means—according to the circumstances of persons, places, times, and culture—that is to say, means that do not involve any grave burden [*aucune charge extraordinaire*] for oneself or another. A more strict obligation would be too burdensome [*trop lourde*] for most men and would render the attainment of the higher, more important good too difficult.[67]

In such reflections it was not improper to consider as well the likelihood of success. In this way, one could come to identify a class of newborn infants for whom treatment would be so costly and so unlikely to succeed that one would be excused from providing or accepting treatment. However, one would not be forbidden to provide treatment as an act of special supererogation. In acts of supererogation one may discriminate. Of the class of children one is not obliged to treat, one may decide to treat only those likely to survive without serious mental or physical handicaps.

The considerations here allow us to go beyond this traditional understanding and to give reasons to show that it is morally proper in such circumstances to omit treatment with the intention that such children will die. In addition, considerations of parental autonomy will weaken the test for seriousness of cost so that the burdens that will justify discontinuing treatment may appear somewhat trivial to many bystanders. There will also not be grounds in principle for objecting to actively expediting death. What is wrong in murder is not the taking of a person's life, but that it is taken without that individual's permission and in addition in many circumstances that it is a maleficent act. Infants are not persons whose autonomy can be violated or entities who can suffer through having their goals thwarted. A painless death through active euthanasia may offer less suffering than passive euthanasia, and at times less pain than life itself. Moral guidelines concerning active euthanasia must thus be fashioned in terms of consequentialist considerations, and not on the basis of appeals to some basic moral distinction between acting and refraining, between active and passive euthanasia.[68]

Our reflections concerning the standing of persons have led us to a reconsideration of our moral rules regarding the active and passive euthanasia of infants born with significant mental and physical handicaps. It is clear that the categorical prohibition of such practices cannot be justified in terms of general moral principles. This is not a view without precedent. The full standing of persons in the social sense has not traditionally been accorded to infants immediately at birth but somewhat later. As I have already suggested in chapter 4, the nexus of obligations, which protects newborns, is not as strong as that which protects children who have already been fully incorporated in the social roles of families and of society. We have somewhat informally acted as the Greeks in delaying full status within the deme until some time after birth.[69] In order to avoid confusions such as those spawned by the so-called Baby Doe regulations from the Department of Health and Human Services, it may be worthwhile more formally to acknowledge these differences.

Fetal experimentation and in vitro fertilization

Current permissive laws concerning a woman's right to secure an abortion can be understood in terms of a recognition of the fetus as not yet a person, the rights of the woman to control her own body, or her rights to make her own reproductive decisions. Most liberal laws and judicial holdings presuppose a balancing of these considerations. The issues of fetal experimentation without therapeutic intent and in vitro fertilization differ in not involving all three of these concerns. In the case of fetal experimentation not focused on improving the capacity of the fetus to survive or to be born healthy, but rather on the acquisition of knowledge, the usual focus on procreative decision making is absent. The fetus is approached as an object through which knowledge will be secured. In the case of in vitro fertilization, reproductive processes occur outside a human body. Claims regarding the privacy and integrity of the woman's body cannot be invoked in order to forbid interference in such undertakings, even if they have a reproductive, not purely scientific, intent.

A general moral understanding within a secular pluralist society of the significance of fetal experimentation and in vitro fertilization must be secured in terms of the status of the fetus. Fetuses are not persons. They are the biological products of persons. They become persons in the strict sense only some time after birth. They may become persons in the social sense if a community ascribes to them some of the fundamental rights to protection usually accorded to persons in the strict sense. Early-gestation fetuses appear to have minimal, if any, mental life. They do not appear to have sufficient mental capacity to suffer as can normal adult mammals. It is for these reasons that this volume has already concluded that their moral status must be understood primarily in terms of their being the special possessions of persons and in terms of our concerns for the persons they may become. The first of these considerations reminds us why we must gain the consent of those who produce an embryo or fetus, or their assignees, before experimenting on or otherwise using an embryo or fetus. The second of these considerations reminds us why we must be concerned about injuring fetuses. If those fetuses are allowed to go to term, so that the harms finally settle on the persons those fetuses become, one will have injured persons in the strict sense.

As a consequence, there will be no sustainable moral arguments in principle against nontherapeutic experimentation with fetuses, or against in vitro fertilization. There may be somewhat persuasive arguments that will establish rules of decorum for such endeavors. But these rules will not be embedded in general constraints to respect the autonomy of persons or to achieve a generally justifiable view of the good life. At best, one will be able to indicate where certain practices may erode the very fabric of respect toward fetuses, infants, or the helpless. However, such arguments are unlikely to be clearly decisive or open to unambiguous articulation. They will depend on various hunches or suppositions regarding the effect of possible future practices on the anticipated activities of humans.

Consider the case of nontherapeutic fetal experimentation done with the permission of the immediate progenitors of the fetus and with reasonable certainty that the fetus will be destroyed if injured, rather than allowed to go to term. The more useful the research, the easier it will be to regard it as a beneficent and warranted act despite the adverse feelings it might evoke in many. A better understanding of fetal development will produce knowledge not only interesting in its own right but also useful toward the end of preventing congenital abnormalities and thus harms to future persons. If fetuses are not persons in the strict sense, it will be difficult to understand why women may seek abortions for any reason but researchers may not engage in fetal experimentation with the very altruistic goal of producing knowledge and well-being. Indeed, as long as the difference between human biological and personal life is borne in mind, such experimentation should be morally edifying. It is an undertaking aimed toward benefiting persons and without the risk of direct harm to anyone.

These reflections lead to justifying a very permissive policy with regard to fetal experimentation. They do not necessarily support a criticism of current restrictive rules that bear on the use of federal funds in fetal experimentation.[70] It is one thing to determine what persons have a right to do with their own resources, and another thing to decide to what extent common funds may be employed to support projects disapproved of by those who contribute to such funds. One may conclude that current state laws that categorically forbid fetal experimentation are without moral justification.[71] The restrictive laws that can be justified will have the same general character as those that would justify interventions to protect the fetus in a woman's womb. Fetal experimentation may be categorically forbidden when it is done with malevolent intent, or without reasonably certain provision for the destruction of the fetus if harmed to such an extent as to make the life of the future person not worth living. In addition, it would be proper to encourage the destruction of all injured or deformed fetuses, because it is better for persons to be free of handicaps. Beyond concerns to protect communal resources from the burden of caring for such individuals, this interest in a better state of persons may be more aesthetic than moral. As long as the existence of those persons is better than no existence at all, one does them a good by engendering them. Yet, as the Greeks underscored, there is a beauty in the healthy and whole mind and body that should be pursued. This sense of should is more embedded in a view of the beautiful life than a view of the good life.

Given this understanding of fetal experimentation, it becomes very difficult to place restrictions on in vitro fertilization done with the goal of producing a healthy child for parents who would otherwise be incapable of reproducing. There have been objections to in vitro fertilization on traditional moral grounds of its being unnatural in presupposing the acquisition of sperm through masturbation or because of the fashioning of human life under direct technological control. As has already been argued in chapter 5, the first contention is difficult to sustain in terms of arguments generally accessible in a secular pluralist context. One would need special premises to show that masturbation, rather than being a morally neutral act that can be engaged in either for recreation or for special procreative goals, violates the laws of nature. The general capacity of humans through rational contrivance to use their physiological capacities in novel ways in order to support their reproductive goals is a capacity produced through natural selection. It has served to maximize the reproductive success of humans. It is natural (in the sense of being a deliverance of evolutionary forces) for humans to use their bodily capacities in unnatural ways (i.e., in unusual ways or in ways that might not occur to lower mammals).

The charge that in vitro fertilization involves an improper objectification of human reproduction has been voiced by a number of thinkers, primarily theologians. The concern has been that the use of technological artifice in the very heart of human reproduction will change its sense and meaning.[72] A classic statement of opposition is provided by Paul Ramsey:

To put radically asunder what God joined together in parenthood when He made love procreative, to procreate from beyond the sphere of love (AID, for example, or making human life in a test-tube), or to posit acts of sexual love beyond the sphere of responsible procreation (by definition marriage), means a refusal of the image of God's creation in our own.[73]

This view is incomprehensible without the provision of special theological premises. Natural circumstances, which are the products of random mutations and natural selection, are far from morally canonical. As the theologian Joseph Fletcher has indicated, rationally planned reproduction is natural to rational beings.[74] The morally interesting issue is whether their rational planning respects the rights of the persons involved and is marked by beneficence.

Human reproduction becomes the object of the intervention of persons because human biology imposes mere factual constraints while persons plan and aspire to goals and purposes that may be realizable only in part through the biological means at hand. There is a recurring tension between humans as persons, as planning, aspiring entities, and humans as bodies, as individuals possessing the idiosyncratic deliverances of a particular biological past. Self-conscious, rational reflection thus engenders an instructive dualism of object and subject. The human body is experienced as an object that only imperfectly embodies the goals of persons. Persons become pregnant at the wrong time, with the wrong person, or not pregnant at the right time, with the right person. These failures of aspiration can be set aside in part through the reasoned interventions of human technology. The use of technology in the fashioning of children is integral to the goal of rendering the world congenial to persons. Such interventions can be seen as in principle improper only by appeal to special theological or ideological premises.

Finally, it will not be possible to condemn in vitro fertilization because it may involve the wastage of fertilized embryos. If early abortion can be chosen without let or hindrance because fetuses are not persons, it follows a fortiori that there is no injury to a person in disposing of excess embryos produced in the process of in vitro fertilization. The fact that one can (1) minimize pain and discomfort to the woman by harvesting a number of ova at one time, (2) avoid the risk associated with the gestation and birth of triplets and quadruplets, by fertilizing all of them but implanting only one or two at a time, and still (3) freeze the extra embryos in the event that further implantations are required to secure a successful pregnancy or a second pregnancy does not render the intervention immoral because defective or unused embryos may be discarded. Embryos are not persons. Moreover, one will need to remember that nature is generally wasteful in the production of offspring. For example, about 60 percent of fertilized human embryos never go to term.[75]

The substantial moral issues in in vitro fertilization are those that involve promises, trust, and commitments. The relations of persons bound together in the production of a child may be complex. In an extreme case, a man A and a woman B may donate an ovum and sperm for in vitro fertilization and implantation in a woman C, who will be the host mother and deliver the child for adoption to a man D and a woman E who are both infertile, the woman without ovaries and a uterus, and for whom the woman C is willing to serve as the host. There will need to be understandings with regard to the qualities of care and attention that will be provided by the in vitro fertilization clinic. There will need to be a web of trust and promises defining the obligations of the host mother C to avoid teratogenic agents or other circumstances that might injure the fetus. One will need to make clear who will accept responsibility for the child if it is born with serious congenital deformities.[76] The limits of the obligations of A and B will also need to be defined. These are important issues, but they are not unique to in vitro fertilization. They are, rather, a part of the web of mutual obligations that generally binds persons together and that is sustained through moral concerns for mutual respect and beneficence.

Most of these issues are not new ones. They have already been raised by practices such as the artificial insemination of the wives of infertile husbands, as well as the artificial insemination of a woman to bear a child for a couple when the wife is infertile. One does not need a complex technology such as in vitro fertilization in order to outline the central moral issues of trust and confidence that such interventions raise. Given the arguments in this volume a moral evil is not involved if all the parties are freely consenting and there is likely to be a positive balance of benefits over harms. Certain religious groups will not agree with this conclusion. Roman Catholics, for instance, will hold such activities to involve not only the moral evil of masturbation but that of adultery as well.[77] Such views require a very particular understanding of the nature of marriage and of proper reproduction, one that cannot be sustained in general secular terms. The general moral focus is instead on a responsible and beneficent involvement of individuals in the important goal of reproduction.

Advances in knowledge and technology will increase such responsibilities. As one comes to understand better what circumstances are likely to injure fetuses, one can become morally responsible for avoiding those circumstances. Even where there are no arguments to justify state force to constrain would-be parents from avoiding noxious circumstances that may injure future persons, there will still be plausible arguments within most understandings of the good life that will make the avoidance of such circumstances beneficent acts, and therefore morally desirable and laudable. As children are no longer seen as the gifts of God or the blind deliverances of biological forces, but rather as the products of biological forces under human control, we confront our responsibilities in their fashioning. This change in perspective is integral to understanding the human predicament where persons are not simply given a nature through evolutionary processes, but provided with a nature amenable at least in part to control and, in the future, to refashioning. We will return to this theme as the final chapter of this volume explores the ethos of a responsible biotechnology. Here it is enough to underscore that in vitro fertilization and techniques that will allow us to study and control human reproduction are morally neutral instruments for the realization of profoundly important human goals, which are bound up with the realization of the good of others: children for infertile parents and greater health for the children that will be born.

The patient as person

Medicine, as opposed to veterinary medicine, is the medicine of persons. It is not aimed at the mere prolongation of biological life. It is undertaken in order to postpone death, to prevent and ameliorate illness and deformity, to cure diseases, to amplify biological and psychological capacities, and to care for the sufferings of persons. Medicine is the agent of persons. It is engaged on their behalf. It is restrained by obligations to respect the wishes of persons and directed by the goal of doing good to persons. It is therefore crucial to recognize when persons begin and when they end in order to know to whom medicine, and health care in general, has its obligations. Physicians, nurses, and allied health workers must know when they are faced with a person whose wishes must be respected and who may set bounds to the desires of physicians and others to realize particular understandings of the good life.

It is for this reason that this chapter explored the issues of brain death and abortion. Such an examination is extraordinarily important for a culture such as ours, which is just coming to terms with a scientific understanding of nature and developing technological capacities to control nature. In over a million years of human history, there have been but a few centuries at most of serious and sustained human investigation of biological processes and what it means to be a person in this world. The distinction between human biological and human personal life is thus often acknowledged with not only intellectual, but also emotional, effort. We must rethink old mythopoetic understandings of the human condition and see what can be sustained for a society of persons drawn from various moral communities, armed with a profound knowledge of their biology and with an ever-growing technology.

For this reason it has been difficult to move from a whole-body definition of death to a whole-brain definition. It is for this reason as well that it will take effort to move to a higher-brain-centers definition, so as properly to draw a line indicating the end of human personal life. However emotionally difficult it will be to take these steps to new understandings, they will be unavoidable, in that it will not be possible generally to justify holding higher-brain-centers-dead but otherwise alive human bodies to be persons. They are not persons. If one kills such an entity, one does not take the life of a person. One may wish, for various considerations, to ascribe special rights to certain human entities in the twilight zone between life and death. However, it must be clear where the serious moral problems exist and where they only appear to exist. What one does to higher-brain-centers-dead but otherwise alive humans, unless it violates prior promises or commitments, will usually not be an offense against the principles of either autonomy or beneficence. It will not be a serious moral issue.

The same must be said about abortion. Despite its capacity to attract major public interest and sustain bitter public debate, abortion is not a serious moral issue. It is not possible to justify, in general secular terms, holding embryos and fetuses to be persons. At the beginning of human life, as at the end of life, one will need emotionally to come to terms with the intellectual realization that human biological life is not coincident with the life of persons.

It is in terms of the lives of persons that the sphere of values and moralities is organized. Intellectually, this will require surrendering the supposed stark contrast between a quality-of-life and a sanctity-of-life ethic. One will need to recognize that both reflect the ways in which persons give value to life that in itself has no value apart from the value it has for those who live it or who benefit from it. Though there is no sanctity of life in the sense of an overriding value of life that can be justified in terms of a general secular ethic, the life of persons has a sanctity in terms of the respect due to those who live it. Persons in terms of the morality of mutual respect can set limits to what can be done with their lives. But this sense of the sanctity of life is still bound up with the notion of the quality of life, for persons determine their actions in terms of the quality of their lives. Moreover, it is persons who determine the comparative values of lives in cooperative endeavors, and who may act on such comparative values insofar as other persons do not set limits. The last clause means that persons may in the end act on the judgment that their life is of significant quality to them to justify continued existence, despite the judgments of others. Quality of life thus has, as we have already noted, an important ambiguity: quality for the person living it and quality for those associated with that life. What may be experienced by others as a totally unacceptable quality of life may be acceptable for the person living it. When one considers the likely quality of outcome of a medical intervention, one must come to terms with the complexity of this concept. How one ought to balance the elements of this concept will be a matter of negotiation among the parties involved. Of course, one can always live one's own life on one's own and with cooperating others in terms of one's own judgment of the quality of one's life. But the cooperation of others may require some agreement on these issues. Consider, for example, the establishment of a cooperative insurance scheme that may give different amounts of support in those cases where medical intervention will restore complete health versus those that will leave individuals blind and quadriplegic. Individuals may cooperatively decide to invest fewer funds to save their lives when the quality will be such as in the second case.

Patients as persons thus meet others who as persons possess different views of proper conduct and of the good life. Patients, physicians, nurses, and other health care professionals must decide how they will cooperate with each other in common understandings and undertakings. The context of health care is an arena where an important community of understanding must be fashioned.

Notes

1. Kan. Stat. Ann., §77–202 (Cum. Supp. 1979) [enacted 1970].
2. Md. Ann. Code, art. 43, §54F (1980) (effective July 1, 1972).
3. Mont. Rev. Codes Ann., §50–22–101 (1978) (adopted April 4, 1977); Okla. Stat. Ann., tit. 63, §1–103 (g) (West Cum. Supp. 1981) (effective April 28, 1975); Tenn. Code Ann., §53–439 (Cum. Supp. 1980) (adopted March 18, 1976); Wyo. Stat., §35–19–101 (Cum. Supp. 1979) (effective Feb. 22, 1979).
4. Colo. Rev. Stat., §12–36–136 (1981) (approved May 21, 1981); I.C., §54–1819 (as added by 1981, chap. 258, §2, p. 549).
5. Conn. Gen. Stat. Ann., §19–139i (West Cum. Supp. 1981): Fla. Stat., §382.085 (1980); Ill. Ann. Stat., chap. 110 1/2, §302 (Smith-Hurd Cum. Supp. 1978) (effective Oct. 1, 1975).

6. St. Thomas Aquinas, *Summa Theologica*, I, Q 118, art. 2, reply to objection 2.

7. I have explored at some length the difference between mental life and mere biological processes and the contrast between the experienced significance of mental life and the presented significance of physical objects. See H. T. Engelhardt, Jr., *Mind-Body: A Categorial Relation* (The Hague: Martinus Nijhoff, 1973).

8. I use the term *principle* here to indicate essential or characteristic constituents. The principles of mental life require as a part of their explication an account of the interiority of that life.

9. Arthur C. Clarke, *2001: A Space Odyssey* (New York: New American Library, 1968).

10. *Black's Law Dictionary*, 4th ed. rev. (St. Paul, Minn.: West, 1968).

11. Roland Puccetti, "Brain Transplantation and Personal Identity," *Analysis* 29 (1969): 65.

12. François Joseph [Franz Josef] Gall, *On the Functions of the Brain and of Each of Its Parts: with Observations on the Possibilities of Determining the Instincts, Propensities, and Talents, or the Moral and Intellectual Dispositions of Men and Animals, by the Configuration of the Brain and Head*, trans. Winslow Lewis (Boston: Marsh, Capen and Lyon, 1835).

13. J. G. Spurzheim, *Phrenology or the Doctrine of the Mental Phenomena*, 2 vols. (Boston: Marsh, Capen and Lyon, 1833).

14. M. J. P. Flourens, *Examen de la Phrenologie*, 2d ed. (Paris: Paulin, 1845).

15. For a treatment of this point, see Robert M. Young, *Mind, Brain, and Adaptation in the Nineteenth Century* (Oxford: Clarendon Press, 1970).

16. See H. T. Engelhardt, Jr., "John Hughlings Jackson and the Mind-Body Relation," *Bulletin of the History of Medicine* 49 (Summer 1975): 137–51.

17. President's Commission for the Study of Ethical Problems in Medicine and Biomedical and Behavioral Research, *Defining Death* (Washington, D.C.: U.S. Government Printing Office, 1981), pp. 13–15.

18. John Hughlings Jackson, "Remarks on Evolution and Dissolution of the Nervous System," in *Selected Writings of John Hughlings Jackson* (London: Staples Press, 1958), pp. 76–91.

19. Ad Hoc Committee of the Harvard Medical School to Examine the Definition of Brain Death, "A Definition of Irreversible Coma," *Journal of the American Medical Association* 205 (1968): 337–43.

20. World Medical Association, "Declaration of Sydney," *Medical Journal of Australia Supplement* 58 (1973): 2.

21. Ad Hoc Committee of the American Electroencephalographic Society on EEG Criteria for Determination of Cerebral Death, "Cerebral Death and the Encephalogram," *Journal of the American Medical Association* 209 (1969): 1505.

22. There have been reports in the press of brain-dead women who have been brought to term. Some may not have been fully brain dead in terms of rigorous whole-brain criteria. Still, one should note that there would be nothing paradoxical in such an event. The living body of a dead woman would have sustained her fetus until birth.

23. Gray et al. v. Sawyer et al., Gray et al. v. Clay et al., 247 S. W. 2d 496, 497 (Ky. App. 1952).

24. President's Commission for the Study of Ethical Problems in Medicine and Biomedical and Behavioral Research, *Deciding to Forego Life-Sustaining Treatment* (Washington, D.C.: U.S. Government Printing Office, 1983), p. 6.

25. Barber v. L.A. Co. Sup. Ct., 195 Cal. Rptr. 484 (Cal. Ct. App. Oct. 12, 1983).
26. Roland Puccetti, "The Life of a Person," in W. B. Bondeson et al. (eds.), *Abortion and the Status of the Fetus* (Dordrecht: Reidel, 1983), pp. 169–82.
27. In re Conroy, 457 A.2d 1232 (N.J. Super. Ct., Feb. 2, 1983).
28. In re Conroy, 464 A.2d 303 (N.J. Super. Ct., App. Div., July 8, 1983).
29. In re Conroy, 486 A.2d 1209 (N.J. 1985).
30. American Bar Association, *Annual Report* 231–32 (1978) (February 1975 midyear meeting).
31. President's Commission for the Study of Ethical Problems in Medicine and Biomedical and Behavioral Research, *Defining Death* (Washington, D.C.: U.S. Government Printing Office, 1981), p. 3.
32. Ibid., pp. 31–4, 37–8.
33. Ibid., p. 40.
34. Immanuel Jakobovits, *Jewish Medical Ethics* (New York: Block, 1959), p. 277; also *Tzitz Eliezer*, 9:46 and 10:25:4, and *Babylonian Talmud, Yoma* 85a, Soncino ed.
35. Planned Parenthood of Central Missouri v. Danforth, 428 U.S. 52 (1976).
36. For a review of the issues raised by tort-for-wrongful-life cases, see Angela R. Holder, "Is Existence Ever an Injury?: The Wrongful Life Cases," in S. F. Spicker et al. (eds.), *The Law-Medicine Relation: A Philosophical Exploration* (Dordrecht: Reidel, 1981), pp. 225–39. Also, G. M. Lehr and H. L. Hirsh, "Wrongful Conception, Birth and Life," *Medicine and Law* 2 (1983): 199–208; and E. Haavi Morreim, "Conception and the Concept of Harm," *Journal of Medicine and Philosophy* 8 (1983): 137–57.
37. Zepeda v. Zepeda, 41 Ill. App. 2d 240, 1963.
38. Williams v. New York, 223 N.E. 2d 849, 1963.
38. Curlender v. Bio-Science Laboratories and Automated Laboratory Sciences, 165 Cal. Rptr. 477 (Ct. App. 2d Dist. Div. 1, 1980).
40. This holding of the court in Curlender has been superseded on appeal and by statute. In a second case involving tort for wrongful life, California courts did not hold that parents would be liable. Turpin v. Sortini, 31 Cal. 3d 220, 643, P.2d 954, 182 Cal. Rptr. 337 (1982). In addition, California precluded by statute suit by children against their parents on such grounds. Cal. Civ. Code, Sec. 43.6 (1982), enacted in 1981. For another tort-for-wrongful-life case that also did not involve recognizing an avenue of recovery against parents, see Harbeson v. Parke-Davis, Inc., 98 Wash. 2d 460, 656 P.2d 483 (1983).
41. The reader will notice here a distinction drawn from the traditions of Catholic moral theology between foresight and intention. This distinction is central to the concept of double effect. Individuals may act foreseeing consequences they do not intend, but that, had they intended, would render the act immoral. Thus, a good Roman Catholic may not directly intend to kill himself. However, if he is engaged in a just war he may throw himself on a grenade that lands in his foxhole to save his comrades. This is permissible as long as he does not intend to kill himself but only to absorb the shrapnel with his body, although he can surely foresee that this will lead to death. One effect is intended (the absorbing of the shrapnel); the second effect (his death) is foreseen but not intended.
   Traditionally, there are four points to the doctrine of double effect: (1) the evil outcome is not intended, (2) the good outcome does not follow from the evil outcome, (3) the action engaged in is not intrinsically immoral, and (4) the good consequences outweigh the bad. In secular moral circumstances these consider-

ations can be employed to distinguish between those circumstances in which one may foresee a harm one is not obliged to avoid, but where it would be immoral (malevolent) to intend that harm.

42. The issue of the emancipation of children will be explored in greater detail in chapter 7. Here it is enough to note that one will need to decide when children are indeed competent. One will need to come to a judgment as to when they understand and appreciate the significance of their choices, such that they must be respected, at least through noninterference. There are limitations on the extent to which parents must comply even under circumstances of competent decision-making on the part of their children. As was argued in chapter 4, children are in certain respects examples of indentured servants who have special duties to their masters.

43. Jessie Mae Jefferson v. Griffin Spalding County Hospital Authority, 247 Ga. 86, 274 S.E.2d 457 (1981). Mirabile factu, Jessie Mae Jefferson delivered her child vaginally and without difficulty. Depending on one's religious convictions or one's views of false positive diagnoses of placenta previa, one may come to the conclusion that attendance at the Shiloh Sanctified Holiness Baptist Church does indeed work miracles. For an account of this case, see George Annas, "Forced Cesareans: The Most Unkindest Cut," *Hastings Center Report* 12 (June 1982): 16–17, 45.

44. Jefferson v. Griffin Spalding, at 460.

45. P. H. Soloff, S. Jewell, and L. Roth, "Civil Commitment and the Rights of the Unborn," *American Journal of Psychiatry* 136 (1979): 114–15. For a review of some court actions and of circumstances that could lead to court actions to force women to accept cesarean sections, see for example Watson A. Bowes, Jr., and Brad Selgestad, "Fetal Versus Maternal Rights: Medical and Legal Perspectives," *Obstetrics & Gynecology* 58 (Aug. 1981): 209–14; J. R. Lieberman, M. Mazor, W. Chaim, and A. Cohen, "The Fetal Right to Live," *Obstetrics & Gynecology* 53 (April 1979): 515–17; Thomas L. Shriner, Jr., "Maternal Versus Fetal Rights—A Clinical Dilemma," *Obstetrics & Gynecology* 53 (April 1979): 518–19; Ronna Jurow and Richard H. Paul, "Cesarean Delivery for Fetal Distress Without Maternal Consent," *Obstetrics & Gynecology* 63 (April 1984): 596–9.

46. Aristotle, *Politics*, in *The Basic Works of Aristotle*, ed. Richard McKeon (New York: Random House, 1941), VII.6.335b, p. 1302.

47. Sextus Empiricus, *Outlines of Pyrrhonism*, in *Sextus Empiricus*, trans. R. G. Bury (Cambridge, Mass.: Harvard University Press, 1976), III. 211, vol. 1, p. 467. For a criticism of Sextus Empiricus's contention, as well as an acknowledgment of the general acceptance of the father's right to expose children, see A. R. W. Harrison, *The Law of Athens: The Family and Property* (Oxford: Clarendon Press, 1968).

48. Soranus, *Soranus' Gynecology*, trans. Owsei Temkin (Baltimore: Johns Hopkins University Press, 1956), p. 80. The Roman fathers' right to kill offspring or at least deformed, handicapped, or weak infants was set aside by Constantine in A.D. 318 (*Codex Justinianus* 9.17.1) and again by Valentinian in A.D. 374 (*Codex Justinianus* 9.16.7). These issues are explored by Darrel Amundsen in "Medicine and the Birth of Defective Children: Approaches of the Ancient World," in R. C. McMillan et al. (eds.), *Euthanasia and the Newborn* (Dordrecht: Reidel, 1986).

49. Anthony Shaw, "Dilemmas of 'Informed Consent' in Children," *New England Journal of Medicine* 289 (Oct. 25, 1973): 885–90.

50. Raymond S. Duff and A. G. M. Campbell, "Moral and Ethical Dilemmas in the

Special-Care Nursery," *New England Journal of Medicine* 289 (Oct. 25, 1973): 890–4. A review of these issues in terms of contemporary law and public policy is provided in R. C. McMillan et al. (eds.), *Euthanasia and the Newborn*.

51. Napoleon A. Chagnon, *Yanomamo: The Fierce People*, 2d ed. (New York: Holt, Rinehart and Winston, 1977). For a study of the challenge of compassing such communities within a state, see Stuart Plattner and David Maybury-Lewis (eds.), *The Prospects for Pluralist Societies* (Washington, D.C.: American Ethnological Society, 1984).

52. H. Tristram Engelhardt, Jr., "Viability and the Use of the Fetus," in W. B. Bondeson et al. (eds.), *Abortion and the Status of the Fetus* (Dordrecht: Reidel, 1983), pp. 183–208.

53. Robert F. Weir, "Sounding Board: The Government and Selective Nontreatment of Handicapped Infants," *New England Journal of Medicine* 309 (Sept. 15, 1983): 661–3.

54. *Federal Register* 48 (March 7, 1983): 9630–2; *Federal Register* 48 (July 5, 1983): 30846–52; final regulations were issued in *Federal Register* 49 (Jan. 12, 1984): 1622–54.

55. American Academy of Pediatrics v. Heckler, 561 F. Supp. 395 (D.D.C. 1983).

56. *Federal Register* 49 (Jan. 12, 1984): 1654. These regulations, as well as the proposed regulations that have followed, outline and suggest the use of infant care review committees. This has led to a growing interest in developing institutional ethics committees. The extent to which such committees will be useful will depend on the extent to which they provide access to special expertise and a chance for the arbitration of disputes or for the diffusion of responsibility. They will not have authority morally to substitute for the agreements of physicians and patients without the consent of those parties. This will be true not only in the case of pediatric care but in health care generally. For a recent history of institutional review committees, see R. E. Cranford and A. E. Doudera, "The Emergence of Institutional Ethics Committees," *Law, Medicine & Health Care* 12 (February 1984): 13–20.

57. American Academy of Pediatrics, "Principles of Treatment of Disabled Infants," *Pediatrics* 73 (April 4, 1984): 559. These principles for treatment were inspired in part by a number of cases in which Down's syndrome children were not treated on the basis of quality-of-life decisions. See George F. Smith et al., "Commentary: The Rights of Infants With Down's Syndrome," *Journal of the American Medical Association* 251 (Jan. 13, 1984): 229.

58. U.S.A. v. University Hospital, No. 83-6343 (2d Cir. February 23, 1984).

59. Pub. L. No. 98-457, 98 Stat. 1749 (1984).

60. Department of Health and Human Services, "Child Abuse and Neglect Prevention and Treatment Program; Proposed Rule. Interim Model Guidelines for Health Care Providers to Establish Infant Care Review Committee; Notice," *Federal Register* 49 (Dec. 10, 1984): 48160-73.

61. Department of Health and Human Services, "Child Abuse and Neglect Prevention and Treatment Program; Final Rule," *Federal Register* 50 (Apr. 15, 1985): 14878–901. The final regulations follow the 1984 amendments to the Child Abuse Prevention and Treatment Act and list as exceptions to when withholding of indicated medical treatment would count as child abuse the following circumstances: "(i) The infant is chronically and irreversibly comatose; (ii) The provision of such treatment would merely prolong dying, not be effective in ameliorating or correcting all of the infant's life-threatening conditions, or otherwise be futile in

terms of the survival of the infant; or (iii) The provision of such treatment would
be virtually futile in terms of the survival of the infant and the treatment itself
under such circumstances would be inhumane." Ibid, p. 14888. The regulations
thus appear to imply that one is obliged to treat a child aggressively, even if one
thought it would die at the age of eighteen months—a conclusion that seems
morally improper. One would hope that parents would be able to choose whether
or not they wish to have their child survive in order simply to die a year later.

62. Pub. L. No. 98-457, 121, 98 Stat. 1749 (1984).

63. *Current Opinions of the Judicial Council of the American Medical Association—
1984* (Chicago: American Medical Association, 1984), p. 10.

64. Ibid., p. 11.

65. Ibid., p. 10.

66. For an overview of the silent acceptance of infanticide in recent times, see W. L.
Langer, "Checks on Population Growth: 1750–1850," *Scientific American* 226
(1972): 3–9. For a study of the generality of the phenomenon of infanticide, see
Glenn Hausfater and Sarah Blaffer Hrdy (eds.), *Infanticide. Comparative and
Evolutionary Perspectives* (New York: Aldine, 1984).

67. Pope Pius XII, Pope, Allocution "Le Dr. Bruno Haid," Nov. 24, 1957, *Acta
Apostolicae Sedis* 49 (1957), pp. 1031. English translation from Pius XII,
"Address to an International Congress of Anesthesiologists," November 24,
1957, *The Pope Speaks*, vol. 4 (Spring 1958): 395–6. For an exploration of the
development of the distinction between ordinary and extraordinary means, see
James J. McCartney, "The Development of the Doctrine of Ordinary and
Extraordinary Means of Preserving Life in Catholic Moral Theology Before the
Karen Quinlan Case," *Linacre Quarterly* 47 (Aug. 1980): 215–24. As McCartney
indicates, the distinction between ordinary and extraordinary care was developed
by Soto in 1582 and Banez in 1595. For further information on the distinction,
see José Janini, "La operatión quirúrgica, remedio ordinario," *Revista Española
de Teologia* 18 (1958): 331–48; Daniel A. Cronin, *The Moral Law in Regard to the
Ordinary and Extraordinary Means of Conserving Life* (Rome: Typis Pontificiae
Universitatis Gregorianiae, 1958); and Gerald Kelly, "The Duty of Using
Artificial Means of Preserving Life," *Theological Studies* 11 (1950): 203–20.

68. The moral significance of the distinction between acting and refraining, and
between active and passive euthanasia, has been explored in a number of articles
in the philosophical literature and elsewhere. See, for example, Natalie Abrams,
"Active and Passive Euthanasia," *Philosophy* 54 (1978): 257–269. Gary Atkinson,
"Ambiguities in 'Killing' and 'Letting Die,' " *Journal of Medicine and Philosophy*
8 (May 1983): 159–68. Jonathan Bennett, "Whatever the Consequences," *Analysis* 26 (Jan. 1966): 83–102. Daniel Dinello, "On Killing and Letting Die," *Analysis*
31 (April 1971): 83–6. P. J. Fitzgerald, "Acting and Refraining," *Analysis* 27
(March 1967): 133–9. James Rachels, "Active and Passive Euthanasia," *New
England Journal of Medicine* 292 (Jan. 9, 1975): 78–80. These issues are reviewed
as well in the very thorough book by Robert Weir, *Selective Nontreatment of
Handicapped Newborns* (New York: Oxford University Press, 1984). See also
Dennis J. Horan and Melinda Delahoyde (eds.), *Infanticide and the Handicapped
Newborn* (Provo, Utah: Brigham Young University Press, 1982).

In terms of the analyses in this volume, distinctions between active and passive
euthanasia can be drawn in terms of which acts involve an invasion of another
person's body or property. Since duties to respect the freedom of others will often
be more easily justified than duties of beneficence, restrictions on active euthanasia will be easier to establish than those bearing on passive euthanasia. However,
agreements or contracts, such as occur through the physician–patient relationship, can create clearly established duties of beneficence. Such fiduciary relation-

ships may preclude passive as well as active euthanasia. The issues become more clouded in the case of infants, who are not yet persons in the strict sense. They do not yet have choices to be respected. Also, though they may be the object of contracts, they cannot yet be party to contracts.

69. Societies often have not accorded full status to infants because of high infant mortality, as well as hesitations to commit full energies to the salvage of children with significant defects. In Judaism, for example, a distinction has often been made between infants who die before thirty days of life and those who die after thirty days of life. See n. 25, chap. 4.

70. See, for example, the federal regulations that require that "no fetus *in utero* may be involved as a subject in any activity covered by this subpart unless: (1) The purpose of the activity is to meet the health needs of the particular fetus and the fetus will be placed at risk only to the minimum extent necessary to meet such needs, or (2) the risk to the fetus imposed by the research is minimal and the purpose of the activity is the development of important biomedical knowledge which cannot be obtained by other means." *Protection of Human Subjects*, 45 Code of Federal Regulations, 46.208(a).

71. See, for example, state laws such as Minn. Stat. §145, 422–3 (1973) and Louisiana tit. 14 §87.2 (1973).

72. Paul Ramsey, "Ethics of a Cottage Industry in an Age of Community and Research Medicine," *New England Journal of Medicine* 284 (April 1, 1971): 700–6; "Shall We Reproduce? I. The Medical Ethics of *In Vitro* Fertilization," *Journal of the American Medical Association* 220 (June 5, 1972): 1345–50; "Shall We Reproduce? II. Rejoinders and Future Forecasts," *Journal of the American Medical Association* 220 (June 12, 1972): 1480–5. For a more general, conservative critique of in vitro fertilization, see Leon Kass, "Babies by Means of *In Vitro* Fertilization: Unethical Experiments on the Unborn?" *New England Journal of Medicine* 285 (Nov. 1971): 1174–9.

73. Paul Ramsey, *Fabricated Man* (New Haven, Conn.: Yale University Press, 1970), p. 39.

74. Joseph Fletcher, "Ethical Aspects of Genetic Controls," *New England Journal of Medicine* 285 (Sept. 30, 1971): 776–83; *The Ethics of Genetic Control* (Garden City, N.Y.: Doubleday Anchor, 1974); *Morals and Medicine* (Princeton, N.J.: Princeton University Press, 1954).

75. John D. Biggers, "Generation of the Human Life Cycle," in W. B. Bondeson et al. (eds.), *Abortion and the Status of the Fetus*, pp. 31–53. An interesting proposal has been made by one Roman Catholic author to avoid at least the embryo wastage that may result when numerous ova are fertilized by in vitro fertilization but only a few are implanted. Though he opposes in vitro fertilization because it "separates human procreation from the expression of conjugal or marital love in sexual intimacy," John R. Connery suggests that couples might host such orphan embryos. He does not comment on the possibility of a single woman offering herself as a host. "Orphan Embryos," *Linacre Quarterly* 51 (November 1984): 310–14.

76. The use of surrogate mothers for in vitro fertilization raises the general problem of creating a contract to govern such endeavors. Though morally such contracts should be binding, they raise a number of important legal issues. See Steven R. Gersz, "The Contract in Surrogate Motherhood: A Review of the Issues," *Law, Medicine and Health Care* 12 (June 1984): 115–17.

77. Gerald Kelly, *Medico-Moral Problems* (St. Louis, Mo.: Catholic Hospital Association, 1958), pp. 228–44; and John P. Kenny, *Principles of Medical Ethics*, 2d ed. (Westminster, Md.: Newman Press, 1962), pp. 90–6.

7

Free and Informed Consent, Refusal of Treatment, and the Health Care Team: The Many Faces of Freedom

Persons have a right to be left alone. This includes the right not to be hindered when joining freely with willing others. Around these expressions of the principle of autonomy the relations of patients, physicians, and other health care workers take shape. These relations include those of association, dissociation, and nonassociation. Patients and physicians weave a web of commitments, as well as boundaries and borders. The fashioning of a physician–patient relationship involves the building of commitments and the setting of limits. It involves as well the mutual understanding of the commitments and limits, the permissions and refusals, that fashion an actual concrete relationship. In health care men and women create a web of expectations and permissions through agreements to being touched and explored by others, through commitments to confidentiality and the keeping of special trusts, and by fashioning common understandings of goals to be jointly pursued. In health care this includes entrusting certain elements of the care and cure of one's body and mind to some but not to others, usually in part, rarely as a whole. As total commitments are rare in everyday life, the same is the case in health care. Few patients commit themselves without reservation to the care of a physician. Usually something is held back, something is reserved; there is some noncompliance with the instructions of a physician. So, too, most physicians do not commit all. There are always limits to the dedication of finite beings.

That which creates the substance of this relationship also fashions its limits: the free choices of individual men and women—patients, physicians, nurses, and others. There is no single way in which the relationship must be structured. Different groups will fashion different relationships given their different needs for independence or acquiescence in the care of others. To understand the variations in this relationship, one is brought to the traditional issues of free and informed consent, confidentiality, paternalism, and the rights of patients to refuse treatment or of physicians not to accept a patient. These must be appreciated in terms of the tensions among the various views of the good life that sustain particular ideals of the patient–physician (or patient–nurse) relationship. These views, which are often in conflict, must then be mediated in the general fabric of a peaceable, secular, pluralist society through the agreement of those involved. In short, competing views of beneficence expressed in competing understandings of the patient–physician relationship will need to be fairly accommodated in mutual respect for the persons participating. Fair procedures of negotiation will form the basis for resolving tensions among competing views of proper actions.

Free and informed consent is central to this procedure. Individuals must communicate and appreciate what each party wishes in order to come to an understanding. The physician–patient contract and the understandings between patients and nurses are the final products of such procedures. These processes of informing and communicating play their central role not simply because they may be valued in their own right (though they may indeed be highly valued), but also due to the lack of common understanding between individuals and across communities. Insofar as there is not one authoritative view of the good life and of the concrete goals of medicine, one will need to create a common understanding. Free and informed consent thus plays its central role not so much out of a commitment to a liberal ideal, but out of a despair regarding the possibility of discovering a concrete view of the goals of health care in a secular, pluralist context. In short, free and informed consent has its current moral significance because of the conceptual difficulties (i.e., inability of reason to establish authoritatively a particular concrete view of the good life) and historical problems (i.e., the historical collapse of the Christian expectation, as well as of the Enlightenment expectation, for all to convert to, or for a general rational argument to establish, a particular concrete view of the good life) that lead to the intellectual problem of gaining moral authority in a secular pluralist society (a point discussed in chapter 2). When such authority cannot be discovered, when one cannot decide what must be done, one must ask the free individuals involved what they want to do and wait for them to come to a common agreement in order to allow peaceable action with moral authority.

As we will see, the amount and character of disclosure and formal agreement will be dependent on the extent to which the physician or other health care professional and the patient share common views of the goals of medicine, the canons of moral probity, and the character of the good life. The more the physician and the patient are strangers to each other's set of values and goals, the more necessary it will be to fashion explicit rules to govern free and informed consent, and for free and informed consent to encompass in detail the matters at stake in treatment. The more patients and physicians share a common view of the goals of health care in particular and of life in general, the less necessary elaborate disclosures will be. However, some disclosures will always be necessary. Friends need to know, even if only implicitly, the character of their joint endeavors. Friends can disagree and become estranged. In the more serious endeavors of medicine it will be necessary at least to anticipate such possibilities.

With the authority to consent comes the right to give oneself over to the care of others and to withdraw from that care, to accept aid and to refuse it. As a result, the topic of free and informed consent is bound to issues of the moral probity of suicide and of aiding and abetting suicide, and to the establishment of lines of authority within the health care team. These various topics are the expression of the freedom of individuals in health care.

The patient–healer relationship

The physician and patient are not alone in the patient–healer relationship. In "Epidemics" Hippocrates enjoins the physician:

Declare the past, diagnose the present, foretell the future; practice these acts. As to diseases, make a habit of two things—to help, or at least to do no harm. The art has three factors, the disease, the patient, the physician. The physician is the servant of the art. The patient must cooperate with the physician in combating the disease.[1]

In addition to the physician and the patient in their confrontation with disease, there is also the art. The art, Hippocrates' *techne*, I will read as the medical profession both as a group of individuals and as a body of skills.[2] The profession attempts to set standards as to what will count as canonical problems and proper medical interventions. This sense of profession transcends national boundaries and can exist without a formal organization of physicians such as the American Medical Association.[3] The very idea of the skilled profession thus reaches into the private exchanges of healers and patients, even before and in addition to the intrusions of state authority through laws, regulations, or requirements of licensure.

To understand the position of healers and patients, one must first turn to the ways in which healers are seen as professionals and regard themselves as members of a profession. The idea of a profession carries with it commitments to particular views of beneficence and proper action. Professions are goal oriented.

The profession

All societies have individuals who play the role of healer, even where the role of healer is not yet fully differentiated from other roles such as that of priest. In societies with an investment in modern science and technology such as ours, the healer often retains magical and priestly roles. This is not unexpected. Healing is sought for concerns that go to the root of human existence: fears of death, deformity, and disability. The healer's role has parallels with that of the lawyer who aids individuals in difficulties with state-recognized powers and that of the theologian or priest who aids individuals in difficulties with the supernatural powers: each is a mediator between individuals and one of the major clusters of potentially adversarial forces. The physician, lawyer, and theologian or priest are engaged in professions that intrude into all elements of human life.

The profession to which the healer belongs is also one of the three traditional learned professions. It is learned in that it requires skill to prevent and control illness, and to forestall death. It is one of the major professions in that pain, deformity, disability, disease, and premature death capture the central attention of both individuals and societies. Such learning and importance set a distance between the healer and the person seeking care. As the skills become complex and intricate, requiring deep knowledge of human nature, physiology, and the mechanisms of disease, a barrier against understanding is erected between the two. This barrier between the expert professional and the layman cannot be overcome by a redistribution of knowledge in the same way that a barrier between the rich and the poor might be overcome in principle by a redistribution of wealth.[4] The very wealth of knowledge that makes the professional able disables communication with the person in need of care. In addition, remnants of magical expectations regarding those who deal with disease and death convey a further sense of distance and importance usually not ascribed to merely mechanical interventions.[5]

As a result, the medical profession takes on an esoteric character. It is a domain of special learning bearing on issues of life and death to which often magical properties are assigned. In fact, part of the traditional placebo power of the physician, the ability of the physician to make the patient feel better by his presence alone is tied to this priestly authority of the healer. This commitment to the esoteric character of the profession is expressed in the Hippocratic Oath where the initiate swears to impart the instruction he will be given only to sons of his teacher and to indentured pupils who have taken the oath, but to no others. The result is the fashioning of a moral and intellectual elite, a group of individuals with a special dedication to (1) aiding those threatened by illness, deformity, and premature death, as well as (2) preserving and increasing the skill of the professional. The first gives a commitment to a set of both moral and nonmoral values. The former values guide judgments about the proper ways in which patients should be treated, and the latter values will include understandings of the levels of disability, pain, and deformity that should be accepted or that should serve as bona fide warrants for treatment. The second not only sets standards for the use of skills but also directs the profession to the acquisition of better skills and greater knowledge. Even without a formal regulatory procedure or membership requirement, the profession is able to recognize who belongs and who lives up to its ideals by appealing to these goals of beneficence and of knowledge. The health care professions either as (1) groups of individuals formally organized into societies or licensed by the state, or (2) groups of individuals informally bound together by commitment to the profession's intellectual and moral goals are self-regulating through appeals to these goals.

These goals not only ennoble the health care professions but also are the basis of moral conflicts as well. Members of the health care professions, as members of a learned profession, are dedicated to the following sorts of goals, not all of which are always in harmony: (1) they serve the health care needs and desires of individuals; (2) they support the health care needs and desires of societies; (3) they engage in their profession to gain income and prestige (professionals are not amateurs, individuals engaged in an undertaking without thought of monetary reward); (4) they aid the profession in being self perpetuating (e.g., in attempting to preserve the art, the members preserve the profession as a special interest group with special privileges and status); and (5) they aim at the acquisition of knowledge. The good of the individual and of society may often be at odds (e.g., reporting requirements with regard to venereal diseases). The pursuit of individual gain not only may financially embarrass individuals and society, but also may lead to undermining the status of the profession. Finally, and here one finds a distinction that marks a learned profession, the pursuit of knowledge may conflict with the interests of the individuals being treated. Here one might think of the remark often said in derogation, but which is nevertheless instructive: "The operation was a success but the patient died." A learned profession is an intellectual joy even apart from its services to others. There is a pleasure in practicing a learned and difficult skill, even when it cannot be of benefit to others.

The pursuit of knowledge, though in potential conflict with the interests of individual patients, is in potential harmony with the long-range interests of future patients and society generally. The acquisition of better knowledge and increased skill should ensure better-quality treatment for individuals in the future. Such use of current patients for the preservation of the art is necessary even apart from high-technology medicine. Skills must be passed from a learned master to an apprentice healer who while in training may lance a boil, set a bone, or treat a fever with less skill than the teacher. If patients do not come into the hands of young apprentices, the skill will die out. In the medical profession everyone must lance his first boil, remove her first appendix, or perform his first cardiac catheterization. This investment of the present on behalf of the future is made even more systematic with the idea of medical progress and with a critical regard of claims about the efficacy of standard treatments. The goals of doing the best for patients, and of avoiding unnecessary harms, lead to the practice of systematic medical experimentation and to the healer not only being one who cares for those in need but also one who studies their complaints and their possible cures. The utilitarian (greatest good for the greatest number) understanding of the obligations of the medical profession becomes intertwined with the focus on individualistic and often deontological obligations to particular patients.

When a patient confronts a physician (or a nurse or other health care professional), the physician is encountered within a complex context of a profession with diverse goals, only some of which are directed to the treatment and care of that patient. If the patient wants what the profession does not usually give or wants treatments that depart from the standards of the profession, the physician must bear the judgment of the profession in mind. Any negotiation with a particular patient will involve the physician in a possible negotiation with the profession. The profession renders judgments (both formally and informally) about which activities are properly medical, about which violate the standards of the profession, and thus about whether the physician or other health care professional in question is in good standing. Even absent formal regulations, organized professional societies, or licensing procedures, there are important sanctions such as the denial of referrals. Patient requests for particular treatments are thus at once put within the context of a community of health professionals with their views of what actions are proper and what interventions are indicated. The interchanges between patient and health care professional are defined not only by these two individuals but also by the health care profession itself. Depending on the view of proper practice held by the profession (or groups within the profession), the profession may even support the physician in telling the patient, "If you want to be treated by me, then you will stop asking all these questions and do what I tell you—that way you will get the best treatment and I will have more time to help other patients in need."

Circumstances are, however, complex, for there is not one unambiguous sense of the health care professions or of the medical profession. Though there will be the possibility for a general abstract understanding of what it means to be a physician or nurse, a concrete understanding will be available only within a particular community of physicians, nurses, or other health care professionals and their view of the morally proper life and of the good practice of their profession. Thus, as patients come to negotiate with health professionals for an understanding about their treatment and a contract for their care, they will need to determine the professional commitments of those with whom they are about to enter into the agreement for care and treatment. A woman of liberal moral persuasions will need to know, for example, whether the gynecologist with whom she is considering developing a patient –physician relationship holds views against sterilization and abortion. So, too, it will be prudent for someone diagnosed with disseminated cancer to know the physician's views regarding the use of narcotics and other drugs in the control of pain. For example, will the physician be willing to give sufficient pain medication on a plan that will avoid the patient's feeling pain instead of relying on minimal amounts of medication so that the patient must request pain medication and experience pain between doses. Similarly, an individual diagnosed with amyelotrophic lateral sclerosis or Lou Gehrig's disease (a fatal degenerative neurological disease) who does not wish to be preserved to the very end will wish to establish a relationship with a neurologist who will support the patient's desires for minimal or no treatment toward the end of the disease's course. In order effectively to fashion a health care contract, the patient will need to know the moral and professional ideals of the physician. So, too, the physician will need to understand the patient's expectations from care.[6]

The patient as a stranger in a strange land

Patients, when they come to see a health care professional, are in unfamiliar territory. They enter a terrain of issues that has been carefully defined through the long history of the health care professions. A patient is unlikely to present for care with as well-analysed and considered judgments as those possessed by health care professionals. Professionals have a community of colleagues to reinforce their views and to sustain them in their recommendations. In addition, the interchange of health care professional and patient is defined by the language of health care. Pains, disabilities, and even fears are translated into the special jargon of the health care professions. The replacement of the ritual and magic of the shaman by the technology and theory of the scientist-healer may have increased, not diminished, the distance between the healer and the person in search of cure and care.

The patient in this context is a stranger, an individual in unfamiliar territory who does not fully know what to expect or how to control the environment. The patient's usual ways of thinking must be put into abeyance or altered in order to accommodate to the theories and explanations of the healer and the routines of the healer's environment. The stranger must adapt to new and alien cultural patterns and expectations. Things no longer happen as usual; they no longer take place in their taken-for-granted ways. As an outsider in a strange culture, the patient always runs the risk of being a marginal person. The stranger, as Alfred Schutz noted, "has to face the fact that he lacks any status as a member of the social group he is about to join and is therefore unable to get a starting-point to take his bearings."[7] To rephrase Schutz's point so as to focus on health care, the patient as a stranger has difficulty even being oriented in the environment of high-technology medicine, much less wielding authority.

Health care professionals attempt to overcome this distance between the patient and the context of health care by altering the set of expectations held by the patient. This is particularly true when the patient and the healer will be in extended contact, as occurs in chronic illness. In such circumstances, the physician and other health care professionals are usually committed to inducting the patient into the life-world of health care. There is an attempt to change and reshape the taken-for-granted expectations of the patient, much as a catechumen is indoctrinated as a part of conversion into a new religion. To treat chronic illnesses such as hypertension or diabetes, the patient must come to see certain diets as forbidden, as medically unclean, much as individuals entering certain religions must come to appreciate certain foods as ritually unclean. Patients must also be taught to regard changes in their bodies in the same way as do their physicians. Shortness of breath, swelling of the feet after a day's work, now become possible signs of medical difficulties that should be reported to the physician. In addition, the patients may learn to measure their own blood pressure and test their urine in order to make inferences about the state of their bodies. Diabetics must calculate their caloric intake, know its source and administer insulin to themselves in carefully measured amounts. Such activities can be understood only within the system of assumptions and theoretical commitments of the physicians and nurses caring for the patient. Patients with a chronic disease become successful participants in their treatment insofar as they incorporate into their assumptions the technological and scientific world view of the physicians and nurses who are treating them. Once the patient has moved into and accepted the life-world of the healer, compliance with treatment will no longer be alien but a part of the new life-world of the patient.

The encounter with the health professional brings profound consequences. To accept a diagnosis is often to be committed to reordering one's very life in terms of the treatments and preventive regimens that the diagnosis warrants. Much of the negotiation between patients and physicians turns on the extent to which a diagnosis should transform a patient's life. In fact, to see a patient with a diagnosis of diabetes as a diabetic, not just a person with diabetes, is an indication of the extent to which a diagnostic label transforms an individual's existence. What is at stake is not simply an external matter concerning how the individual is to be regarded but it touches on how the individual should regard himself. The physician may be arguing that the individual's continued well-being is dependent on his seeing himself as a diabetic. He may want to avoid accepting a diagnostic label that will so throughly transform his life, in part because he does not wish to control his diabetes as strictly as the physician demands, and because he does not wish to acknowledge the changes in expectations the diagnosis brings, from the possibility of blindness, impotence, and kidney failure to early death. Health care professionals attempt to transform the patient from a stranger in a strange land into a permanent resident alien in the world of medical expectations and interventions.

Strangers and friends

Edmund Pellegrino and David Thomasma have argued that the physician and the patient meet as friends dedicated to the good of health.[8] He does this following arguments provided by Plato in the *Lysis*.[9] It is plausible to see the physician (or nurse or other health care professional) and the patient as friends, rather than strangers, only insofar as they are not set apart (1) by the possibly conflicting interests of the health care professions and those of patients, (2) by conflicting views of the goals of health care, (3) by differing understandings of the canons of moral probity, and (4) by differing views of health and disease. Health care professionals may differ from patients (1) in being specially dedicated to the long-range survival and security of their professions and to the development of knowledge for the aid of future patients, (2) in their views regarding the control of pain and the establishment of proper human abilities and form (e.g., how much medication should be given for the control of anxieties, the extent to which homosexuals should receive treatment not to change their sexual orientation, but to give them success in it), (3) in their judgments regarding the concrete character of the canons of moral probity (e.g., regarding the morality of allowing newborns with severe mental and physical handicaps to die), and (4) in their views of good medical treatment (e.g., regarding what amount of chance for a cure for a patient's cancer is worth what amount of disfigurement).

The more physicians and patients share a common view of the good life, the more plausible it will be that they meet as friends. A common view of the good life provides both moral and nonmoral values so that those who share that view know what ought to be done, what risks are prudent, and what actions should be avoided. When individuals share a common view of the good life, they live within a common fabric of mutual understandings and of commitments to common goals. In such circumstances, consenting to common endeavors often requires very little explicit communication, for communication has already taken place through the web of tacit understandings that fashions the common view of the good life. When this occurs, health care professionals and patients do not meet as strangers, but as individuals who are committed to a set of common goals.[10]

Individuals can come from widely differing communities and still be friends. In fact, as Aristotle notes, there may be an advantage to friendship with a foreigner, in that one thus avoids conflicts about personal advancement in the same polis.[11] But friendship with a foreigner is possible only insofar as one does share commitments to certain goals and goods. One way of reading Aristotle's remark for bioethics is that it may be easier for a physician to have a friendship with a patient than with another physician, because physicians are in competition with each other for patients or for advancement within the community of physicans. What is at stake here in distinguishing between friends and strangers is the extent to which health care professionals and patients either (1) share a common understanding that does away with the need for a great deal of formal disclosures and consent procedures, or (2) fail to possess such common commitments so that formal procedures of disclosure and consent are necessary to avoid serious misunderstandings.

Much of the formal bureaucratic structure for disclosure and consent in countries such as the United States is a function of the fact that in peaceable, secular, pluralist societies health professionals and patients recurringly meet as strangers. They are not simply strangers in that they often do not share the same set of professional commitments and scientific and technological understandings. They are strangers as well because their views of the good life are drawn from radically different communities of belief. When devout Roman Catholic physicians encounter Marxist women seeking abortions, or when liberal gay physicians encounter conservative Baptist patients in need of advice about treatment for their sexual dysfunctions, much cannot be taken for granted regarding a common understanding of the goals of health care and the canons of civil probity. Pellegrino's proof text passage from Plato for the argument that physicians and patients are friends presumes an unambiguous sense of health.[12] But as chapter 5 has shown, this is not the case. One might even wish to speak of health in the plural to indicate the diverse views of human well-being that motivate health care from the termination of unwanted pregnancies to the achievement of various sexual lifestyles. The woman who would rather have a less invasive therapeutic procedure to treat her breast cancer than the one preferred by the physician (in whose judgment the latter treatment offers a greater chance of long-range survival) engenders a dispute over the goals of health care and the composite sense of health (including physical intactness as well as chances for long-range survival) that should motivate therapeutic interventions.

Bureaucratic mechanisms for disclosure of information by physicians to patients and for the acquisition of free and informed consent are an essential part of the moral life of societies where individuals do in fact meet as strangers in the sense of not sharing the understanding and the moral commitments that often bind friends. Patients do not encounter physicians as they do religious counselors, pace Pellegrino.[13] One chooses a religious counselor in great measure because one shares with the counselor a rich web of moral and metaphysical commitments. However, the believing Christian may seek an oncologist, not because that oncologist is a fellow believer, but because of the technical abilities of the oncologist. Because physicians and the abilities of medicine are often sought for their efficaciousness as instruments toward the realization of important personal goals, conflicts arise when the goals of individuals do not accord with the value commitments of the physicians and other health care professionals. This is not a problem simply for medicine and the biomedical technologies, but for applied sciences generally, where there are conflicts between those who seek the applications of science and the scientists needed to effect the applications.

Physicians are often cast into a role analogous to those of bureaucrats in a large-scale nation. They must come to terms with the moral commitments and views of individuals from various moral communities while preserving the moral fabric of a peaceable, secular, pluralist society. It is for this reason that Hegel identified civil servants as the universal class (in contrast to Marx, who assigned this role to workers). Civil servants are committed to the general realization of freedom in the nation according to Hegel.[14] Civil servants must provide their services to citizens, whether the citizens are Catholics, Protestants, Jews, atheists, Marxists, or libertarians.[15] Letter carriers must deliver mail to all on their routes and not discriminate against some on the grounds of their religious or political commitment. The post office should accept the magazines of believers or nonbelievers, magazines of erotica and pamphlets against the reading of pornography. To ensure that this takes place, one may need bureaucratic rules that clearly establish what will be done, for whom, and under what circumstances. Physicians and other health care professionals are often in the position of civil servants, in that they must make clear to patients what will be done for them, to them, and under what circumstances. When health care professionals and patients meet as strangers, such disclosures and safeguards must be explicit and often detailed. On the other hand, physicians will need to know what services they have committed themselves to provide. By entering into a particular physician–patient relationship without sufficient warning to the patient about the physician's goals and moral viewpoints, the physician may have made an implicit commitment to provide services in emergency circumstances in ways that conflict with the physician's value commitments (e.g., a physician who has failed to make such disclosures and who cannot transfer a patient to another physician may be morally committed to perform an abortion to save the life and health of a woman, even if that conflicts with the physician's particular moral commitments). The same will occur, but even in nonemergency circumstances, if the physician joins a health service committed to providing particular forms of health care (e.g., including abortion).

Something is surely lost when patients and health care professionals must meet each other through a maze of bureaucratic rules and formal systems of mutual protection. There is also the danger that such rules and formal constraints will be turned into a fetish through which governments will intrude into all elements of the personal life of physicians and patients. Such rules and regulations should exist only as protections against individuals' imposing their understandings of the good life on unwilling others. They are not to be sought for their own sake. There are also many areas into which they should not intrude, such as the private choices of individuals about themselves and their willing associates, as well as in decisions of parents regarding defective newborns, as explored in chapter 6. As Robert Burt laments in *Taking Care of Strangers*, there is a price to be paid for government by "laws not men."[16] There are many circumstances in which one should not be a merely disinterested applier of formal rules. Still, in the life lived outside communities constituted out of a common commitment to a concrete view of the good life, one needs a disinterested application of the rules to protect against misunderstandings and to guard against abuses of power.[17] In its place there is much to be gained from the rule of laws, not men.

Medical care from passing strangers

A great number of patients do not have personal physicians on whom they rely. They have very little, if any, experience with the idealized physician–patient relationship, often portrayed in terms of the dedicated family practitioner or general practitioner, who knows a patient and his or her family over the span of a number of years. Instead, patients come to health maintenance organizations or to public clinics where the relationship with a particular physician or nurse is often episodic and transitory. In place of a personal physician–patient relationship, patients under such circumstances develop a health care receiver relationship with an institution rather than an individual. Even those who have a personal physician with whom they have a longstanding relationship may still find that in time of serious illness they are examined by numerous consultants. If hospitalized, they may come under the care of residents and attending physicians who rotate through a service on a monthly basis. As a result, even the most affluent patients will share in some of the experiences of the indigent who meet different physicians each time they come for treatment in a clinic or a hospital. Rules and regulations may in these circumstances give a character to an institution. They can indicate to the patient the commitments of the institution from which the patient is seeking treatment. Moreover, in the very fashioning of the rules an institution fashions its character; it comes to understand its commitments and to articulate them for those who come for care.

Free and informed consent

The practice of free and informed consent is justified both out of respect for the freedom of individuals as well as to achieve their best interests.[18] One must remember that the practice is a heterogeneous one. It involves gaining consent not only from individuals about to be treated, but also from the guardians of individuals not able to consent for themselves. The first case concerns individuals able freely to choose their own destinies and from whom authority must be gained for common endeavors. The second case concerns those who are in authority over others or who are considered for various reasons to be proper authorities regarding their best interests.

In the case of competent individuals, one can give a complex justification for the practice of free and informed consent: (1) it respects the freedom of the individual involved and provides authority for common endeavors; (2) it recognizes that individuals are often the best judges of their own best interests; (3) even if they are not the best judges, it acknowledges that the satisfaction of choosing freely is often preferred over having the correct choice imposed by others; and (4) it reflects the circumstance that the patient–physician relationship may often be such as to bring about a special fiduciary relationship that creates an obligation to disclose information. One can thus give a justification for the practice of free and informed consent on the basis of the principles of autonomy and beneficence. This complex justification leads to moral tensions, since individuals often choose in ways contrary to their own best interests. The same obtains in true proxy consent. If an individual appoints a proxy to choose, either according to specific instructions or according to the general instruction, "Do whatever you want," the second individual is a moral extension of the freedom of the first. Here one may encounter conflicts between respecting the capricious choices of the designated proxy and securing the best interests of the ward.

Most guardians do not act on the basis of advance directives that convey moral authority to and offer instruction for the proxy's choice. When guardians speak on behalf of individuals who have never been competent or who did not, while competent, leave instructions or convey authority to others, the place of the guardian is radically different from the appointed proxy.[19] Such guardians are not the extension of another individual's freedom. Instead, they may be in authority over their ward as a parent is over an infant by virtue of either having produced that individual or through a form of indentured servitude that arises through a minor's receiving parental support while not seeking emancipation. One might think here of parents refusing treatment for their severely defective newborn on grounds of hopelessness, or cosmetic surgery for their ten-year-old child on religious grounds. In addition, such guardians may be in authority to choose particular understandings of an individual's best interests in terms of the values embraced by the community within which the ward lives and to which, it can often be presumed, the ward will or would subscribe. One might think here of Jewish parents requesting that their son be circumcised. Or the guardian may be an authority regarding the incompetent individuals, proclivities, interests, and wishes. As such, the guardian becomes a substitute for an advance directive. One asks the guardian how that individual would have wanted to be treated with the presumption that the guardian may aid in choosing the treatment the individual would have found most appropriate. The guardian attempts to reconstruct what that individual would have wanted. Finally, guardians may simply play the role of choosing as rational and prudent persons choose on behalf of an individual who has left no instructions and who is not integrated within a particular community. Here one might imagine someone choosing among different treatment options for a ward of the state. In short, proxy consent is a composite of practices: (1) the choice by an authorized agent on behalf of an authorizing individual; (2) the choice by parents (or their assignees) on behalf of infants they have produced; (3) the choice by guardians on behalf of unemancipated minors whom they are rearing; (4) the choice by guardians in terms of the best interests of another as understood within a particular moral community; and (5) the choice by a guardian in terms of the best interests of another as understood with reference to what a rational and prudent person would choose.

The various practices of free and informed consent raise questions about what constitutes informed choice (e.g., how likely does a risk need to be in order to warrant describing it to a patient?), who is competent to choose, who is free to choose (e.g., when may adolescents choose their own medical treatment?), who is in authority to choose on behalf of another (e.g., as a designated proxy or through a status such as being a parent), and who is a good judge of the best interests of others (e.g., are parents any better judges of the best interests of their children than dispassionate outsiders?). We will need to examine the rights of individuals to determine their own treatment and the circumstances under which they may determine the medical treatment of others.

The right to be left alone

One of the ancient presumptions of English law is that individuals should be secure in their bodies against the unauthorized touching of others.[20] This right to the forbearance of others has its roots in ancient pagan Germanic traditions.[21] The presumption against unauthorized touching in the law extends to interventions by physicians from at least the eighteenth century. One finds in a 1767 decision, *Slater* v. *Baker and Stapleton*, that "it is reasonable that a patient should be told what is about to be done to him, that he may take courage and put himself in such a situation as to enable him to undergo the operation."[22] This decision does not underscore an autonomy-based right but rather suggests why it would be *useful* to gain consent. However, a bold finding in favor of the patient's right to consent to and refuse treatment based on the autonomy of the patient is found in Justice Cardozo's 1914 opinion in *Schloendorff* v. *Society of N.Y. Hospital*: "every human being of adult years and sound mind has a right to determine what shall be done with his own body; and a surgeon who performs an operation without his patient's consent commits an assault, for which he is liable in damages."[23] This opinion can be taken as setting the character of the debate about free and informed consent. The opinion strongly underscores the right of individuals to consent to treatment; yet it qualifies this right by acknowledging it only in individuals of sound mind and adult years. As we shall see, it was not easy for the courts to accept this right without qualification even for competent adults.

The right to free and informed consent includes the rights (1) to have sufficient information to be able to participate in treatment, as well as (2) to withdraw from treatment in whole or in part. *Slater* v. *Baker and Stapleton* underscores free and informed consent in the first sense, as a means for more effective collaboration between physician and patient in order to secure more effective treatment of the patient. Justice Cardozo's ruling in *Schloendorff* underscores the second. This second theme becomes prominent in twentieth-century reflections on individual rights and is at times captured simply as the general right to be left alone. One might think here in particular of the dissent written by Justice Brandeis in *Olmstead* v. *United States*:

The makers of our Constitution . . . sought to protect Americans in their beliefs, their thoughts, their emotions and their sensations. They conferred, as against the Government, the right to be let alone—the most comprehensive of rights and the right most valued by civilized men.[24]

Both Brandeis's opinion and Cardozo's decision raise the issue of whether one need respect all decisions of individuals or only those that appear sound and well reasoned. Need one respect the decisions of competent individuals, even if the decisions themselves appear foolish and ill reasoned. If a decision is competent only if it is well reasoned from well-established, firm premises, the range of patient wishes to be respected will be markedly restricted. If a decision is competent because it is the free choice of a competent individual (i.e., an individual who generally understands and appreciates his circumstances in the world and the general significance of his decision), then the range of decisions that must be expected will be much greater.

This issue reaches into health care decisions generally. Individuals who hold that the existence of God should be accepted by all rational individuals may conclude that medical and other decisions made on nontheistic presumptions are irrational, moved by passion, prejudice, or ignorance. On the other hand, individuals who do not judge such theistic presumptions to be well founded, or who do not find that particular religious faiths show the marks of rational defensibility, may conclude that medical decisions made on such theistic presumptions are irrational. This issue was addressed by Chief Justice Warren Burger while a member of the Circuit Court of the District of Columbia when he wrote a dissenting opinion to the denial of a petition for rehearing a request by a woman wishing to refuse a lifesaving blood transfusion on religious grounds. Justice Burger developed his opinion as a gloss on Brandeis's dissent in *Olmstead*:

Nothing in this utterance suggests that Justice Brandeis thought an individual possessed these rights only as to *sensible* beliefs, *valid* thoughts, *reasonable* emotions, or *well-founded* sensations. I suggest he intended to include a great many foolish, unreasonable and even absurd ideas which do not conform, such as refusing medical treatment even at great risk.[25]

According to Burger, individuals should be acknowledged to have the authority to refuse treatment, even if their choices are based on premises and understandings of the world that most would judge to be wrong and foolish.

The principle of autonomy gives a foundation for a right to be left alone, a right of privacy, a right to refuse the touchings and interventions of others. This right is central to the very notion of a peaceable community bound together by mutual respect. It sets a boundary against the interventions of others in the sense that they must show their authority to constrain the actions of other moral agents. The sense of this right has been captured in legal decisions that have affirmed the right both to consent and to refuse treatment. The court in *Natanson* v. *Kline*, for example, gives what is both a gloss on and a development of Cardozo's rule in *Schloendorff*:

Anglo-American law starts with the premise of thorough-going self determination. It follows that each man is considered to be master of his own body, and he may, if he be of sound mind, expressly prohibit the performance of life-saving surgery, or other medical treatment.[26]

The court endorsed a right to be left alone.

To justify successfully the right to be left alone in one's choices, one need only show that the choice does not involve unconsented-to force against the innocent and that the choice is one of a moral agent: a rational, self-conscious individual, who freely chooses a particular action or omission. To be a choice made by such an agent, the content of the choice need not be rationally grounded or argued for. It is sufficient if the individual understands and appreciates the general circumstances of the choice and in this sense affirms and endorses it. It will be enough if the choice is embraced by the agent within a general context in which choices are freely made and within which the chooser can at least advance the following justification: "I enjoy choosing capriciously, even about risky matters." Such a choice may be one for which the agent knowingly takes responsibility and is responsible. In this sense a choice is a competent choice because it flows from an accountable and therefore competent agent, even if that agent has chosen to choose poorly.

This analysis takes seriously the fact that moral agents often choose willfully. They choose in ways that are perverse and morally improper, not simply out of intellectual error, as many Greeks and Scholastics thought, but because of a desire to be free of others, and for the immediate exhilaration of breaking free from constraints. Etymologically, capricious actions are goat-like actions. Moral agents at times choose undisciplined frolicking over the careful reflections of a systematically analyzed life. This sense of rebellion for its own sake is captured in the classic statement of Satan in Milton's *Paradise Lost*, "Evil be thou my Good" (IV, 110). Freedom to choose includes as well the freedom to commit oneself to a particular belief no matter how absurd, or even because it is absurd. One might think here of the phrase, at times attributed to Tertullian, "I believe because it is absurd" (Credo quia absurdum est).[27] The fact that religious individuals commit themselves to beliefs that transcend reason or even conflict with reason does not impeach the competency of the individuals or their right to have their choices respected. The fact that individuals' choices are troublesome, bizarre, and tragic does not of itself mean that one may use force to stop them.

Three senses of freedom

The notion of choosing freely in free and informed consent includes at least three senses of freedom: (1) being able to choose, (2) being unrestrained by prior commitments or justified authority, and (3) being free from coercion.

FREEDOM TO CHOOSE. For valid consent, the agent must be free in the sense of being able to choose freely as a moral agent; the individual must be able to understand and appreciate the meaning and consequences of his or her actions so as to be imputable and responsible for those actions. The requirement of understanding and appreciating the significance of one's action is no more than the requirement that the behavior be an action, a behavior undertaken by a moral agent, rather than simply caused by neurological and psychological processes. Choices that will fail to meet this test will include behaviors of the acutely psychotic, the severely senile, the very young, the very drunk, the delirious, at times the very neurotic, and others who are not able to understand their own behaviors or to require others to respect them in the pursuit of their goals.

Even such individuals may be able from time to time to make competent decisions. To borrow a phrase from Heinz Hartmann, there are islands of ego autonomy. Some of these islands may be above the water only at low tide but be completely inundated by the high tides of stress and illness. One must avoid judging individuals to be either fully competent or incompetent. Different individuals in different times and circumstances will be competent or incompetent in different areas and to different degrees.[28] Competence, the ability to understand and appreciate the consequences of one's actions, and thus also the responsibility for one's actions, is neither a global nor a binary phenomenon. However, while partial incompetence may partially excuse, partial competence can be an absolute moral bar against the interventions of others insofar as there is an understanding and appreciation of the significance of refusing such interventions.

UNRESTRAINT BY PRIOR COMMITMENTS OR JUSTIFIED AUTHORITY. There is a second sense of freedom at stake as well: that of being unencumbered by preempting commitments to others. The very freedom of persons allows them to give or barter away their freedom to choose in general and in health care in particular. A requirement for joining an army might be ceding the right to refuse vaccinations, surgical procedures, and other treatments required to maintain battle readiness. In such forms of indentured servitude, individuals may transfer to others a right that was theirs. As we noted in chapter 4, something of this sort occurs in the relationship of children with their parents. By accepting parental support and failing to emancipate themselves, children may accept their parents as prima facie authorities regarding their medical best interests. Parents may also make commitments to their children that will preclude the parents' refusal of lifesaving treatment for themselves.

This last issue was raised in the case that occasioned Warren Burger's gloss on Brandeis's dissent in *Olmstead*. The Circuit Court of Appeals of the District of Columbia denied the patient's request to refuse transfusion because, among other reasons, her death would lead her to abandoning her seven-month-old child.[29] One should note that in another case the fact that a parent had financially provided for his children's well-being defeated this consideration.[30] The extent to which being a parent leads to an obligation to support the child will vary from community to community, as will the opportunities to transfer the obligation to other individuals or the community in general. One might note that there are in fact groups who force children to fend for themselves at very early ages. Here the Ik, who were mentioned in chapter 2, may again serve as an example. Ik children are put out of the home and begin to forage for themselves in groups at the age of about three or four.[31]

By committing a crime one may also lose the right to refuse treatment; thus, prisoners in general or those awaiting execution in particular may as a part of their punishment lose the right to refuse treatment. Their commission of the crime would count as their ceding their right to refuse treatment and being kept alive may be part of their punishment. This and other cases show that individuals who are free to consent in the sense of being competent may not be free to consent because they are restrained by prior commitments or the valid authority of others (e.g., that of parents, military officers, and prison wardens).

FREEDOM FROM COERCION. Finally, even if individuals are able to choose freely and are free of prior constraints, they may still find themselves in coercive circumstances. Since the very fabric of morality depends on mutual respect, any agreements extracted under coercion will not be binding. The person who uses coercion to secure an agreement cannot consistently appeal to the notion of a moral community to claim that the person coerced ought to be forthcoming. Valid consent must be acquired without the use of tactics that reduce the consenting individual to a mere means, that is, that set the consent aside. Thus, not only outright threats of violence but deception, threats to break contracts, or the failure to provide information owed will count as unconsented-to and unjustified force against the innocent. Such interventions are forbidden because they violate the principle of autonomy, which supports the minimal notion of the peaceable community. It follows from this basis for these prohibitions that force, deception, and breach of contract are not wrong in and of themselves. They are wrong only when they are used against the unconsenting innocent. Those who employ unjustified force cannot consistently complain when others defend themselves with whatever means necessary, from force of arms to deception.[32] Since in most cases patients must be considered innocent persons, the use of force in medicine is usually forbidden. Still, the use of force or deception is morally justified in order to control a patient who is without warrant threatening health professionals.

One will need in medicine, as in everyday life, to distinguish between acts of coercion and those of peaceful manipulation. If one understands coercive actions as those that place or threaten to place a patient in a disadvantaged state without justification, and if one defines peaceable manipulation as those actions that place or offer to place a patient in a advantaged state to which the patient is not entitled, coercions will be forbidden and peaceable manipulations will be allowed. The first violates the morality of mutual respect by violating the free choice of innocent persons, but the second does not. In fact, peaceable manipulations undergird the very process of peaceable negotiation through which individuals fashion peaceable agreements. People become friends, lovers, marriage partners, in part at least because they please, delight, and satisfy each other.[33] Any and all incentives will in principle be permissible, from offering financial inducements and honors to sexual satisfaction and other sensual pleasures, as long as the offer or maneuver does not make rational choice impossible.[34] One may wish in certain communities to avoid particular forms of excessive offers or offers of a particular sort. However, there will not be general arguments to show that such are in principle wrong through violating the very notion of mutual respect, as long as the individual being manipulated can still act, that is, choose, and be held responsible.

Though the distinction between coercions and peaceable manipulations may on the surface appear clear cut, this is far from the case. As Robert Nozick and others have indicated, what may appear at first to be a peaceable manipulation may under closer examination be shown to be a hidden form of coercion.[35] If, for example, a physician exaggerates risks and unduly frightens a patient so that the patient will agree to the form of treatment offered by the physician, coercion has been employed. So, too, if a physician threatens to withdraw promised supportive treatment unless the patient agrees to a particular intervention, which the physician deems to be indicated, coercion is involved. Either instance would be an example of the physician's placing the patient in a disadvantaged circumstance through a form of unconsented-to force (in the first case through force of words, i.e., deception, and in the second case through threatened breach of contract).[36] These considerations lead to the question of how much information is owed to a patient so that he or she can be properly advantaged for giving consent.

Three senses of being informed

The ability of patients to choose with effective liberty will depend on how much they know about the likely benefits and risks of the treatment they are considering and its alternatives. Depending on what physicians or other health care professionals disclose to a patient, and how it is disclosed, the patient will be inclined to refuse or to accept a treatment. A physician can make the use of almost any drug appear ill advised, if not risky. For example, the published warnings concerning penicillin include possible fatal allergic reactions, as well as hemolytic anemia, leukopenia, and neuropathies. If the likelihood of these risks is not put in terms of the likelihood of the benefits, a patient may decline a lifesaving treatment.

It is for this last reason that physicians have traditionally been concerned about the disclosure of too much or the wrong information to patients. The fear has been that, as strangers in an alien land, patients are likely to miscalculate the prudent balance of benefits and risks and as a result decline a treatment that would likely be effective with few real costs. Medicine in particular and health care in general are goal-oriented undertakings. They are focused on curing and preventing diseases and on caring for the worries, pains, and anxieties of patients. Only in very particular circumstances has medicine been focused on increasing the freedom of individuals to choose.[37] As the court in *Nishi* v. *Hartwell* affirmed, "The doctor's primary duty is to do what is best for the patient. Any conflict between this duty and that of a frightening disclosure ordinarily should be resolved in favor of the primary duty."[38]

This dedication to choosing and effecting the best treatment for the patient leads to collisions with the wishes of the patient to understand the nature and risk of treatment. Moreover, the dedication is not a purely altruistic one. Disclosures to patients can be time-consuming and vexatious, in addition to perhaps foreclosing the choice of the treatment deemed best by the physician. These various conflicts of interest between physicians and patients reach into the beginnings of Western medicine. Consider the description given by Plato of the difference in the amount of information disclosed to freemen and slaves.

> *Athenian*: . . . You agree that there are those two types of so-called physicians?
> *Clinias*: Certainly I do.
> *Athenian*: Now have you observed that, as there are slaves as well as free men among the patients of your community, the slaves, to speak generally, are treated by slaves, who pay them a hurried visit, or receive them in dispensaries? A physician of this kind never gives a servant any account of his complaint, nor asks him for any; he gives him some empirical injunction with an air of finished knowledge, in the brusque fashion of a dictator, and then is off in hot haste to the next ailing servant—that is how he lightens his master's medical labors for him. The free practitioner, who, for the most part, attends free men, treats their disease by going into things thoroughly from the beginning in a scientific way, and takes the patient and his family into his confidence. Thus he learns something from the sufferer, and at the same time instructs the invalid to the best of his power. He does not give his prescriptions until he has won the patient's support, and when he has done so, he steadily aims at producing complete restoration to health by persuading the sufferer into compliance.[39] (*Laws*, 4.720b–e)

Plato endorses a form of respect he takes to be due to free individuals. He also indicates that apart from any consideration of mutual respect, it may be useful to provide patients and their families with that amount of information that will allow patients to be effective collaborators in their treatment. Seen in this light, Plato does provide a critique of the attitude of many physicians: physicians underestimate the usefulness of disclosure for the compliance of patients with treatment. This element of Plato's critique can be harmonized with the general concern of physicians to treat effectively the diseases of their patients.

The more difficult issue is coming to terms with patients' demands to know, not simply in order better to cooperate with their physicians, but so that they may choose for themselves, even if those choices undermine what the physicians would hold to be the best or the most effective therapeutic approach. To what extent are physicians bound to disclose information when they believe that such disclosures are not likely to be useful in the treatment of the patient? One should note here that the right to consent is not equivalent to the right to be informed. Innocent, free individuals have a right not to be forced into being the patients of physicians. But do they have a right to become patients on their terms rather than on the physician's terms? Why may not a physician state that in return for treatment, which he or she is not obliged to offer, the patient must agree to be contented with whatever information the physician judges to be in the best interests of the patient's treatment?

Such a demand by a physician that a patient be contented with the level of disclosure a physician judges to be in the patient's best interests will not violate the morality of mutual respect. It may be contrary to certain cultural ideals of promoting individual autonomy or encouraging individuals to see themselves, and to be regarded by others, as self-determining. It may increase risks of fraud and duress on the part of physicians and be in violation of legal requirements. It may fail to encourage self-scrutiny on the part of physicians and rational decision making on the part of patients.[40] However, physicians as free individuals may count the goods to be pursued through limited disclosures to outweigh such possible harms.

The question of the proper balance between physicians' interests in effectively and successfully treating patients and patient and societal concerns for self-determination and scrutiny of physician recommendations has led to various legal standards for disclosure. Though there are serious questions to be raised about the authority of the state to impose a particular test for disclosure, the different standards offer concrete portrayals of the different possible compromises between these competing goals and interests.

THE PROFESSIONAL STANDARD. The traditional approach in the law has been to presume that patients should receive that amount of information usually provided by physicians in their community. Physicians were required to make those disclosures of information "which a reasonable medical practitioner would make under the same or similar circumstances."[41] This standard was defended on the grounds that only a physician can accurately determine (1) what amount of disclosure will not have an adverse effect on the patient so as to jeopardize treatment, and (2) what information is actually relevant to the patient's choice. As the Supreme Court of Missouri held in 1965,

The question is not what, regarding the risks involved, the juror would relate to the patient under the same or similar circumstances, or even what a reasonable man would relate, but what a reasonable medical practitioner would do. Such practitioner would consider the state of the patient's health, the condition of his heart and nervous system, his mental state, and would take into account, among other things, whether the risks involved were mere remote possibilities or something which occurred with some sort of frequency or regularity. This determination involves medical judgment as to whether disclosure of possible risks may have such an adverse effect on the patient as to jeopardize success of the proposed therapy, no matter how expertly performed.... After a consideration of these and other proper factors, a reasonable medical practitioner, under some circumstances, would make full disclosure of all risk which had any reasonable likelihood of occurring, but in others the facts and circumstances would dictate a guarded or limited disclosure. In some cases the judgment would be less difficult than in others, but in any event, it would be a medical judgment.[42]

In short, the use of the professional standard was justified on the grounds that the decision about the amount of information disclosed is a medical judgment, one requiring expert knowledge.

Though one might dispute, as other courts have, whether such a judgment is a medical judgment, one can morally defend the professional standard in terms of the principle of mutual respect. Unless otherwise warned, patients may reasonably expect that practitioners will give that amount of disclosure customary for members of that profession, school, or group (e.g., as is given by family practitioners, Jungian psychoanalysts, and members of the Libertarian Medical Society). To give less than that amount of disclosure without prior warning would constitute a form of deception. It may also breach a duty the practitioner has regarding the patient to the profession, school, or group of which the practitioner is a member. To give more than a reasonable medical practitioner would give may presuppose a hierarchy of values different from that endorsed by the profession or school. Such an increased disclosure might require a special warning to the patient of the following sort (appropriately expanded and altered): "I am willing to tell you things that most members of my profession [school or group] hold ought not to be disclosed. The risks of the disclosure are likely to be anxiety, worry, and so on. Do you want to hear the information?"

Unless individuals have taken steps to create special expectations and/or special requirements, the professional standard meets the principles of autonomy and beneficence. It does not violate the morality of mutual respect, as long as the patient knows of the general limits on disclosure. If it is pursued in a reasonable and well-intentioned fashion, the professional standard is also an example of an endeavor to achieve the good of others. The difficulty is that many individuals value self-determination and autonomy more than they do a worry-free and efficient treatment of their diseases. They may value freedom so highly that they will become anxious if they are not allowed to be self-determining. In addition, they may judge that only they could anticipate the likely significance for their lives of different therapeutic choices and their possibly adverse significance. Since there is an important difference between freedom as a value and freedom as a side constraint, the proper ranking to be given to free and informed choice is more to be created than discovered.

THE OBJECTIVE STANDARD. For more than a decade courts have been departing from the professional standard in order to embrace a standard of disclosure based on a duty to explain to a patient the procedure about to be undertaken and "to warn him of any material risks or dangers inherent in or collateral to the therapy, so as to enable the patient to make an intelligent and informed choice about whether or not to undergo such treatment."[43] In order for a patient to make such intelligent, informed choices, it became the duty of physicians to acquaint patients with all material risks, where a material risk is understood as a risk that "a reasonable person, in what the physician knows or should know to be the patient's position, would be likely to attach significance to in deciding whether or not to forego the proposed therapy."[44] The standard for disclosure thus became the patient's need for information.

The scope of the physician's communications to the patient, then, must be measured by the patient's need, and that need is whatever is material to the decision. Thus, the test for determining whether a potential peril must be divulged is its materiality to the patient's decision.[45]

Because this standard depends not on what would influence a particular individual, but what would influence reasonable and prudent individuals, it can be termed an objective standard. Instead of relying on the particular subjective concerns of a particular individual, one is to make disclosures on

an objective basis: in terms of what a prudent person in the patient's position would have decided if suitably informed of all perils bearing significance. If adequate disclosure could reasonably be expected to have caused that person to decline the treatment because of the revelation of the kind of risk or danger that resulted in harm, causation is shown, but otherwise not.[46]

These court decisions have made the standard for disclosure that amount of information necessary for the effective choice of a reasonable and prudent person, rather than that amount of information necessary for achieving what would be in the profession's view effective treatment.

This switch from using the judgment of reasonable members of the professional community as the standard to that of reasonable and prudent individuals can be justified if the medical profession is under the moral authority of society. However, in the absence of specific agreements and understandings, that is not the case. Members of a profession are as much entitled to their views regarding proper standards of disclosure as are members of the general public. A reasonable compromise between the two viewpoints is to be achieved, if at all, through negotiation. Even before the use of the objective standard, the professional standard could be seen as a point of departure for agreements that could bind physicians to make disclosures by an objective or subjective standard.

THE SUBJECTIVE STANDARD. A commitment to the values of self-determination can lead not only to an objective standard, but also to arguing that physicians should supply whatever information is material to a particular individual's choices. If a patient had a neurotic concern about developing cancer or becoming paralyzed, a physician would be obliged to provide information on these risks, even if they were so remote that they would not count as material considerations for a reasonable and prudent person. Alexander Capron sees the possibility of interpreting the standard embraced in *Cobbs* v. *Grant* as a subjective standard, since the court held that the physician's need for information "must be measured by the patient's need, and that need is whatever information is material to the decision."[47] At law, such an interpretation would constitute a severe burden for physicians who would need to show they had satisfied the worries of particular patients. There would always be the temptation for a patient to consider after the fact that the physician had not dealt with all of the patient's special concerns.

Even if one concluded on pragmatic grounds that this is not a standard to use in the courts, one might still embrace it as a moral ideal because of an autonomy-oriented view of the good life. If one is concerned with autonomy more than successful treatment, a subjective standard would be morally attractive. Or one might also hold that individuals can effectively choose so as to maximize their best interests, even if they are in part based on special or even neurotic concerns, only if they can determine their treatment. One might hope that individual physicians would ascertain the special worries and concerns of patients and then disclose to those patients enough information for them to make choices in terms of their special concerns. This would allow even neurotic patients to choose effectively within the context of their obsessions. The extent to which one would see this as desirable would depend on one's comparative ranking of the value and usefulness of self-determination versus objective or professional determinations of effective treatment.

One should realize that the professional standard did not in principle foreclose giving that amount of information that a reasonable and prudent person would want or that a particular patient with special concerns would want. The professional standard was rather premised on the fact that the disclosure of such information was often in fact detrimental to the effective treatment and to the good of the patient, and that it thus ought not to be provided.

THE RIGHT NOT TO BE INFORMED. In developing the objective standard for disclosure, a special subjectively grounded exception has been incorporated. Particular patients, if they decline such knowledge, need not be told what rational and prudent individuals usually need to know in order to make a reasonable decision. Both *Cobbs* v. *Grant* and *Sard* v. *Hardy*, for example, explicitly underscore the fact that a physician is not obliged to disclose risks where the patient requests not to be informed.[48] The right to be informed is not an obligation to be informed. Nor does it create an overriding obligation on the part of the physician to inform. It rather requires offering to the patient the opportunity to acquire information. Here again respect of freedom serves as a side constraint, not a value. The goal of free and informed consent should not be to force patients to be autonomous, but rather to give them the opportunity to be autonomous in their choice of medical treatment.

This underscores the fact that different individuals seek quite different sorts of physician–patient relationships. Some wish to be full collaborators in their treatment, if not directly in control of it. Such individuals see physicians as agents of their already well-formed wishes. For such individuals anything but a robust subjective standard of full disclosure may be too weak. On the other hand, many wish to entrust their care to a physician in whom they have faith. Such individuals wish last and least of all to be obliged to listen to all the risks and possible harms to which they may be subjected. They would rather repose their confidence in their initial choice of a physician and see the physician's major duty to be that of shouldering the fears, anxieties, and hesitations that go with making important choices in circumstances of uncertainty. The opportunity to waive disclosure allows patients to fashion a relationship with physicians that will meet the patients' needs. It allows patients to request that the standard of disclosure be the professional standard or one that provides even less information than the reasonable and prudent physician would offer. But what if the physician deems that it is in the patient's best interests to have certain material disclosed anyway? May the physician require the patient to agree to the disclosure as a condition for treatment? Despite the constraints of the law, the physician should possess that right in terms of the principles of beneficence and autonomy, unless the physician through prior agreement has waived the right to require disclosure as the condition for treatment, or has failed to warn the patient in advance of these sorts of requirements so that the patient could engage a different physician.

THE THERAPEUTIC PRIVILEGE. Even in court rulings that have upheld the objective standard, a qualification has been introduced for circumstances when the disclosure would so distress the patient as to make rational choice impossible or in fact to harm the patient. In *Canterbury* v. *Spence*, for example, the court recognized that "patients occasionally became so ill or emotionally distraught on disclosure as to foreclose a rational decision, or complicate or hinder the treatment, or perhaps even pose psychological damage to the patient."[49] In such circumstances physicians were not to be bound by the objective standard but rather the disclosure could be limited to

that required within the medical community when a doctor can prove by a preponderance of the evidence he relied on facts which would demonstrate to a reasonable man the disclosure would have so seriously upset the patient that the patient would not have been able to dispassionately weigh the risks of refusing to undergo the recommended treatment.[50]

In taking this position the court affirmed a view already developed in the literature,[51] namely, that disclosures that seriously alarm the patient could in fact constitute bad medical practice.[52]

The therapeutic privilege can be interpreted as a form of emergency. Physicians have generally been excused from gaining consent in emergency circumstances when delaying to obtain such consent would lead to death or permanent bodily and perhaps mental harm.[53] Instead, they have been allowed to provide that form of treatment that is medically required to save life and limb or avoid permanent bodily harm. Bona fide cases in which the therapeutic privilege is invoked are similar to emergencies if the patient is not able to be consulted because communicating the requisite information would itself make the required choice impossible (i.e., the communication would so distress the patient that competent choice would be impossible). Unless there were some prior agreement or disclosure, the physician may in good conscience provide care according to the standards of the profession, even though it may later become clear that the patient would have wished to be treated differently. If the disclosure is likely to harm the patient, one may similarly presume that the patient would not in fact wish to be harmed, and thus garner a moral justification for the use of the therapeutic privilege.

Moral problems surface if one highly values freedom. Those passionately interested in self-determination may wish to have full disclosure, even if it is likely to harm them. They may value their opportunity to be autonomous more highly than a long life or freedom from pain, deformity, and disability. From a moral point of view, such patients should be free to make agreements with willing physicians to be informed no matter what. Such patients should be able to waive the benefits of the therapeutic privilege.

PLACEBOS AND BENEFICENT DECEPTIONS. There are many circumstances under which individuals implicitly consent to minor deceptions. They may simply be seeking reassurance, even against and despite the facts. We often need a gentle hand that will assure and not necessarily remind us of the harsh realities of life. It would not be morally improper, for example, for a physician to stress the positive aspects of the results of plastic surgery after a serious burn. Under the circumstances, it is unlikely that the patient would expect a physician to do otherwise. The role of the physician here traditionally has been to bolster spirits, not to state bluntly that some will find the patient's appearance distasteful, if not disturbing. On the other hand, the physician should not attempt to convince the patient to enter a beauty contest, if that is not warranted. Nor should a physician fail to speak the unvarnished truth when that would be helpful and the patient is willing to listen. To decide where support ends and true deception begins requires not only clinical experience but thorough self-knowledge on the part of the physician. It is easier to be the bearer of good news than of bad news.

Many important social relationships in fact presume other than truthful answers. Some questions, such as "How are you doing?" are not usually meant as an invitation for a brief history of one's recent medical problems. Indeed, games such as poker presuppose mutual consent to active deception. Similarly, there may be circumstances under which it is unreasonable to presume that individuals want full disclosure of information. If in an emergency one does not have pain-killing drugs on hand, it is not deceptive to begin an intravenous drip with a glucose solution while solemnly declaring, "As this fluid enters your veins, the pain will begin to diminish." There is a reasonable expectation that the placebo effect will diminish the pain, even though the drip has nothing to do with this directly, but is rather part of the ceremony and ritual through which physicians over centuries have calmed patients and controlled pain. In short, it is not a false statement. It is unreasonable to expect that the patient would want anything but relief of the pain (except in certain bizarre situations in which one might encounter individuals who were known to have committed themselves to truth at all costs and in all circumstances). To provide a preliminary lecture on the placebo effect and ask for permission to employ it would be not only self-defeating but absurd. Not only is such disclosure not required by the principle of autonomy, but it would violate the principle of beneficence.

Such emergencies where a presumptive permission to deceive is clearly available grade into areas where some general explicit consent to deception is required. In programs designed to wean a patient slowly from an addiction through substituting nonactive ingredients, it may be necessary to indicate that unspecified beneficial forms of deception will be integral to the therapeutic regimen. At other times it may be enough simply to state, "If you take this drug, you will begin to feel better and your anxieties will diminish." Again, given the placebo effect, such a statement is not deceptive and in most circumstances further information need not be given unless the patient specifically requests it. Even if the patient requests it, the physician may morally respond, "If you want to be treated by me, take the medicine I give you and trust me."

Negative placebo effects are more problematic. What of drugs that have as possible side effects symptoms that others may suffer as much from suggestion as from the drug? One might think here of nausea, headaches, or impotence. If the physician believes that the patient is suggestible and is more likely to suffer from the symptoms because of the suggestive force of the disclosure than because of the actions of the drug, should a disclosure be made? The answer depends in part on how remote the risks from the drug are and in part on the kind of relationship the physician has with the patient. A close relationship fashioned in trust may enable the physician to know the extent to which the patient would presume that the physician would make such disclosures. On the other hand, if the risks are real and the physician cannot presume such an implicit consent for partial disclosure, then the facts must be stated. Part of being a free competent individual is that one must take the risk involved in the stewardship of one's own destiny. The answers to the moral questions regarding the use of placebos and beneficent deception can be found only in a careful examination of the physician–patient relationship and the moral community in which it develops. All deception and all truthtelling are contextual, and medicine is no exception.

FASHIONING THE PHYSICIAN–PATIENT RELATIONSHIP. In general, physicians and patients meet as free individuals. Each in terms of his or her own views of proper action should participate in fashioning the character of the physician–patient relationship. It is the case that particular patients may be more in need of the care of a physician than particular physicians will need to provide care to a particular patient. This is especially true in situations of acute care. But most physicians and patients meet because of chronic health care needs or because of the everyday vexations of life that do not require immediate or emergency treatment. Under such circumstances, there are opportunities for patients both individually and in groups to shape the character of health care. One must remember that it is patients and potential patients who possess the majority of the resources of all societies. Without recourse to the coercive force of the state, they can influence the ways in which health care is delivered by setting standards of disclosure required on the part of physicians who receive reimbursement through insurance policies, use community-owned hospitals, or receive salaries through community-owned health maintenance organizations.

One can agree wholeheartedly that a paternalistic medicine, one that decides what patients should or should not know, may be not only oppressive and vexatious, but in the long run injurious to the health of patients by not encouraging patient responsibility, and still hold that the use of state force is not justified to impose either a subjective or objective standard of care. Even apart from the constraints on the use of force by the principle of autonomy, there may be advantages to be derived from setting standards for disclosure through multiple negotiations by various groups of physicians and patients. Individuals vary greatly in their desires and abilities to shoulder the responsibilities for dealing with medical decision making. One might imagine a scheme in which subscribers to insurance programs were asked to check which standard of disclosure they wished used in their treatment; they might also be asked to review their choices semiannually or annually. The opportunity to consider in advance and review whether one wishes either to be autonomous in decision making or to convey trust to a physician may best allow patients to realize with freely cooperating physicians their views of a proper patient–physician relationship.

Making choices for others: three forms of paternalism

The *Oxford English Dictionary* defines paternalism as "the principle and practice of paternal administration; government as by a father; the claim or attempt to supply the needs or to regulate the life of a nation or community in the same way as a father does those of his children." Patients often regress under the stress of disease and come to be treated and want to be treated as children by health professionals. Informal requests for paternalistic care occur as a matter of course in health care because patients are in a strange environment. Like many travelers in unfamiliar lands where the language is in part a barrier to communication, they may look for others to lead them. Consider the ways in which individuals who visit foreign countries as part of a package tour embrace a form of paternalism. They trust the tour guide and company to have selected the reasonable places to see. In a similar fashion, patients often look to their physician for guidance and direction.

Often paternalism cannot or at least should not be avoided. One must treat infants in a paternalistic fashion. The very senile must be similarly treated, often leading to tensions as children and parents radically reverse their social roles. The moral issue is the extent to which paternalism in health care is allowable and desirable. To address this issue one must first recognize the different forms of paternalism, each of which raises different moral issues.[54]

PATERNALISM FOR INCOMPETENTS. In the case of individuals who have never been competent, such as infants, young children, and those profoundly or very severely mentally retarded from birth, paternalism is unavoidable. Others must choose on their behalf. Others must determine their best interests. Paternalism in which parents protect and foster the best interests of their incompetent children is a good example. It is justified in terms of the principle of beneficence. This form of paternalism also plays a role in the choices made on behalf of individuals who were once competent and who failed to direct in advance how they were to be treated, should they become incompetent. In the absence of specific instructions, others must choose on their behalf either by appeal to a standard of a reasonable and prudent person or by an appeal to a standard articulated by a particular community of individuals committed to a particular set of standards and values. As we will see, each standard has its own problems. The more one attempts to establish the best interests of a ward by appeal to what a reasonable and prudent individual would choose, the less content such standards have. On the other hand, the more one appeals to concrete understandings of best interests fashioned in particular moral communities, the more divergent judgments become.

One is then pressed to ask who should determine which standard to use, and on what basis. These two points are obviously closely intertwined. If one allows a guardian to choose in terms of the guardian's particular moral community (e.g., as an Amish, Jehovah's Witness, or Christian Scientist), one has already decided to allow the pursuit of a particular interpretation of best interests. If one constrains the guardian to choose as a reasonable and prudent person would choose, to what sense of reasonableness and prudence ought one to appeal? One returns here to the problems raised in chapters 2 and 3 with regard to discovering concrete standards for proper beneficent actions. There will also be conflicts about who is in authority over an incompetent and thus free to choose the standard. As has already been argued, parents come to be in authority over the infants they produce. Similarly, individuals who care for and nurture formerly competent people come to be in authority over them, for such persons can no longer possess themselves and therefore can come into the possession and authority of others. Within certain restrictions, which we will explore further in the section on proxy consent (as well as those already examined in chapters 4 and 6), those in authority can be accepted as proper judges of the best interests of their wards because they have a form of property right in their wards as masters have in their indentured servants. As we saw in chapter 4, humans who are not persons cannot possess themselves. They are most plausibly held to be possessed by those who produced them or care for them. As a result, those in authority over others may choose for their wards not simply to achieve their best interests, but also in order to control and direct their lives. For example, many of the choices made by parents for their children are made not to achieve the best interests of the children (nor necessarily in order to thwart their best interests), but in order to achieve parental goals and values not directly related to the children's care. If no one is an authority, beneficence would dictate choosing a guardian who appears best able to determine the ward's interests. When the ward is a member of a particular community, the choice is properly made by an appeal to that community's standard, not to that of reasonable and prudent persons generally, whatever that might mean. This is particularly the case when the person was previously competent. The best-interests standard of the previously competent person's community most likely represents that individual's prior preferences.

FIDUCIARY PATERNALISM. The appointment of another individual to choose on one's behalf justifies paternalistic actions in terms of mutual respect. The appointed individual may determine the best interests of the ward, not simply because he or she is a good judge of those interests (which may or may not be the case), but by virtue of having been placed in authority by the explicit choice of the ward. Fiduciary paternalism occurs in two forms.

1. *Explicit fiduciary paternalism.* Patient–physician relationships are often explicitly paternalistic. When a patient tells a physician, "You decide what you think is the best form of treatment," authority is conveyed to the physician and a paternalistic relation is created. The physician must then attempt to use professional judgment to determine what forms of therapeutic intervention would maximize the patient's best interests. To some extent, all patient–physician relationships that involve complicated and technical interventions require such a fiduciary paternalism, unless the patient is also a physician expert in that area. Otherwise, even physicians who are patients must repose their faith in another. The liberty of the physician to choose on behalf of the patient will be determined by the patient's wishes in the matter, including the extent to which the patient has formed a judgment regarding the issues at stake. "Doctor, I wish I could make up my mind whether to have

a coronary bypass operation. I really would rather you tell me what you would do in this circumstance."

The extent to which it is sensible to speak of advance directives establishing a fiduciary paternalism will depend on the extent to which paternalism requires that another determine the best interests of the ward. Thus, it would seem implausible to speak of explicit advance directives appointing a particular individual to effect them as creating a fiduciary paternalism. Not all agents act paternalistically on behalf of the individuals who appoint them. Rather, because authorized agents effect the wishes or carry out the orders of those who appoint them, those who appoint them are not simply wards, even when they are no longer competent. However, when an individual is appointed to care for another and is given latitude in deciding the criteria for proper care, a paternalistic relation has been established. One might imagine such being effected through an instrument establishing a durable power of attorney. The most extreme example of explicit fiduciary paternalism would be the instruction, "Please do what you think best over the course of the treatment, even if I lose heart and ask you to stop. You just keep doing what you think is right."

2. *Implicit fiduciary paternalism.* Even though patients have not explicitly appointed others as their surrogate decision makers, it is often argued that there is an implicit presumption that others will make certain sorts of decisions on their behalf.

Minor, *short-term* paternalistic interventions are often justified on the ground that reasonable and prudent individuals would not mind and do in fact want such interventions if they are undertaken when there is some doubt whether the individuals are competent or well informed. These forms of intervention are often seen as instances of the weak paternalism justified by John Stuart Mill.

Again, it is a proper office of public authority to guard against accidents. If either a public officer or any one else saw a person attempting to cross a bridge which had been ascertained to be unsafe, and there were no time to warn him of his danger, they might seize him and turn him back, without any real infringement of his liberty; for liberty consists in doing what one desires, and he does not desire to fall into the river. Nevertheless, when there is not a certainty, but only a danger of mischief, no one but the person himself can judge of the sufficiency of the motive which may prompt him to incur the risk; in this case, therefore (unless he is a child, or delirious, or in some state of excitement or absorption incompatible with the full use of the reflecting faculty), he ought, I conceive, to be only warned of the danger; not forcibly prevented from exposing himself to it.[55]

In such paternalistic intervention the right of individuals to choose capriciously, indeed, recklessly, is not denied. Rather, it is assumed that individuals would wish to be protected against errors that are not integral to their plans or choices when such protection involves only a minor intrusion.

Such considerations may morally justify not only preventing suicide when it is not clear that the individual is truly incompetent, but also in fact civilly committing the individual for a brief period of time to allow for an evaluation of his mental health. For example, California enacted a code to allow civil commitment for seventy-two hours in order to evaluate individuals thought to be mentally ill and a danger to themselves.[56] The code also provided for an additional fourteen-day commitment when there is an imminent threat of an individual's committing suicide.[57] The extent to which such further commitment would be morally justified will depend on how seriously one doubts the competence of the would-be suicide.

One should note that requiring greater certainty of competence when an individual's choices are likely to be dangerous is a form of weak paternalism. If a patient consents to a standard treatment with few and negligible risks and with considerable promise of benefit, physicians or nurses rarely question the validity of the consent, even if the patient is only marginally aware of the significance of the choice.[58] This may be justified on the principle that most individuals choose what rational and prudent persons choose and that consent, however enfeebled, suggests that the individual in question has no objections. In addition, where there is little risk and much good to be achieved, there appear to be few grounds to intervene to protect the best interests of the patient by special determinations of competency. So, too, if a patient refuses a treatment when there is little chance of success or of significant benefit, there is little ground for not accepting the patient's apparent competence. For instance, if terminal patients appear fairly competent, there is little ground for a careful assessment of competence prior to accepting their decision to refuse treatment. However, when the patient wishes to choose a risky treatment or refuse clearly beneficial treatment, physicians should establish clearly that the patient is competent. Such patients can be seen on the analogy of Mill's individual approaching the bridge and may be hindered in their decisions until it is clear that they are choosing competently. When there are no well-founded doubts concerning competence, one may not interefere in bizarre and risky undertakings of others without offending against the principle of autonomy.

Some have also argued that citizens of a society have implicitly agreed to paternalistic interventions as a form of insurance against unwise or dangerous actions.[59] This view is difficult if not impossible to defend if one takes freedom of individuals seriously, that is, distinguishes between freedom as a value and freedom as a side constraint. Even if one held that many agreed to such interventions, individuals while competent could explicitly declare their nonparticipation in such paternalistic insurance schemes.

BEST-INTEREST PATERNALISM. This form of paternalism is also termed strong paternalism: the contention that under certain circumstances one may override the competent refusal of an individual in order to achieve the best interests of that individual. Since this is the most morally problematic form of paternalistic intervention, some have had this form of paternalism in mind when they have spoken of paternalism in general. Thus, Bernard Gert and Charles Culver provide the following five conditions, which they take to be necessary and sufficient for paternalism (best-interest paternalism or strong paternalism in our terminology):

A is acting paternalistically toward S if and only if A's behavior (correctly) indicates that A *believes that*:
    (1) his action is for S's good
    (2) he is qualified to act on S's behalf
    (3) his action involves violating a moral rule (or doing that which will require him to do so) with regard to S
    (4) he is justified in acting on S's behalf independently of S's past, present, or immediately forthcoming (free, informed) consent
    (5) S believes (perhaps falsely) that he (S) generally knows what is for his own good.[60]

There are difficulties with this analysis.[61] The central moral difficulty lies in the problem of establishing the priority of duties of beneficence over duties of autonomy. As chapter 3 has shown, outside particular moral communities, where individuals have already agreed to a particular ordering of goods and harms that will place successful medical intervention higher than liberty interests, it will be morally blameworthy to engage in such paternalistic actions.

Proxy consent and the emancipation of minors

As we saw in the beginning of the section on free and informed consent, individuals may plausibly claim on quite different grounds to have the right to choose on behalf of others: (1) a guardian may have been explicitly authorized by the ward while the ward was still competent; (2) guardians may be in authority over the ward because they produced the ward (i.e., parents); (3) a guardian may be in authority over the ward because of the indentured servitude that develops between parents and children, between those who care for others and those for whom they care; (4) a guardian may be a good judge of the best interests of the ward as seen within the community to which the guardian and ward belong; (5) a guardian may be a good judge of the best interests of the ward in terms of what reasonable and prudent persons would choose. In the first three cases guardians claim the right to choose because they are in authority, not necessarily because they are good authorities, as in the last two cases.[62]

This tension between those in authority and those who are authorities is closely tied to the tensions between the applications of the principles of autonomy and beneficence. Those in authority claim the right to be respected in their choices, whether or not they are the best choices, because others do not have the authority to intervene in their persons, possessions, or actions. The authorized guardian is the extension of the ward and can express the ward's desires to be left alone and justify choices on the basis of the principle of autonomy. In the second and third cases the ward is in the possession of the guardian and may not be touched without the guardian's consent (see chapter 4). Those who are authorities (as opposed to being in authority) claim the right to decide because they know what is best, as in the fourth and fifth cases. They claim the right to intervene on the basis of the principle of beneficence. In chapter 6 we examined elements of proxy choice with respect to fetuses and newborns. There the objects of our concern were not yet persons in the strict sense nor yet bearers of all the special rights that can be accorded to persons in the social sense. In addition, as in the case of cesarean and fetal surgery, interventions to protect the best interests of the fetus could involve intrusions into the mother's very body. The issues are further complicated when the individual is a person in the social sense, or even in the strict sense, and thus a bearer of special rights.

There are a number of legal exceptions to the right of parents and guardians to choose health care on behalf of their wards. First and foremost is the exception of need or emergency. When death or permanent bodily harm would result from delaying so as to gain consent, physicians and others may presume that the person in need would wish to be treated in the ways in which reasonable and prudent individuals would choose. Here the physician becomes a proxy in the fifth sense, as a good judge of what reasonable and prudent individuals would want. The physician may operate in that role until a guardian arrives who has authority to choose treatment on some other basis (e.g., a Jehovah's Witness with a durable power of attorney from the Jehovah's Witness patient demanding that all blood transfusions for that patient be stopped).

Other exceptions have included (1) concerns with public welfare, which have allowed minors to consent to the treatment of venereal disease and drug addiction, (2) areas of privacy such as the choice to secure an abortion or use contraceptives, and (3) circumstances under which minors have emancipated themselves from their guardians.[63] The first two of these exceptions may simply be particular instances of the third: areas where minors have in part come into their own authority and have been recognized as able and free to choose on their own behalf. They may involve as well circumstances where society for various public policy reasons may not wish to enforce parental rights over children. Society may recognize the moral right of parents to enforce their own views on their children, as far as they are able, but not wish to expend the resources of society in this endeavor because of the costs involved, including the problem of determining when children become fully emancipated in the moral sense. For example, parents are generally considered to be at liberty to indoctrinate their children in various political and religious viewpoints. They may attempt to bring up their children as revolutionaries or to instill in them the view that the slightest lascivious thought will lead to eternal damnation, for as long as they can get their children's attention. They must pursue these goals, however, without state assistance, since such goals fall outside the interests of a neutral, peaceable, secular pluralist state.[64]

It is plausible that children come into their own possession incrementally, as they gain the capacity to understand and appreciate the significance of their actions and as they assume authority over and support of themselves. There are no sharp boundaries between competence and incompetence, or between being under one's parents' authority and being free of it. The concept of the mature minor underscores the circumstances under which minors, though they are not emancipated through living apart and supporting themselves, are partially freed from parental authority in areas where they understand and appreciate the significance of decisions having substantial bearing on the future character of their lives (e.g., reproductive choices) and which decisions do not require parental subvention. It is plausible to hold that children in different circumstances and different areas may thus come partially into their own possession by being morally responsible for such choices. In such circumstances (e.g., concerning decisions bearing on the future existence of the child) either the scope of the indenture to parents does not include ceding the right to choose in such important areas affecting one's future life, or even if it does involve such a cession of rights, the state may not be interested in protecting parental rights because of the costs involved in affording such protection (e.g., the difficulty of determining the extent to which such rights have plausibly been ceded to parents).

How is one to balance the right of those in authority to choose and the interest of authorities to protect the best interests of wards? How is one to strike a balance between the right of guardians to be left alone in making their choices regarding their wards, and the right of wards to be free to make choices in areas where they have an emerging authority to control their own lives. Given the arguments to this point, it seems plausible to state the principle for intervention on behalf of a ward and against the wishes of a guardian in the following fashion.

PRINCIPLE FOR INTERVENTION ON BEHALF OF A WARD

Out of considerations of beneficence or concerns for the autonomy of wards, one may use (but, because of countervailing significant costs, not be obliged to use) force to rescue a ward from a guardian in authority who by at least clear and convincing evidence (given the uncertainties in ethical decisions, the test for certainty must be strong) is acting or failing to act in ways that are significantly contrary to the best interests of the ward (as determined by reasonable and prudent persons), if and only if:

    i. The guardian's actions or omissions injure the body or mind of the ward to a degree significantly contrary to the best interests of the ward, as determined by the standard of a reasonable and prudent person, and which harms are the sort to which the ward in the future by at least clear and convincing evidence will not consent. This condition is set aside when the ward does competently agree (as might occur with the moral equivalent of a mature minor). Where the harm to the ward results from the guardians' failure to provide a costly service to the ward, the intervener must be willing to assume the costs of providing the service; or

    ii. The child asks for rescue and is competent;

    iii. The injury is malicious; or

    iv. The actions or omissions are contrary to agreements made with the ward before the ward became incompetent.

The principle sets the limits of a guardian's authority and establishes the realm of a rescuer's authority.

Significant interests of the ward must be at stake to warrant an intervention because of the importance of family and other caring units for the protection of those who cannot defend or support themselves, and because interventions may undermine this defense and support. Whatever values a rescuer might hold, that individual will need to determine that the goods to be achieved outweigh the costs involved in the rescuer's intrusion. To warrant a rescue where the person is not competently asking for aid nor where the injury is in violation of a prior agreement, the injury must involve significant and direct physical or mental harm to count as a direct use of force against a future person. One is not constrained, absent prior agreements or a special view of the good life and beneficence, to live in ways that will maximize the advantage of present, much less future, persons. As has already been observed, it is difficult to protect future individuals from being used as means. Circumstances must be quite clearly spelled out in order to show that a guardian is using a future person as a means *merely*, that is, in ways to which it is unlikely that the person will consent. To be at the mercy of the wisdom and vision of past persons is the predicament of future persons. Future persons have the right to expect that past persons will not have acted in ways that directly use force against them without their presumed permission. It is plausible to hold that harming the minds and bodies of others through positive actions or omissions, in the case of guardians who have special fiduciary responsibilities, may be an unconsented-to use of force against such individuals. Because interpreting an outcome as an injury depends on a complex set of values and understandings of the world, one will need to be very certain that the ward will in fact interpret the guardian's interventions as injuries. One runs the risk of falsely interpreting as a harm what will be received as a beneficence and therefore groundlessly interfering with the authorized actions of actual persons. The appeal to a reasonable and prudent person standard here underscores the need for certainty, rather than reliance on a particular hierarchy of values: the appeal should have as much generality as possible in order to have a sufficient likelihood of identifying a true injury. The appeal to future likely consent allows "idiosyncratic" views to set the reasonable and prudent standard aside. However, when the child is competent and asks for rescue, or when the injury is malicious or in breach of contract and therefore against the principle of autonomy, one need only consider the likely balance of harms versus risks involved in the rescue.

Obviously it is very difficult to make clear and certain judgments in these matters. The rearing of children and the caring for wards take place in the embrace of visions of the good life and of beneficence. The very vitality of the visions often leads to conflicts that are insoluble, TEYKU. What, for example, ought one to make of ritual or other mutilations of the bodies of incompetent individuals? One might think here of male circumcision, which rarely has medical indications and which is usually performed for religious or vaguely traditional reasons.[65] The foregoing analysis suggests that it is permissible under the assumption that the individual will not object when he in the future becomes competent. This assumption is an especially well-grounded one in the context of a religious community. The same argument will support the tattooing and scarification of individuals that are a part of the tradition of particular communities. Those who will likely live out their lives in such a community will likely affirm the action as beneficent. But what of female circumcision, which is performed to contain female sexual desire and to increase male pleasure in intercourse? This practice is a major source of morbidity and mortality in northern Islamic Africa.[66] The practice has been so pervasive that it has been adopted by some Christian Copts as well.[67] What of the widespread attempt among groups in the West to instill sexual guilt in children for harmless activities such as masturbation? What of those who would wish to send their children to schools that would encourage early sexual play and fondling?

It seems unlikely that one can decide with any certainty whether future individuals will be pleased or not regarding their strict or licentious sexual upbringing. In such circumstances there is unlikely to be authority to rescue. Issues of serious mutilation, such as those involved in female circumcision, are less clear. If the individual will live out her life in the closed context of a traditional society, she may with great likelihood be pleased with having been circumcised. Judgments will need to be made in terms of likely future outcomes and circumstances. Even if, under special circumstances, one will forgo rescue, it does not follow that one may not at the same time attempt to change such practices through showing the virtues of a different set of values and of a different view of the world.

Issues are even more complicated when wards have not established advance directives regarding their care, and when they are unlikely ever again to be competent. If they were once competent, their guardians should, as far as possible, use substitute judgment in order to respect the wishes of these individuals who were at least once competent. One should try as far as possible to act on prior preferences. One may often presume that current wishes of those irreversibly incompetent still express their prior competent choices, except where following such wishes would lead to significant harms. One might think here of honoring a refusal of treatment or food by even a very senile individual. The difficulty lies with those who have never been competent; that is, never in any of the areas of their lives have they been persons in the strict sense of moral agents. When individuals have not in advance stipulated their desires for care, these analyses lead to a great but not absolute latitude of choice for parents and other guardians of incompetents. For example, when a guardian wishes to choose a course of action that will lead to death, as for example when a Jehovah's Witness refuses blood transfusions for a child, how can one speak of a future possible concurring permission as required by the principle of proxy consent? It might be suggested that one should examine the extent to which adult Jehovah's Witnesses are true to their faith, even to the point of refusing blood transfusions and dying. However, that would be to miss the point. If a Jehovah's Witness refuses a blood transfusion for an infant, that child never becomes a future person to be injured, as occurs with women subjected to radical circumcision. In addition, the general obligations of beneficence due to sentient nonpersonal life will protect only against malevolent acts and thus will not serve to forbid infanticide for which nonmalevolent grounds are given in justification. Where it is implausible that the actions are non-malevolent, one may use force to protect the infant.

As we have seen from chapter 4, forbidding such actions must depend on the extent to which the social sense of person confers a commitment to provide treatment and care for humans who are not yet persons in the strict sense. In exchange for treatment in hospitals and clinics supported by communities not in agreement with the Jehovah's Witnesses or similar beliefs, one could envisage such hospitals and clinics, and their physicians, making any care conditional on the acceptance of whatever care is required to preserve life and limb. However, if Jehovah's Witnesses were like the Amish or the Yanomamo and retreated into communities closed off from the rest of society in order to ensure that their children would receive only that amount of health care consistent with their religion, there would be no grounds for intervention, except to rescue competent children who wished treatment.[68]

Research involving human subjects

Research is integral to medicine as a science. It is a part of the disciplined knowing of the health care professions. All health care professions, as has already been observed, treat patients not only for their own good, but for the good of the profession. At the very minimum, skills must be passed on from one generation of practitioners to another, and the patient serves as a medium. As members of learned professions, physicians and nurses seek not just to maintain their skills, but also to increase them. A systematic scrutiny of the encounters between health care practitioner and patient is needed in order to learn more so as to be able to treat better. The result is a tension between the health care professional's roles as healer and scientist. This conflict between roles has been at the root of traditional criticisms of human experimentation. In the late Middle Ages, increased experimentation by physicians and surgeons led to warnings by the Christian Church.[69] Bartolomaeus Fumus, in his *Summa Armilla* of 1538, stated that physicians sin "if they supply a doubtful medicine for a certain one, or do not practice in accord with the art, but desire to practice following their own stupid fancy, or make experiments and such like, by which the patient is exposed to grave danger."[70] A similar suspicion that experimentation was equivalent to rash treatment of the patient continued even in American law until recently.[71]

These hesitations have been combined with a view that experimentation on human subjects involves a morally questionable use of persons. As Hans Jonas argues,

[The] compensations of personhood are denied to the subject of experimentation, who is acted upon for an extraneous end without being engaged in a real relation where he would be the counterpoint to the other or to circumstance. Mere "consent" (mostly amounting to no more than permission) does not right this reification. Only genuine authenticity of volunteering can possibly redeem the condition of "thinghood" to which the subject submits.[72]

On the basis of these concerns, Jonas sets very stringent criteria for authentic volunteering and equates most consent with a form of conscription.[73] Jonas endorses these high standards to overcome what he contends is a central moral problem in research using human subjects. "What is wrong with making a person an experimental subject is . . . that we make him a thing—a passive thing, merely to be acted upon . . ."[74] These general concerns regarding the moral probity of research involving human subjects have been vindicated at least in part by the history of the abuse of humans in experimentation. Though the atrocities reviewed at Nuremberg may come most quickly to mind, there were considerable abuses before the Second World War, as Jay Katz's review of experimentation indicates.[75] The Tuskegee syphilis study in the United States also demonstrates the need for the special protection of human research subjects.[76] One would need to add that the mere publication of codes and laws does not appear to be sufficient to protect human subjects. As Hans-Martin Sass has shown, quite exacting and in many respects progressive rules for the protection of human subjects were in fact enacted in Germany in 1931 and were theoretically in force until 1945.[77]

The use of human subjects in research is thus tied to the need to afford special protection for free and informed consent so as to ensure that adequate knowledge is communicated and that consent is free of coercion. Because of the conflicts between roles, subjects may often confuse research without benefit for them with treatment that could in fact improve their health. Moreover, students, prisoners, and other special populations may be both overtly and covertly coerced to participate in human research. The principle of autonomy requires that, as a condition of mutual respect, individuals be protected against both deception and coercion. The principle of beneficence requires that there be a net benefit to others. Here one must note that biomedical research is directly and indirectly tied to benefits for patients. Indeed, one's moral concerns regarding the practice of human experimentation will in part depend on one's view of the safety of health care in the absence of rigorous research. One need not only fear the reckless use of humans in medical research. One should also fear the costs of reckless treatment—treatment not based on adequate research. The other side of the concern to protect human subjects is the concern to protect patients against untested and ill-founded treatments.

RESEARCH AS BENEFICENCE. People have an impulse to do things to help those in need. Throughout history and across cultures individuals have devised various means to prevent illness and cure disease. The difficulty is that a great number of these interventions, from trepanning and bleeding to blistering, purging, and clystering, usually do more harm than good. Much of the history of well-intentioned medical treatment is the history of useless suffering. Even the most superficial analysis of that history would suggest that more individuals by many magnitudes have suffered from ill-founded treatments than have suffered from the side effects of research. If one abandons the notion that standard or accepted treatments are good simply because they are standard and accepted, one is confronted with the recurring question whether any of the accepted modalities of medicine do more harm than good.

This question has been a part of the development of modern scientific medicine. One must recognize the chaotic state of the materia medica until quite recently.[78] It was a collection of various treatments, only some of whose uses were well founded. As a result, there was a search for a *methodus medendi*, a methodical or systematic approach to treatment. Such an approach requires research involving humans. As Thomas Sydenham put it, one needed a system of care "approved by numerous experiments."[79] The advances in modern medicine came both through developments in the basic medical sciences, as well as through systematic and statistical assessments of standard means of treatment. They depended on a growing skepticism regarding traditional means of treatment. One might think here of the classic study by Louis in 1835 to show that blood letting did not in fact have, as was supposed, a beneficial effect on inflammatory diseases.[80] One is brought to a general suspicion of all treatment that has not been systematically assessed. One has substantial grounds for fearing that untested treatments will do more harm than good.

Research bears in different ways on the possible treatment of actual patients. One can distinguish among (1) research that is likely to be of direct benefit to the subject; (2) research likely to benefit individuals with the same disease or disorder as the subject; (3) research that is likely to establish whether particular treatments are on balance beneficial or harmful; (4) research focused on developing new treatments; and (5) fundamental research directed to basic understandings of biology and the disease processes. All five forms of research lead, whether directly or indirectly, to the abandonment of previously established treatment modalities when they are shown to provide more harm than benefit compared with alternative treatments or with no treatment at all. Systematic and careful research in medicine is integral to controlling and directing the impulse to cure so that it does less harm and more good. Research is integral to a beneficent medicine. Research is not simply a part of the knower's interest in knowing, nor is it simply tied to a pursuit of some future state in which there will be perfect treatments for all diseases and disorders. It focuses, in addition, if not first and foremost, on particular patients who may be benefited, as well as contemporary individuals who will be aided in the future by the abandonment of old treatments and the establishment of better treatments. The risks involved in the use of subjects in human experimentation can be realistically assessed only against the background of the risks involved in a medicine unguided by systematic research. One finds here yet one more application of the Socratic adage that the unexamined life is not worth living, namely, that medicine unexamined through systematic research may be a danger to patients. In this light, the role of research subject is not that of a "thing" co-opted into the service of alien goals, but of an individual cooperating in an important social goal of importance to that individual as well.

RESPECTING SUBJECTS, PROTECTING SUBJECTS, AND TOLERATING DAREDEVIL RESEARCH. Because of the misunderstandings that individuals are likely to have about the nature and significance of medical research, researchers will usually have a moral obligation to use special care in gaining the consent of would-be subjects. One will need to avoid all forms of deception to which the subject does not consent, and one will need to eschew all forms of coercion. A good example of the attempt to achieve such protection is found in the American Code of Federal Regulations for the Protection of Human Subjects. There, informed consent is clearly spelled out in terms of the need to warn would-be subjects of the circumstances of the research and of the opportunities for both refusal and participation. Research subjects are strangers in a strange land, and like patients will need to be shown how to orient themselves in order to choose freely. The Federal Code gives the following account of informed consent through requiring, among other things, that a subject be provided with:

1. A statement that the study involves research, an explanation of the purposes of the research and the expected duration of the subject's participation, a description of the procedures to be followed, and identification of any procedures which are experimental;
2. A description of any reasonably foreseeable risks or discomforts to the subject;
3. A description of any benefits to the subject or to others which may reasonably be expected from the research;
4. A disclosure of appropriate alternative procedures of courses of treatment, if any, that might be advantageous to the subject;
5. A statement describing the extent, if any, to which confidentiality of records identifying the subject will be maintained;
6. For research involving more than minimal risk, an explanation as to whether any compensation and an explanation as to whether any medical treatments are available if injury occurs and, if so, what they consist of, or where further information may be obtained;
7. An explanation of whom to contact for answers to pertinent questions about the research and research subjects' rights, and whom to contact in the event of a research-related injury to the subject; and
8. A statement that participation is voluntary, refusal to participate will involve no penalty or loss of benefits to which the subject is otherwise entitled, and the subject may discontinue participation at any time without penalty or loss of benefits to which the subject is otherwise entitled.[81]

In addition to requiring strict criteria for free and informed consent, the regulations require that the risks to the subject be at least reasonable, considering the possible benefits. "Risks to subjects [must be] reasonable in relation to anticipated benefits, if any, to subjects, and the importance of the knowledge that may reasonably be expected to result."[82] These, along with other protections, are designed to secure subjects of federally funded research against abuse.

All of these restrictions are not required by the principle of autonomy, or by the principle of beneficence if a high value is given to liberty. They rather express a particular understanding of the proper conduct of research endorsed by the federal government. For example, if it is morally proper for individuals freely to volunteer for service in the armed forces, it should be morally proper as well to volunteer for service in research forces. In fact, one might very well imagine why it would be useful to have a stable population of individuals highly paid and highly motivated to participate in human research.[83] Such individuals might be forbidden by their contract from withdrawing from particular forms of research, just as individuals, once they have joined the armed forces, have ceded their right to decline to participate in or to withdraw from certain activities. Such an approach to research would be in violation of current regulations, as one can see from section 8 of the passage on consent quoted from the Code of Federal Regulations.

There is also a wide range of research endeavors that is unlikely to be approved by the institutional review boards established to review research in institutions receiving federal research support, but which research would not be in violation of the principles of autonomy and beneficence.[84] Here one would find research ranging from that which is extremely dangerous to that for which high rates of pay are offered. There is nothing wrong in principle in allowing individuals to volunteer freely for risky research, especially if it promises great benefit to others. One generally approves of such research in the case of autoexperimentation. One might think here of the Nobel Prize winner Werner Forsmann, who catheterized his own heart.[85] As we have seen from the examination of the nature of peaceable manipulation, there is also nothing wrong with offering individuals as much money as is required to attract their services, as long as the offer does not itself render them incompetent. So, too, there will be no grounds in principle for forbidding research that most would think to be both boonless and harmful. One might think here of advocates of laetrile or other nonorthodox approaches to health care, privately funding and conducting trials of their therapies. Such endeavors need not and ought not be supported by those who hold them to be harmful or ill advised. However, if the individuals involved understand and appreciate the risks, their choices should be tolerated. One should be as tolerant of martyrs for unconventional understandings of science as one is of martyrs for what others may hold to be unconventional religious viewpoints (e.g., an adult Jehovah's Witness deciding to die rather than accept a blood transfusion, or a devout Roman Catholic deciding to die rather than accept a direct abortion to protect her from heart failure due to the strain on her heart with serious mitral valve disease).

RESEARCH ON SPECIAL POPULATIONS. To a great extent we have already explored the moral limits to experimentation on humans who are not persons in the strict sense. Fetal experimentation has already been discussed in chapter 6, and in the previous section we have examined the range of allowable proxy consent. Though the principle of proxy consent gives fairly broad latitude to the guardian, concern for the good of wards and fear of exploitation are likely to support limits on the amount of risk to which incompetent subjects may be exposed.[86] One might think of the requirement by the Code of Federal Regulations that federally funded research involving children not involve greater than minimal risk to the subjects if it has no prospect of directly benefiting the individual subject, unless it is likely to yield generalizable knowledge about the subject's disorder or condition.[87] Even then, such research is not allowed unless the risk represents only a minor increase over the minimal risk, except in circumstances where the research offers an opportunity to understand, prevent, or alleviate a serious problem affecting the health or welfare of children.[88] Minimal risks are understood as those that "are not greater, considering probability and magnitude, than those ordinarily encountered in daily life or during the performance of routine physical or psychological examinations or tests."[89] These restrictions on the use of federal funds express a well-wrought ethos of beneficence. Though the regulations ostensibly apply only to research involving children, they could with moral propriety be applied to the mentally ill and others incapable of giving consent for themselves.

Questions of consent to research arise as well with regard to individuals who agree to participate under coercive circumstances. One must include here not only prisoners but also students, who may fear that their future will be determined in part by their willingness to participate in research programs. Given the history of the exploitation of prisoners, there is much to be said for the protection afforded by federal regulations to prison populations.[90] These restrictions, which for practical purposes forbid using prisoners in any federally funded research not directed to the treatment of individual prisoners or the understanding of diseases and conditions bearing on prisoners, also remove the prisoners' opportunity to contribute to society and to recapture a sense of moral dignity through such altruism. In so completely protecting prisoners against coercive pressure to participate in research, one further lowers the dignity and moral capacity of prisoners. Finally, one must observe, as Hans Jonas has indicated, that there is nothing intrinsically wrong with forcing prisoners to participate in human experimentation, if it is a part of their punishment.[91] Aside from concerns about the possible abuse of such an opportunity to use prisoners, and the change in ethos such activities might entail, the central question is whether such compulsion has clearly been made part of the punishment. One might imagine punishments for various crimes including specified periods of serving as a subject of research of a particular sort. Committing the crime would entail consenting to the research. Here one also finds part of the answer regarding the use of students as subjects. Unless participation in research is part of a course elected by a student, special protections against coercion may be needed.

DECEPTION IN RESEARCH. As we have seen, there is a moral impetus to do research in order to protect individuals from well-intentioned interventions that will in fact do more harm than alternative treatments and in some cases than no treatment at all. It is hard to know truly in medicine because of (1) the problem of random remissions and spontaneous cures; (2) the remembrance by physicians of their therapeutic triumphs more clearly than their failures, thus distorting their judgment of a treatment's efficacy;[92] (3) the placebo effect, which aids even intrinsically inefficacious treatments in benefiting patients; and (4) the psychology of discovery that leads individuals to see what they anticipate.[93] As a result, it has been hard to determine when conservative versus surgical treatment of coronary artery disease offers greater benefit,[94] or if radical mastectomies offer a greater chance of survival than simple mastectomies.[95] Though one might think that such a clear outcome as being alive or dead after a period of time would lead to easy assessment, the various distortions of observer bias have made judgment difficult.

Much of modern medical research depends on not disclosing to subjects what drugs they are actually receiving, or which treatment they will receive, in order to compensate for distorting forces. For example, often both the investigator and the subject-patient are not informed which of a set of drugs the subject-patient is actually receiving. Instead, the investigators and the patients involved in the study are informed that the subjects will be receiving one of two or more drugs through a random assignment in order to compare their relative efficacy. Such double-blind random clinical trials, which are employed because of the history of observer bias, are not immoral for employing such deception unless the prospective subjects are not warned of the deception. Here again the model of poker is instructive. In playing the game the participants agree to certain forms of mutual deception, but not others (e.g., poker bluffs but not hidden cards). So, too, in random clinical trials subjects must be informed (or at least be offered information about) what kinds of information will not be disclosed, what form of randomization will occur, why it will take place, what information will be provided, and when. Since the amount of certainty required to hold that a trial has been completed is arbitrary, subjects will need to be informed of when and under what circumstances codes will be broken to indicate that one treatment has been shown to be more useful than others.[96] What is essential is that subjects be offered sufficient information to allow them to decide whether to accept the risks and benefits of a research protocol. The principle of mutual respect does not require that individuals be protected against deception, but only that they not unwittingly be subjected to deception.[97] There is no violation of the principle of beneficence either, if in the end the good is accomplished.

THE DEMOCRATIZATION OF SCIENCE AND THE PARTNERSHIP OF KNOWLEDGE. To recognize individuals as free and able to consent or refuse to participate in research is to see science as the collective endeavor of a great number of free men and women. Those who govern its course are not only scientists, physicians, surgeons, and nurses, but patients and research subjects as well. Medicine will not be able to extend its skills from one generation to another if current patients are not willing to allow their bodies and minds to be explored by students and young physicians and nurses who are acquiring the skills necessary to care for and if possible cure the complaints of patients yet to come. So, too, when patients and others freely participate in research, they join in the collective endeavor of individuals concerned to avoid treatments that do more harm than good, to acquire treatments that cure better and with fewer costs, as well as in the general cultural aspiration to the better understanding of man and the human condition. The principle of autonomy defines the character of this interaction; the principle of beneficence supports the altruistic dedication of some to the good of all.

Confidentiality

The fabric of health care is sustained by trust. Patients bare their bodies and minds to physicians, and physicians treat patients in all of the vulnerable moments of their lives, from copulation and birth to disease and death. In order to ensure adequate care for the concerns of patients physicians need to know what is bothering them and how they understand their problems. As a result, a bond of confidentiality has protected physician–patient relationships since the beginnings of modern Western medicine. One might think here of the famous passage from the Hippocratic oath, "And whatsoever I shall see or hear in the course of my profession, as well as outside my profession in my intercourse with men, if it be what should not be published abroad, I will never divulge, holding such things to be holy secrets."[98] In matter of fact, communications to either priests or physicians are not as secure as the client–lawyer privilege, which is near to being absolute. In theory, priests can be compelled to testify in many jurisdictions regarding supposedly confidential disclosures made in the confessional.[99] In addition, physicians have a special duty to inform public authorities that their patients have contracted sexually transmitted diseases, have sustained gunshot wounds, have abused children, or otherwise have been associated with problems regarding which the state demands disclosure. For instance, there has been an increasingly recognized legal duty of health care professionals to disclose to third parties a possible danger from a patient under treatment.[100]

The principle of autonomy makes it morally permissible to create such special exclaves secure against such requirements for disclosure. The particular individuals who might be benefited by the disclosure have no right to the physician making a disclosure that will protect them, even though they may have a moral claim on the patient for such disclosure. Moreover, the fact that a priest or a physician comes to know that an individual is dangerous does not in itself increase the dangerousness of the individual. Silence on the part of the priest or physician is not itself a direct injury against those who may be the individual's victims. Holding oneself out as an individual to whom one can speak in absolute confidentiality does not in and of itself constitute an injury against others just because one might come to know of possible dangers to others. In addition, there may be special advantages from both priests and physicians offering strict confidentiality. The capacity of physicians or priests to function in their special roles, which have social value, may be undercut by the notion that compelling state interests could force disclosure of their private communications. Priests provide a secure exclave where one may speak without hindrance or hesitation about one's sins and guilt. So, too, the Hippocratic commitment to confidentiality offers an opportunity to speak fully of one's medical concerns, which may also be tied to sins and legal infractions. This not only may lead to a more adequate treatment of patients, but also will underscore the special value of recognizing exclaves of privacy secure against state intrusion.

Arguments such as the latter lie behind the client–lawyer privilege, which is nearly absolute. This privilege has been justified, inter alia, on the grounds that a defendant has the right to at least one confidant who will champion that individual's interests against the powers of the state.[101] One need not stand alone against the state. The same considerations support a privilege for both physicians and priests. A physician is often an individual's sole confidant in defense against the blind forces of illness. So, too, priests are seen as an individual's special refuge from personal guilt and for defense against the wrath of the Almighty.

Whether it will on balance be desirable to endow the patient–physician or the priest–penitent relationship with the absolute confidentiality usually given to the lawyer–client relationship will depend on the usefulness of the role. One must note that even the history of the priest–penitent relationship shows that an unqualified seal of confession did not always exist. Many argued, for example, that those who confessed heresy need not be guaranteed any such special privilege.[102] In the end, the notion of an absolute obligation to maintain confidentiality developed even to the point of protecting the disclosure of sins one intended to commit in the future. The priest could at best give a general warning to those endangered, but could not disclose the identity of the sinner.[103] The ground for this absolute protection lay in the fear that any exception to the seal of confession would deter individuals from shriving and thus saving their souls.

The same argument is available against the legal duty of physicians to report to the state or third parties the fact that a particular patient has either a sexually transmitted disease or constitutes a possible danger to others. The more one has grounds for suspecting that such disclosures prevent individuals from seeking treatment or hinder them from seeking treatment in a timely fashion, the more one will suspect that the requirements of disclosure will do more harm than good. It is considerations such as this that have traditionally led physicians to underreport sexually transmitted diseases even when required, and to the establishment of clinics in some cities, which have treated the sexually transmitted diseases of homosexuals with a commitment to absolute confidentiality, given the danger of disclosure for the careers of such patients. So, too, it might be one thing for physicians to agree to disclose child abuse discovered in the course of treating children, and another thing to require physicians to disclose such abuse when the parents seek treatment for it. The clear and certain threat of disclosure is likely to hinder such parents from seeking timely treatment, thus leading to further abuse and injury to their children. Even the requirements to disclose abuse discovered in the course of treating a child brought by a parent who is then willing to receive treatment may be unwise. Similarly, a careful examination of the costs and benefits involved in requiring disclosure to third parties that a patient is possibly dangerous may show that once this requirement is well known, dangerous patients who could have been adequately treated will not seek treatment in a timely fashion. The fact that a particular disclosure of a patient's dangerousness could have saved the life of a particular third party should not obscure the fact that a general rule requiring disclosure may in fact lead to the deaths of more individuals. If such costs are involved, a rule providing for such disclosure is not the sort that prudent men and women ought to adopt. One may be brought to establishing the same absoluteness for patient–physician communications as for client–attorney communications. But even the ill-considered actions of free men and women must be tolerated. Some may weigh the possible danger to identifiable individuals greater than the danger to statistical individuals, leading to a rule for disclosing danger to identifiable third parties, even when such a rule will harm more individuals in the long run.

One should recognize how widespread both formal and informal rules for disclosure are. Physicians in the armed forces, company physicians, or physicians employed by schools may have special duties to disclose information to third parties in ways unassociated with the treatment of a patient. As a result, there are numerous areas for possible conflict between the goals of treatment with patient confidentiality and the special goals of the organizations employing the physicians. In principle, this conflict is no different from the conflict between the physician as healer committed to confidentiality and the physician as public health officer committed to reporting sexually transmitted diseases. It should receive the same solution. Students, workers, and members of the armed forces should be given notice of the extent to which such physicians will depart from the usual practices of physician–patient confidentiality. If individuals generally come to know that the disclosure of information will not be protected by confidentiality, there is no violation of the principle of autonomy and perhaps not even the principle of beneficence, given the special weighting of the harms and benefits.

Finally, one must stress the complexity of health care relationships and the difficulties of maintaining confidentiality. Even in the private physician's office, the confidentiality of communications may be eroded when the patient applies for insurance or in other circumstances voluntarily releases information. Most patients often underappreciate the extent to which they are disclosing personal information to third parties not directly involved in their care. Individuals may need to act collectively to seek ways of persuading insurance carriers and others to accept more limited access to patients' records. Such limitations will surely not be without cost to those seeking insurance under such conditions.

Restrictions on the disclosure of information will become more desirable from the point of view of patients as medicine is able to determine distant future risks of developing diseases, including diseases in the workplace. Employers and schools may not hire or admit individuals with a high future probability of developing a serious disease. A better understanding of the genetic mechanisms of illnesses and occupational diseases will increase the need for individuals to protect the confidentiality of their medical records. However, many forces work against the preservation of confidentiality. The very enterprise of coherent health care in a large hospital setting, including the dedication to high-quality health care, presupposes that many individuals, not just physicians, come to see the records of patients. The protection of confidentiality will require a systematic commitment, not only to guarding information in general, but to sequestering particular areas of information concerning the patient.

Suicide, euthanasia, and the choice of a style for dying

There is much talk of the choice of a style of life, for the principle of autonomy underscores the right of free men and woman to choose their ways of living. In fact, the principle of beneficence gains content only in terms of such choices, for they fashion the concrete vision of meaning and purpose. Death requires similar choices. The good death, as the good life, requires forethought and planning. It is unlikely to happen by accident. There was much made of this in the late Middle Ages under the rubric of the *ars moriendi* literature.[104] This concern can be captured in contemporary terms. One must write one's deathbed speech while in good health and make careful plans, for it is unlikely that one will have the opportunity either to write it or to deliver it in the modern intensive-care unit. Such forethought may include the use of advance directives, through which competent individuals plan for their treatment when in the future they may be seriously ill and/or incompetent.[105]

The modern era has departed in radical ways from traditional views of death. The medieval Christian prayed "A subitanea et improvisa morte, libera nos, Domine" (From a sudden and unprovided-for death, deliver us, O Lord).[106] Many members of contemporary societies hope, instead, to die without warning, painlessly in their sleep. However, since such painless deaths are not the rule, even we in contemporary societies must fear an unprovided-for dying, one that will occur under circumstances that will vex us and boonlessly use our resources. Technologies that can save our lives and postpone death also underscore the need to decide when to accept death and to prolong dying no longer. They raise the ancient question of when individuals should take their own lives or be aided in their suicide. In increasing our effective range of free choice, new medical technologies have here as elsewhere established new responsibilities. Individuals who would have died in the past now survive, often in circumstances that few would find acceptable, and often with major burdens for their family and society.

These circumstances make death no longer the mere outcome of fate or the decision of the gods. When it occurs and under what circumstances is increasingly the choice of individual men and women who employ technologies to postpone death. The human responsibility in this matter, however, has been avoided through the presupposition that one should maximally treat so as to extend human life as far as possible. Many physicians and families of patients have acted under the supposition that medicine has been traditionally obliged to save life at any cost. This, however, is false. Medicine

traditionally avoided treating hopeless cases. The unrestrained commitment
to treat individuals at any cost in order to save life of any quality is a modern
peculiarity without classical roots.[107] A responsible use of our limited
resources both communal and private will require choosing when in fact to
prolong life and when not. Such choices will need to be made against a view
of the good death and the good life. Thinking in this way may return
individuals to a Stoic appreciation of individual responsibility for one's own
death. One might think here of Seneca's remark that no one can complain of
life or of suffering, because if the pains are too great, suicide is always
available.[108] If one suffers, according to Seneca, it is no one's fault but one's
own. In this vein, we are led to deciding which lifesaving treatment we will
accept, which we will refuse, and when if ever suicide is a morally appropriate
option.

One must wonder whether the determination of some to prolong life at any
cost does not spring from the loss of a theodicy of suffering and of a belief in
an afterlife. Some appear to have concluded that, if one lives only once, life at
any expense is worth it (evidence from experience with the technological
prolongation of dying notwithstanding). One should note how this view
contrasts with that of the believing Christian or Jew who sees his or her life as
only a journey to a final destiny with God. For those who truly believe, it is
difficult to understand why they should hold tenaciously to this life at great
cost, when the resources could instead be used for the poor, while they
accepted death and met their Maker. An element of the technological
obsession that leads to intensive care units functioning as high-intensity care
hospices must be understood in terms of this peculiar idolatry of our fleeting
life, even under those circumstances when that life is of little value, if any, to
those who are living it. One must suspect that communities that use
substantial medical resources in such circumstances, or that construe the
right to life as a duty to stay alive under all circumstances, suffer from
confusions consequent on the collapse of the Judeo-Christian heritage. Such
communities may have lost sight of a traditional element of what it means to
be a good Christian or Jew and not yet learned what it is to be a good pagan.

The right to be left alone and the context of death

If one possesses the right to free and informed consent, it follows that one
should possess the right to refuse treatment, even lifesaving treatment. Here
again the ruling in *Natanson* v. *Kline* is pertinent. The court stated that
"Anglo-American law starts with the premise of a thorough-going self
determination. It follows that each man is considered to be master of his own
body, and he may, if he be of sound mind, expressly prohibit the performance

of life-saving surgery."[109] The recognition of the right to be left alone, not to be touched without one's permission, has come only with controversy. A great deal of the controversy has been associated with the requests by Jehovah's Witnesses to refuse lifesaving blood transfusions. Though in most cases the request has been honored, where the individual refusing treatment was neither pregnant nor the guardian of dependent minors,[110] a number of courts have held that such refusal could be tantamount to suicide, which if not illegal was at least against public policy.[111]

Such refusals, which were in the past more restricted to individuals declining treatment on religious grounds, have been extended to individuals refusing treatment because they no longer see life to be a benefit. Consider the individual who, suffering from amyelotrophic lateral sclerosis (Lou Gehrig's disease), an irreversible and ultimately fatal neurological disease, sought to discontinue further life-prolonging treatment. He requested that the respirator, which was maintaining his breathing, be disconnected. His family members did not raise objections to his request, and no minor children were involved. The Florida Supreme Court unanimously confirmed a previous appeals court decision, which recognized this patient's right to refuse treatment. The decision, however, was a very narrow one. It held closely to the facts of the *Perlmutter* case, namely, that a competent, terminally ill individual with no minor dependents could refuse life-prolonging treatment with the concurrence of the family.[112]

What would have been such an individual's fate, had a family member disagreed? Does a family member have a right to require a competent individual to prolong the process of dying? An individual should indeed be allowed under such circumstances to refuse all treatment unless a prior, explicit commitment had been made to a particular family member or some other individual.

Opposition to the refusal of lifesaving treatment is closely bound to the Christian condemnation of suicide, which came to be expressed in Western law. In Anglo-American law suicide was traditionally forbidden because "the suicide is guilty of a double offence; one spiritual, in invading the prerogative of the Almighty, and rushing into his immediate presence uncalled for; the other temporal, against the king, who hath an interest in the preservation of all his subjects."[113] These interests came to be imbedded in a wide range of concerns by the state for the would-be suicide and for third parties. The state's right to prevent suicide came to be derived from compelling state interests to (1) prevent citizens from committing an offense against God and/or good public morals, (2) protect the state's interests in the productivity of its citizens, (3) preserve respect for life because of the utility of this practice in assuring decent care for individuals, (4) enforce the obligations of individuals to support their dependents, discharge their debts, and to fulfill their contracts, and (5) protect individuals from imprudent choices, even when they are dangerous only to themselves.[114]

Given the arguments in chapter 4 regarding the limited authority of states, and those in chapter 3 regarding the rights of individuals to noninterference under the morality of mutual respect, the contentions in favor of state force weaken. A state does not have the right to employ force to protect the rights of the deities, nor to establish a particular concrete moral point of view (beyond those enforcements that depend for their justification on the principle of autonomy). One might recall here the arguments of the New York Court of Appeals, which held that laws against sodomy could not be enforced because they reflect a particular moral point of view.

We express no view as to any theological, moral or psychological evaluation of consensual sodomy. These are aspects of the issue on which informed, competent authorities and individuals may and do differ. Contrary to the view expressed by the dissent, although on occasion it does serve such ends, it is not the function of the Penal Law in our governmental policy to provide either a medium for the articulation or the apparatus for the intended enforcement of moral or theological values. Thus, it has been deemed irrelevant by the United States Supreme Court that the purchase and use of contraceptives by unmarried persons would arouse moral indignation among broad segments of our community or that the viewing of pornographic materials even within the privacy of one's home would not evoke general approbation.... The community and its members are entirely free to employ theological teaching, moral suasion, parental advice, psychological and psychiatric counseling and other noncoercive means to condemn the practice of consensual sodomy. The narrow question before us is whether the Federal Constitution permits the use of the criminal law for that purpose.[115]

This argument, with appropriate changes, applies against the state's contention that it has a right to forbid suicide because of its offense against good public morals. With some alterations, it applies as well to the notion that states own their citizens and therefore have a right to their productivity. As the arguments in chapters 2 and 4 have shown, individuals create and possess their states, not the reverse.

The contention that one may forbid suicide or the refusal of treatment because it would undermine the sanctity of life receives a similar rejection. Competent individuals possess a right to pursue as far as is possible with consenting others the realization of their particular view of the good life and the good death. With this right comes the right not to join with others. If that in fact leads to a lower evaluation of life than would occur with the cooperation of those individuals, one has discovered one of the prices of freedom, not grounds for compelling cooperation. Free individuals are not responsible for the free actions of others, though they must live with the consequences of others' free choices. The world might be better in general if

people had married spouses other than the ones they chose. From that, no
state interest follows to compel individuals to marry only ideal partners at
ideal times. So, also, free individuals should be able to die freely as they
choose, even if they do not choose ideal times.

The objection to suicide on the basis of enforcing contracts carries the
greatest weight. A state may properly use force to compel an individual to
pay debts or discharge obligations before quitting this life. It would seem
very plausible that the armed forces might require officers to promise not to
commit suicide, save under very delimited circumstances. Other contracts,
which may not be as explicit, would need to be examined in great detail and
with great care. It is plausible that dependent children would have a right to
veto the suicide of their parents, insofar as those parents have promised
support of a certain sort. However, the extent of such commitments would
clearly vary from culture to culture and family to family. Moreover,
individuals should be able to circumvent such restrictions by acquiring
special suicide insurance to allow them, should they ever choose, to commit
suicide and to create an endowment for their children's support. Such
policies should be conceived as insurance against the cost of being in a
circumstance where suicide is a reasonable option. One might note that many
insurance policies pay even with suicide, once they have been in force for a
certain period of time. As long as such policies were engaged early in life, and
as long as the frequency of suicide was not that high, the costs would not be
great. Finally, one must note that the closer the individual refusing treatment
and choosing suicide comes to death, or the more disabled the individual is,
the less plausible it is that enforced continuance of life will lead to the
discharge of duties.

The contention that the state has a right to protect free individuals from
their own misguided choices finds little support from the arguments in this
volume. The treatment of paternalism in section two of this chapter and of
the limited authority of the state in chapter 4 supports the strong autonomy
rights that were sketched in chapters 2 and 3. Being free means having the
right to choose tragically and in a misguided fashion. On the other hand,
individuals may establish special paternalistic relations. Individuals who are
concerned about their reactions in times of despondency would be well
advised to establish some form of advance directive for a psychiatrist or
other person to compel treatment or to impede suicide under specified
circumstances. Finally, one must stress that the duty to respect freedom does
not include a duty to respect the unfree choice of death by mentally ill
persons. When an individual does not competently choose to refuse treatment or to commit suicide, there is no freedom to respect and one is instead
bound by the principle of beneficence to achieve the good for that person,

rather than to conform to statements that reflect mental illness, not free choice.

These reflections lead to generally supporting the right of individuals to refuse treatment, even lifesaving treatment, and to commit suicide. Insofar as individuals possess this right for themseves, they should have as well the right to be aided by others. It is an element of the right to be left alone: the right to be left alone in one's free association with consenting others. One might note that Texas, which unlike other Anglo-American jurisdictions never forbade suicide, did not in fact criminalize aiding and abetting suicide until 1973. The argument was that if suicide was not a crime, it could not be a crime to aid others in a noncriminal activity. In taking this position, Texas departed from most, if not all, American jurisdictions.[116]

It may be a violation of morals and ethics and reprehensible that a party may furnish another poison or pistols or guns or any other means or agency for the purpose of the suicide to take his own life, yet our law has not seen proper to punish such persons or such acts.[117]

Here it is useful to read the Texas court as distinguishing between the moral authority of Texas as a peaceable, secular pluralist state, and the moral commitments of particular communities, which might disapprove of suicide or of aiding and abetting suicide. It will be very difficult for a secular, peaceable, pluralist state to interfere with moral authority in the free choices of individuals and of those who assist them in refusing treatment or committing suicide. We will return to the issue of suicide and assisted suicide in a later section after examining one of the major Christian approaches to the issue of refusing treatment and expediting death.

Here it is enough to note that, given the arguments in this book, the central evil in murder, in terms of a secular morality, is not taking the life of an individual, but taking that life without the individual's permission. Old Texas law can furnish another example. In the first days of the republic, neither suicide nor aiding and abetting suicide nor dueling was a crime.[118] The republic took seriously, as few other nations have, the notion that with consent there is no harm, *volenti non fit injuria*.[119] This view was not shared by the Judeo-Christian heritage. Within those traditions it has been important to determine whether one intends or simply foresees the likely death of an individual. Intending to kill an innocent individual would be an offense against God; however, in many circumstances, foreseeing but not intending that one's actions would lead to a death would not be the basis for justified blame.

Intending death, foreseeing death, and refusing treatment

In the area of refusing treatment and expediting death one finds an important application of the principle of double effect, mentioned in passing in chapter 6. This principle, which was originally fashioned primarily for moral judgments in wartime (e.g., in a just war foreseeing but not intending the death of innocent noncombatants could excuse one from moral blame), came to be applied to medical issues as well.[120] The principle held that one could engage in actions likely to harm or even kill another, as long as (1) the physical evil was not intended (e.g., a good Catholic soldier could shoot arrows over a city's walls, foreseeing but not intending that innocent civilians might be killed); (2) the good sought from the actions did not follow directly from the harms (e.g., the city would not be brought to surrender because of the death of the innocent civilians); (3) the action was not in itself intrinsically evil (e.g., one could indirectly kill noncombatant children, but not commit adultery in order to take the city); and (4) there was a proportionate good to be derived (e.g., the likely benefits would outweigh likely harms).[121] This principle has provided a framework to allow devout Catholics not only to engage in actions that have as their foreseen but not intended effect sterilization and contraception, but also to provide a basis for discontinuing treatment or even providing pain control likely to bring an earlier death.

One could properly decide that further investment of resources in prolonging life was not obligatory because it constituted an inordinate or extraordinary drain on the resources of a family or society, or because such an investment offered little probability of doing anything beyond extending the process of dying. Ordinary means for preserving life were defined as "all medicines, treatments, and operations, which offer a reasonable hope of benefit for the patient and which can be obtained and used without excessive expense, pain or other inconvenience."[122] In this way Catholic theologian Gerald Kelly held that providing digitalis or intravenous glucose for a comatose ninety-year old with cardiorenal disease would be extraordinary treatment.[123] In the past, at least, a severe inconvenience was taken to include having to travel from one's native town or village for treatment in a distant city.[124] In short, one could stop all extraordinary treatment and allow the patient to die, as long as one did not intend to kill the patient, but simply foresaw that the choice not to prolong death or to misinvest resources might lead to an earlier death. So, too, this moral analysis also allows giving a patient dying of cancer pain-controlling medication that is likely to increase the chance of the patient's dying earlier, as long as the death is not intended, the pain is not controlled through killing the patient, and there is significant pain.

The principle of double effect, which permitted individuals to engage in actions that they foresaw would lead to death as long as they did not intend the death, and the principle of ordinary versus extraordinary treatment, which set limits to the obligation to provide treatment or to be treated, allowed Christians within very conservative moral viewpoints both to refuse life-prolonging treatment and to engage in activities that might hasten death. This should not be unexpected. If one believes in an afterlife, it would be morally incongruous to employ all available resources to cling tenaciously to this life. Indeed, given religious beliefs in an afterlife, it may appear idolatrous of physical existence or at least disproportionate to use ICU resources to prolong life when there is no hope of recovery. It may not be an accident that the ethos of providing every chance of clinging to this life emerged as religious belief and the certainty concerning an afterlife waned.

These reflections take much of the bite out of the supposed distinction between active and passive euthanasia, between killing and letting die. For the devout traditional Catholic, the distinction between acting and refraining is not central to the moral debate; what is central is whether death is intended or simply foreseen, and whether the treatment forgone is ordinary (i.e., obligatory treatment) or extraordinary (i.e., nonobligatory treatment). For an argument set in secular, pluralist terms, what will be at stake is the consent of the individual, any prior agreements and obligations that might morally limit the indivdiual's choices, as well as whether the refusal or the prolongation of life is in the best interests of that person. Since concrete understandings of the best interests of persons can be articulated only within a particular, concrete view of the good life, such will be context dependent. If one tries to take the wishes of individuals seriously, one will be able to come to terms with many of the issues raised by the dying without stepping outside the traditional constraints of Western society.

A major difficulty is the reluctance of physicians to take competent individuals seriously. Even well-intentioned and well-disposed physicians appear to have great difficulty in asking individuals about the extent of treatment they wish or under what circumstances they would want to be resuscitated. A recent study has shown that even physicians who believe that patients should participate in decisions about resuscitation avoid discussing the matter with them.[125] In fact, of twenty-five survivors of cardiopulmonary resuscitation interviewed to determine whether they wanted to be resuscitated, eight stated unequivocally that they had not desired resuscitation and they did not wish it in the future.[126] One will need to develop policies aimed at respecting the wishes of competent individuals regarding their further treatment and/or resuscitation.[127] In addition, one will need to give a greater weight to actions that likely express the residuum of competent judgments. One might think here of demented individuals in nursing homes who repeatedly refuse food and fluid by hand. Under such circumstances it is plausible that such refusals express the sentiment that further life is not worth the undertaking and that tube feeding should not be instituted to preserve life ever further.[128]

Advance directives, proxy consent, and stopping treatment on the incompetent

If competent individuals can personally refuse treatment, there should be no moral objection in principle against their doing it through an agent or through some advance directive. Such is the moral foundation of both durable powers of attorney and living wills as instruments for individuals to control their treatment when they are no longer competent. From a moral point of view, one should be able not only to appoint others to choose among treatment options as reasonable and prudent custodians of one's future treatment, but also appoint them to choose in special ways or simply capriciously (a liberty that appears at present not to be available through the law), even to the point of refusing lifesaving treatment. The need for such directives is found in the precarious nature of life, which is fraught with the risk that one may become incompetent and debilitated for a considerable period of time before one's death. As a result, prudent and thoughtful individuals, out of concern for their own well-being and that of their families and society, have sought ways to ensure that their present wishes with regard to nontreatment will be honoured when they are no longer competent.

Those concerns have led to the drafting of so-called living wills, instruments that direct a physician to discontinue treatment under specified circumstances.[129] Such instruments have inspired natural death statutes, which have turned out to be at best unwieldy and at worst obstacles to free men and women controlling the circumstances of their own death. Such laws have provided less than was hoped. The California law, for example, allows one to execute such a living will only if one is terminally ill, and even so, the instrument does not go into effect for fourteen days. It provides only for the refusal of artificial means of life support.[130] But there is a wide range of treatments individuals may wish to direct that they not receive, even before they are terminally ill. Individuals should have the right to tell others to leave them alone, either personally or through a written directive, even if they are not yet suffering from a terminal disease. One might wish to direct that certain treatment not be provided if one has had a serious stroke of a certain sort, even if at the time that one writes the directive one is in good health. Even if one did not have a terminal disease, one might not wish to be treated so as to be able to live out a long life as a mentally incompetent cripple in a nursing home. The most one can say for statutes such as the California

Natural Death Act is that they protect physicians against civil liability, and thus encourage their acceptance by physicians, though many laws provide no sanctions for disobeying such a directive.[131] One should instead move to laws that unequivocally protect the right of free competent individuals to refuse treatment. One might think here of the model act for the refusal of treatment proposed by the Legal Advisors Committee of Concern for Dying.[132]

An actual written advance directive is not necessarily required in order legally to decide the proper treatment one ought to receive when competent. In a New York case a religious brother had his wish not to have his life prolonged via extraordinary means respected, not because of a durable power of attorney or a statutorily recognized living will (i.e., an instrument recognized under a state natural death statute), but because he had communicated his wishes to a priest-friend.[133] Individuals appear to be able to reach out to control their future treatment through the use of (1) durable power of attorney statutes, (2) natural death statutes, and expressions of their wishes to others that may be (3) written (i.e., informal living wills not recognized through statute), or (4) oral. Such is as it should be from a moral point of view because of both the concern to respect the freedom of individuals and the concern to achieve their best interests.

Here one must stress that prolonging life is not always in an individual's best interests. Even in the absence of an advance directive or previously established views on the matter of terminating treatment, the circumstances of life may be so boonless or threatening as to justify refusing treatment because it would be more of an injury than a benefit. One might take as an example of such a proxy decision to refuse treatment the case of Joseph Saikewicz, a severely retarded individual suffering from acute myeloblastic monocytic leukemia. There was a moderate chance for remission but a serious risk that because of the individual's mental incapacities he would misunderstand attempts at treatment as a violation of his body and a form of torture.[134] Proxy decision makers may thus morally refuse treatment not only on the basis of the principle of autonomy, because they represent good reporters of the treatment that individual would have chosen (since Saikewicz had always been incompetent, there were no prior wishes to report), but also on the basis of the principle of beneficence, because as reasonable and prudent men and women they may judge that the prolongation of life, or what would be involved in the prolongation of life, would be more a harm than a benefit.

Morally such guardians may also take costs into account, for costs defeat duties of beneficence. Even the traditional distinction between ordinary and extraordinary care suggests that guardians may decide that the further investment of resources and time in the extension of life is simply too costly. Individuals in particular and society in general may set bounds to the amount of resources available, even for the extension of life, because no duty of beneficence is absolute. No individual, even if competent and alert, has the right to be a six-million-dollar man or woman. When the capacity to appreciate the benefits of such treatment dims, the claim against such resources surely dims as well, because the good one could achieve decreases. One's concerns for entities that are not and will not be persons in the strict sense may properly be less than for persons in the strict sense.

As a result, guardians may morally not only make quality-of-death decisions, but quality-of-life decisions regarding irreversibly incompetent wards, who while competent had expressed no contrary judgments. For the most part, courts have seen the first to be a proper province of proxy decision makers. Yet they have retreated from allowing quality-of-life decisions, decisions that life under certain circumstances is not worth living. The arguments in chapter 6 regarding quality-of-life decisions should apply here as well.

$$\frac{\text{Strength of duty}}{\text{of beneficence}} = \frac{\substack{\text{Chance} \\ \text{of} \\ \text{success}} \times \substack{\text{Quality} \\ \text{of} \\ \text{outcome}} \times \substack{\text{Length} \\ \text{of} \\ \text{life}}}{\text{Costs}}$$

One should also note that duties of beneficence are usually greater to individuals who have been brought fully within the social role of persons than to neonates.

When individuals have not made use of an advance directive, it may be very difficult to determine who is the best authority regarding the best interests of an incompetent individual. Such circumstances of ambiguity may at times lead to conflicts among family members about who is in authority regarding the incompetent's best interests. A spouse may choose not to treat, but a guilt-ridden estranged child may insist that all treatment be provided. To avoid such difficulties it may be best to establish clearly by law, as many jurisdictions have, who is presumptively in authority (i.e., given their consent to act in the role): a spouse, the parents, the sibling closest in age. Individuals could always defeat that presumption by a specific advance directive establishing a different individual as able to choose according to a best-interests test. If such lines of presumptive authority are not established, the hesitations of family members not close to the patient may lead to the boonless prolongation of the process of dying. With such lines of authority in place, one can clearly know who is responsible, and who should be held responsible for treatment decisions. The importance and cost of dying are likely to force a better clarification of who is in charge. In fact, costs may make it appropriate to give insurance discounts for those who enact a living will. One might envisage Medicare requiring all recipients at least to review a living will. We cannot responsibly possess powerful and costly technologies without carefully determining their proper uses.

Suicide and assisted suicide

In a number of circumstances, merely refusing treatment may not be enough. The decision to stop treatment in order not to prolong the process of dying may not lead to an easy death. An individual with amyelotrophic lateral sclerosis who decides not to have further respiratory support may be faced with hours of agonizing struggle for breath as death intervenes, unless someone provides a sufficient dose of some narcotic or other medication to render the patient unconscious. Similar decisions will face individuals who decide not to prolong treatment for their cancer. Even if pain can be controlled, the various debilities consequent on disease and the treatment of disease, ranging from anal and urinary incontinence to exhaustion, may make any further life unacceptable. Suicide may be the most reasonable choice under such circumstances, and the aid of others may be needed.

An example is provided by the death of Sigmund Freud. After sixteen years of struggling with cancer, and after thirty-three operations, he lay on his deathbed in London at the age of eighty-two. When he saw that prolonging life would in fact be boonless, he asked his personal physician to ease his way. "My dear Schur, you remember our first talk. You promised me then you would help me when I could no longer carry on. It is only torture now and it has no longer any sense."[135] Ernest Jones, Freud's biographer, records: "The next morning Schur gave Freud a third of a grain of morphia. For someone at such a point of exhaustion as Freud then was, and so complete a stranger to opiates, that small dose sufficed."[136] Freud had evidently considered such a remedy from the time of the first diagnosis of his illness.[137] A similar judgment was made by the physicist–philosopher and Nobel prize winner Percy Bridgman (1882–1961). In July 1961, he had a disseminated malignancy and faced the possibility of considerable pain and the loss of what he had in his youth termed intellectual integrity.[138] He wrote, "I would like to take advantage of the situation in which I find myself to establish a general principle, namely, that when the end is as inevitable as it now appears to be, the individual has a right to ask his doctor to end it for him."[139] On August 20 of the same year he took his own life and left the following note: "It isn't decent for Society to make a man do this thing himself. Probably this is the last day I will be able to do it myself. P. W. B."[140]

These actions reflect a well-established philosophical view that rational suicide is not only allowable but in certain circumstances laudable. This view underscores the fact that life is not a good in itself, but rather life takes on value through the goods it allows to be realized. It is a view that, under certain circumstances, tenaciously clinging to life at all costs indicates a lack of moral integrity, as much as does the embrace of suicide as an easy escape from the duties and vexations of life. As Seneca argued in his letter on suicide, "Living is not the good, but living well. The wise man therefore lives as long as he should, not as long as he can. . . . He will always think of life in terms of quality, not quantity."[141] Thus Seneca argued that when "one death involves torture and the other is simple and easy, why not reach for the easier way? . . . Must I wait for the pangs of disease . . . when I can stride through the midst of torment and shake my adversaries off?"[142] Seneca, who took his own life in a famous scene recorded by Tacitus, could see no justifiable grounds against suicide where a prolonged and tortuous death awaited.[143] The philosopher David Hume even saw it in terms of a duty to oneself. "That suicide may often be consistent with interest and with our duty to ourselves, no one can question, who allows that age, sickness, or misfortune may render life a burthen, and make it worse even than annihilation."[144]

Those following the views of Seneca and Hume must be tolerated in terms of the principle of autonomy. One might think here of the fact that up until 1973 the use of force against a rational suicide or the aiders of a rational suicide would have counted as assault and battery in the state of Texas. The use of force against rational individuals committing suicide or those aiding them in suicide would involve an unconsented-to use of force against the innocent, unless the suicide was being prevented in order to allow the discharge of prior duties (e.g., paying one's VISA bill, grading one's students' papers, establishing a trust to support one's children). Individuals should be secure in their rational choices with themselves and consenting others, no matter how reprehensible they may seem.

One might raise the issue of whether there can be a duty to die, a duty not only to refuse treatment, but under certain circumstances to have one's death expedited. One can imagine special circumstances where, for example, joining the CIA obligates one to agree to commit suicide to avoid compromising a delicate mission. One can freely create special circumstances in which one promises to take one's life so that one is morally obliged to do so. The moral foundations for this position become clear once one distinguishes freedom as a constraint on human actions from freedom as a value. Kant condemned suicide because he saw it as a rejection of the basis of the moral community. "To destroy the subject of morality in his own person is tantamount to obliterating from the world, as far as he can, the very existence of morality itself; but morality is, nevertheless, an end in itself."[145] Kant here confuses the conceptual conditions for the possibility of being blameworthy or praiseworthy with the material conditions for having *a* moral community. If one or all rational agents decided to commit suicide, they would not be choosing in a way that would contradict the very *concept* of a community based on mutual respect, though they may be setting aside the possibility of the *existence* of a moral community. Further, it is not possible, pace Kant, to use oneself as a means merely, for one always consents to the uses one makes of oneself.[146] The character of Kant's argument leads to forbidding not only suicide but masturbation[147] and selling or giving one's organs to another, because such would involve using one's self as a means. Kant contends that "to give away or sell a tooth so that it can be planted in the jawbone of another person . . . [is] partial self-murder."[148] The analyses in this volume of the principle of autonomy undercut this line of argument and lead, as we have seen, to holding that murder is a moral offense primarily because it involves taking the life of another individual without that individual's consent. Competent suicide or taking another's life at that person's request does not violate the moral principle of autonomy, unless there are prior agreements to the contrary (e.g., agreements not to commit suicide or engage in dueling or obligations to discharge debts).

Whether killing another at that person's request or suicide violates the principle of beneficence will depend on the ranking of harms and benefits and on the circumstances. When the individual to be killed is in severe pain, beneficence-based arguments may indeed make it morally laudatory if not obligatory to hasten death. If the individual is ill and debilitated, obligations to support dependents or discharge debts may have become moot and no longer plausibly hinder the choice to die. Death may even be laudatory. Consider Hume's suggestion that suicide under certain circumstances would be an act of social responsibility. "But suppose that it is no longer in my power to promote the interest of society; suppose that I am a burthen to it: . . . In such cases my resignation of life must not only be innocent but laudable."[149] One might imagine a patriotic citizen with a debilitating terminal disease committing suicide in order not to encumber further the Medicare fund. At least, failing to take the time to leave instructions for others about the level of treatment one wishes should one become irreversibly and seriously demented may count as a form of moral and social truancy, insofar as such unclarity commits family and society to forms of treatment the individual would not have wanted. It may even be important to leave instructions regarding the circumstances under which one ought to be killed (presuming, naturally, that laws have appropriately been changed).

The prospect of an ever-developing technological capacity to extend life under circumstances that are costly and at times of little enjoyment to the individual underscores the issues of treatment refusal, suicide, and voluntary euthanasia. Though for many these issues necessarily raise the specter of a dictatorial state enforcing involuntary euthanasia, there is little to support this concern. The fact that Texas, which for over 130 years had no law against suicide or against aiding and abetting suicide, easily avoided dangerous slippery slopes, shows that such policies do not necessarily lead to abuse if pursued in a society that takes the freedom of individuals seriously.[150] In order effectively to use the resources at our disposal for the benefit of those who wish to live, it may not only be necessary to recognize the rights of competent individuals to commit suicide, but proper to remind individuals that stopping treatment, taking their lives, or instructing others to kill them may be a reasonable solution to the final debilities and decrepitudes of life. We will need to reexamine themes already articulated by the ancient Greeks and Romans.

Here it is necessary to emphasize that a defense of the moral right of competent individuals to refuse treatment or take their own lives is not an endorsement of tolerating suicide generally.[151] Clearly, the majority of individuals who seek to commit suicide do so because of mental disorder. They should receive psychiatric treatment, not aid in committing suicide. In addition, a great proportion of the competent individuals who choose suicide may do so on ill-considered grounds or because of circumstances that can be remedied through the kindness and compassion of others. Such individuals should be the subject of peaceable persuasion aimed at preventing suicide. However, there are debilitating diseases and final stages of decrepitude where competent men and women may reasonably decide that enough is enough. One may not wish to live out the last few weeks of a death from cancer complicated by multiple metastases and multiple organ difficulties. One may not wish to be warehoused in a nursing home or other facility where one will have very little, if any, conscious awareness of the circumstances of one's life. One might think of cases where the individual is so obtunded as to have little experience of the environment. Finally, one need not commit physicians to being the terminators of life. One must note that the so-called Hippocratic oath, which was more likely written by a group of neo-Pythagoreans than by Hippocrates, did not represent Greco-Roman medical practice as a whole.[152] Many physicians of that time probably did give advice regarding how to achieve a quick and painless death. There may be benefits rather than serious moral consequences from physicians being able at least to advise patients on the best means for avoiding a protracted death.

These suggestions obviously would require substantial revisions of the laws bearing on suicide and murder. A number of states still hold suicide[153] or attempted suicide[154] to be a crime. Even under the old law of the state of Texas, which tolerated aiding and abetting suicide, death had to be effected by the person committing suicide. If another pulled the trigger or placed poison in the suicide's mouth, that person became a murderer, not an abettor of suicide. For many individuals with severely debilitating diseases, more help would be required than the old law allowed, and which the new Texas law completely proscribes.[155] One might think again of the individual dying of amyelotrophic lateral sclerosis who wishes to refuse further respiratory support but does not wish to die gasping for breath. That individual might reasonably want to be assisted in dying, but because of the disease would need not simply passive facilitation but active help. We will need to discover ways in which we can respect the free choices of individuals to aid others in ending their lives. Uruguay, for example, has allowed judges to forgo any punishment when the individual aiding the suicide has previously been honorable and is responding to the repeated requests of the suicide, and the Netherlands have allowed physicians to respond to requests of patients to have their suffering ended through aiding their death. Through this the Netherlands have taken a significant step toward acknowledging the rights of individuals to determine the character of their deaths.[156]

These issues will be inescapable as we extend life expectancy without a dramatic compression of morbidity in old age. The risk of growing older, only to be severely mentally and physically debilitated, may be more than society in general or individuals in particular will wish to bear. In the future there will be an ever-increasing risk, as more individuals live beyond the age of eighty-five, not only of suffering the minor debilities of old age, but of spending months, if not years, requiring comprehensive nursing care. That risk can be avoided if individuals are allowed to direct that they should be painlessly killed under certain specified circumstances. One would not need fear growing old to the point at which life would be an indignity to oneself and a burden to others. Not only would such a policy remove this substantial fear, but it would also free resources to protect the health and augment the pleasures of life when it still can be lived with reward. Even reflecting about such a policy grates against many of the elements of contemporary Western mores. One finds here another example of technology expanding responsibility, where the capacity to do more, in this case live longer, raises vexing moral questions: when one ought to live and when one ought to die.

Euthanasia

If life is not always better than death, it may be beneficent to expedite death rather than to let "nature take its course." This is the case even when the death is not freely chosen, either personally or in advance, by the dying individual. If there is no difference in principle between intending someone's death and merely allowing it, there will be no absolute moral bar against hastening death once one has decided that prolongation of life would be harmful. In fact, we have already seen that active euthanasia of severely defective neonates, who are not persons in the strong social sense, may be morally endorsable. The principle of autonomy itself does not bar terminating the life of an individual who was once competent and (1) who is not competent and (2) will not again be competent, (3) where it appears by clear and convincing evidence that the person would have wished not only to be allowed to die but to have death expedited in the circumstances in question. Given the widespread nonacceptance of assisted suicide and euthanasia in our culture, the burden of proof to establish such hypothetical consent would be quite high. One must presume that most individuals who have not explicitly directed that their death be expedited have no interest in such a remedy. However, instances of *protracted* and *severe* pain and suffering in the absence of contrary religious or other beliefs may make it plausible to hold that the individual would want as quick a relief as is available, even if this involves expediting death. One may even require a noncompetent assent by the individual for whom one is considering expedited death. I will term such a practice euthanasia where there is no actual competent consent but only presumed consent, in order to distinguish it from suicide and even assisted suicide, where a competent individual dying effects death, either alone or through the agency of another. Even effecting death on the basis of an advance directive will thus be a special case of assisted suicide.

Among the considerations to be raised in allowing the practice of euthanasia will be prudential and utilitarian ones, including the possible misuse of the practice were it to be established. Though such fears are often evoked as an argument against euthanasia, it is hard to determine how seriously they ought to be taken. As indicated earlier, the experience in the state of Texas suggests that a practice grounded in respect of free individuals does not lead to disasters. Any reasonable consideration of the matter will need to balance current, actual costs and sufferings involved in the care of individuals, against the possible costs from establishing a limited policy of euthanasia.

As has been noted, allowing euthanasia as well as aiding and abetting suicide will require changes in the law. Until such changes are effected, it is likely that moral duties of beneficence to expedite the death of those dying in pain will be defeated by the risks of legal prosecution and of civil liability.[157] In the end, a sustained and serious moral examination of a revision of policy in these areas will be unavoidable. We will need to examine carefully the ways in which men and women ought to come to terms with dying and the range of choices that must be tolerated.

The health care team

The character of health care is defined by a web of exclusions and inclusions shaped by the various values that direct the free choices of patients, physicians, nurses, and allied health professionals. Decisions to be left alone, to refuse treatment, or to be less than fully compliant with medical recommendations, as well as requests for care, cure, and support, reflect often competing views of good health care. So, too, do decisions of physicians and nurses regarding what care they will provide and under what circumstances. Provision of coherent care is complicated by the number of men and women involved. They determine the character of health care through numerous free choices. In addition, the decisions of insurers, hospitals, and other third parties shape the character of care. But even in terms of the physicians involved, the matter is complex. When a patient is admitted to a referral hospital, there may be not only an admitting physician, but also an attending physician, a resident, and an intern, who may change every month. In addition, consultants will be engaged to provide opinions regarding specific problems or particular forms of treatment. The greatest continuity of care may be provided by the nurses involved in the care of the patient.

To speak of this coterie of individuals as a health care team may suggest more coherence and organization than in fact exists. Allied to the problem of organization is a problem of deciding who directs the team and with what authority. Traditionally, the attending physician has been seen as the captain of the team. Here one might recall stronger metaphors, such as the notion of the physician as the captain of the ship.[158] Such metaphors have been weakened by the increasing independence, and in some cases independent licensure, of nurses, as well as by the increased emphasis on the rights of patients. If authority to treat the patient comes from the patient directly or through the patient's family, is the patient more the captain of the ship, and the physician the pilot? Insofar as patients or their families want to take charge of the course of treatment, they can come to be those centrally responsible and accountable for the direction of care. They may insist that consulting physicians report not simply to the attending physician, but to the patient and/or family. Insofar as patients or their families pay consultants directly or through their insurance, such is a legitimate request. Patients and their families may insist that they themselves direct the treatment. In that patients control the funding of health care, it is not unreasonable to suppose that radical changes can be realized. Though such changes could be achieved, they would involve major alterations in the ways in which physicians traditionally have supported and cared for patients and their families. Quite bluntly put, a pursuit of the activist goals of patient autonomy will be undertaken at the price of the traditional trust, reliance, and comfort afforded by putting oneself or one's family in the hands of a worthy physician. Those involved will need to judge for themselves what costs and benefits should be pursued or avoided.

Much is often made of the model of the trusted family physician from whom one receives treatment over a large span of years. Though many never have the opportunity to come under the care of such physicians, either because of financial barriers or because of the mobile character of modern life, the ideal offers an individual with whom one can frame a personal understanding of what treatment should or should not be provided under different circumstances. Such discussions can be conducted in a nonacute care context and without the press of emergency decisions. In such circumstances, very little may need to be written out in the form of living wills or other instructions. The physician can come to know the patient and his or her family and can direct care as the patient would wish, should the patient be hospitalized. In such happy circumstances one will have found a physician as a friend, an individual who can safeguard one's understandings of good health care and of the good death.

The more medical care is given outside such a personal relationship, the more one will need explicitly to spell out one's wishes in order to give direction to one's care-givers. One will need to indicate in some detail what kind of care one will want, should one become incompetent. Here one should underscore that the sparse character of living-will instruments will rarely be sufficient to indicate adequately what treatment is to be provided or forgone.[159] Indeed, the less one lives within the embrace of traditional communities and personal relationships, the more one will need to fashion formal understandings. Not simply for legal reasons, but to avoid feelings of guilt and misunderstandings on the part of family members, one may need to have relatives sign a living will as a moral commitment to honor the requests of the patient. When the patient is sent to a referral hospital where physicians may rotate monthly in providing care, the patient and family will need to take special steps to ensure that the wishes of the patient (and of the family of an incompetent patient) are clearly known and understood. Formal written directives may offer the only reliable safeguard against being provided treatment or being resuscitated against one's wishes because a new attending physician, resident, or intern did not know of the prior decisions of the patient or family. Patients and their families must captain the direction of health care if such outcomes are to be avoided. Still, even when patients take such an interventionist role (which many patients may not wish to shoulder), the physician remains inescapably the pilot, the individual who knows where wishes can go aground and hopes shipwrecked. One must not forget that the physician is the one who knows the intimate geography of possibilities in setting a course through dangerous waters.

The structure of the health care team will depend on the extent to which patients seek to captain their destiny and the extent to which physicians, nurses, and others believe that charting a particular course is necessary for good health care. Physicians may insist that consultants report to them, not directly to the patient. They may insist that nurses not inform patients of their judgments regarding care and prognosis but defer to physicians in this matter. Whether consultants speak directly to patients or primarily to the

320   THE FOUNDATIONS OF BIOETHICS

attending physician, whether nurses will have independent areas in which
they can communicate decisions regarding the medical treatment and prognosis of the patient, or the extent to which nurses and other allied health
care professionals function as physician assistants will in the end depend on
the balancing of the wishes and interests of all involved. The fact that the
profession of physician's assistant[160] developed as nurses withdrew from
being physician extenders may show that there is a persistent and important
role for such individuals.[161]

The point is that the character of health care is to be created, not
discovered. There is no single orthodox or canonical ranking of values that
will dictate the role of physicians, patients, nurses, and others. Each can
surely withdraw or refuse to participate. However, none may compel the
uncritical services of the other. No one may independently and unilaterally
fashion the concrete character of health care. Each depends on the free
agreement of the others to participate in the complex endeavors of health
care. There are surely opportunities for patients and others to create
opportunities for the realization for particular sets of values. Just as there are
hospitals established by Seventh Day Adventists and Roman Catholics, one
may establish special libertarian or paternalist hospitals that would allow the
participants to have the special character of care they seek.

The opportunity to realize such special structures will depend not only on
the free choices of these individuals but also on the availability of resources.
One will need to know what treatments individuals may refuse to receive or
to give, as well as who has a right to the positive provision of health care or a
duty to provide health care and under what circumstances. The character of
health care will be determined not just by rights and duties of forbearance,
but also by rights and duties of beneficence.

Notes

1. Hippocrates, "Epidemics" I, XII.10–15, in *Hippocrates*, trans. W. H. S. Jones
   (Cambridge, Mass.: Harvard University Press, 1962), vol. 1, p. 165.
2. The body of skills and knowledge possessed by members of a learned profession
   constitutes a conceptual structure that guides and defines the community. See,
   for example, Karl Popper's treatment of ideas as a world of quasi-platonic
   objects: Karl R. Popper and John C. Eccles, *The Self and Its Brain* (New York:
   Springer, 1977), pp. 36–50.
3. At the time of Hippocrates (c. 460–377 B.C.) there was no formal association or
   lobby group such as the American Medical Association. There was also little
   formal control of the medical profession. See, for example, the Hippocratic
   treatise "Law". However, there were avenues for the equivalent of malpractice
   suits against physicians in ancient times. Darrel W. Amundsen, "The Liability
   of the Physician in Classical Greek Legal Theory and Practice," *Journal of the
   History of Medicine and Allied Sciences* 32 (April 1977): 172–203; "The Liability

of the Physician in Roman Law," in H. Karplus (ed.), *International Symposium on Society, Medicine and Law* (New York: Elsevier, 1973), pp. 17–30: "Physician, Patient and Malpractice: An Historical Perspective," in S. F. Spicker et al. (eds.), *The Law-Medicine Relation: A Philosophical Exploration* (Dordrecht: Reidel, 1981), pp. 255–8.

4. Alfred Schutz provides a very helpful treatment of the problems associated with the social distribution of knowledge and how this bears on the differences among experts, laymen, and well-informed laymen. Alfred Schutz and Thomas Luckman, *The Structures of the Life-World*, trans. R. M. Zaner and H. T. Engelhardt, Jr. (Evanston, Ill.: Northwestern University Press, 1973), pp. 304–31.

5. There is a certain awe involved in the intervention with powerful mechanical devices, such as the space shuttle. There may be a special sense of awe or respect for those who repair such devices, which in part depends on the complexity of the mechanism being repaired.

6. An exploration of the problem that patients face in anticipating the moral and professional commitments of physicians is provided by Alasdair MacIntyre, "Patients as Agents," in S. F. Spicker and H. T. Engelhardt, Jr. (eds.), *Philosophical Medical Ethics: Its Nature and Significance* (Dordrecht: Reidel, 1977), pp. 197–212.

7. Alfred Schutz, "The Stranger: An Essay in Social Psychology," in Arvid Brodersen (ed.), *Collected Papers* (The Hague: Martinus Nijhoff, 1964), vol. 2, p. 99.

8. Edmund D. Pellegrino and David C. Thomasma, *A Philosophical Basis of Medical Practice* (New York: Oxford University Press, 1981), pp. 64–6, 72, 86, 187, 200.

9. Plato discusses the issue of the patient being a friend to the physician for the sake of health in *Lysis*, 218d–219d.

10. Pellegrino and Thomasma's interpretation of this passage is dependent on Plato's assumption that there is a univocal sense of health and that both the physician and the patient have a common understanding of the good of health to be achieved through medicine.

11. Aristotle, *Magna Moralia*, 2.12115–16.

12. "The sick man, as we just now said, is a friend to the physician. Is he not? He is. On account of sickness, for the sake of health? Yes." Plato, *Lysis*, 218e, in Edith Hamilton and Huntington Cairns (eds.), *The Collected Dialogues of Plato* (Princeton, N.J.: Princeton University Press, 1969), pp. 162–3.

13. Pellegrino and Thomasma, *Philosophical Basis of Medical Practice*, p. 72.

14. G. W. F. Hegel, *Philosophy of Right*, trans. T. M. Knox (London: Oxford University Press, 1965), sec. 303.

15. Ibid., sec. 270, with Zusatz. In this section Hegel criticizes the anti-Semites of his day and gives what can be interpreted as an argument for a religiously neutral tolerant state.

16. Robert A. Burt, *Taking Care of Strangers* (New York: Free Press, 1979), p. 19.

17. Even within communities bound together by a concrete view of the good life, there is a place for the rule of law, not that of men: the law should always be a source of protection for persons against unconsented-to force. In many communities this will not require bureaucratic rules. The more the community is a face-to-face community, the less need there will be for elaborate formal regulations.

18. For a review of some of the issues raised by free and informed consent in the law, see Alexander M. Capron, "Informed Consent in Catastrophic Disease Research and Treatment," *University of Pennsylvania Law Review* 123 (Dec. 1974): 340–438; Donald G. Hagman, "The Medical Patient's Right to Know: Report on a Medical-Legal-Ethical, Empirical Study," *UCLA Law Review* 17 (1970): 758–816; Leslie J. Miller, "Informed Consent: I," *Journal of the American Medical Association* 244 (Nov. 7, 1980): 2100–3, "Informed Consent: II," *Journal of the American Medical Association* 244 (Nov. 21, 1980): 2347–50; "Informed Consent: III," *Journal of the American Medical Association* 244 (Dec. 5, 1980): 2556–8; "Informed Consent: IV," *Journal of the American Medical Association* 244 (Dec. 12, 1980): 2661–2; Marcus L. Plante, "An Analysis of 'Informed Consent,'" *Fordham Law Review* 36 (1968): 639–72; M. L. Plante, "The Decline of 'Informed Consent,'" *Washington & Lee Law Review* 92 (1978): 91–9. J. R. Waltz and T. W. Scheuneman, "Informed Consent to Therapy," *Northwestern University Law Review* 64 (1970): 628–50. These articles provide an introduction to some of the legal issues raised by this volume's analysis of free and informed consent. The reader should bear in mind that this volume focuses on the analysis of conceptual issues, not directly on issues raised in the law.

19. Natalie Abrams, "Medical Experimentation: The Consent of Prisoners and Children," in S. F. Spicker and H. T. Engelhardt, Jr. (eds.), *Philosophical Medical Ethics* (Dordrecht; Reidel, 1977), pp. 111–24.

20. The Magna Charta (June 15, 1215) gave a general protection against unjustified governmental use of force against individuals. "No freeman shall be taken or imprisoned, or disseised, or outlawed, or banished, or any ways destroyed, nor will we pass upon him, nor will we send upon him, unless by the lawful judgment of his peers, or by the law of the land" (sec. 39).

There were also grounds for action against individuals who beat others without justification. Thus, William Blackstone gives the following commentary regarding battery:

> The least touching of another's person wilfully, or in anger, is a battery; for the law cannot draw the line between different degrees of violence, and therefore totally prohibits the first and lowest stage of it: every man's person being sacred, and no other having a right to meddle with it, in any the slightest manner. And therefore upon a similar principle the Cornelian law *de injuriis* prohibited *pulsation* as well as *verberation*; distinguishing verberation, which was accompanied with pain, from pulsation, which was attended with none...

William Blackstone, *Commentaries on the Laws of England* (1765), Book III, p. 120. Blackstone originally published his work between 1765 and 1769. Earlier commentaries give a more restricted notion of battery, as that provided by Thomas Wood (1661–1722): "A *Battery* is any Injury done to the Person of another in a Rude or Angry Manner; as by Striking, Pushing, Jostling, Catching by the Arm, Filliping upon the Nose, Spitting in the Face, Pulling of a Button in a Rude and Insolent Manner, *etc.*" *An Institute of the Laws of England* (London: Nutt and Gosling, 1724; reprinted 1979), p. 423. This might be compared with the Texas penal code, which holds that a person commits the offense of assault if he "intentionally or knowingly causes physical contact with another when he knows or should reasonably believe that the other will regard the contact as offensive or provocative." *Texas Penal Code Annotated*, sec. 22.01(a) (3)

(Vernon Supp. 1982). Modern codes have developed the views of Cornelian law regarding assault and battery, to which Blackstone alluded.

21. Free individuals were immune under ancient Germanic law from the torture regularly used in the Mediterranean world and later in the Christian world. It was a crime to use violence against a free individual. Consider the following passage from a classic treatise on torture: "For the cringing suppliant of the audience chamber, abjectly prostrating himself before a monarch who combines in his own person every legislative and executive function, we have the freeman of the German forests, who sits in council with his chief, who frames the laws which both are bound to respect, and who pays to that chief only the amount of obedience which superior vigor and intellect may be able to enforce... This personal independence of the freeman is one of the distinguishing characteristics of all the primitive Teutonic institutions." Henry Charles Lea, *Torture* (Philadelphia: University of Pennsylvania Press, 1866; reprinted 1973), pp. 24–5.

22. Slater v. Baker and Stapleton, 2 Wils. 359, 95 Eng. Rep. 860 (Kings Bench 1767). There were severe limits to the amount of information that needed to be disclosed for patient consent. Consider Justice Oliver Wendell Holmes's remark: "... the patient has no more right to all the truth than he has to all of the medicines in the physician's saddlebags." Quoted in Eugene M. Hoyt, "Mandatory Disclosure Standards or Informed Consent—Texas Style," *Texas Medicine* 79 (Oct. 1983): 56.

23. Schloendorff v. Society of N.Y. Hospital, 211 N.Y. 125, 105 N.E. 92, 93 (1914). This decision was anticipated, for example, by Mohr v. Williams, where the court ruled that a procedure undertaken by a physician without a patient's consent should count as a tort. Mohr v. Williams, 95 Minn. 261, 104 N.W. 12 (1905).

24. Olmstead v. United States, 277 U.S. 438, 478 (1928) (Brandeis, J., dissenting).

25. In re President & Directors of Georgetown College, Inc., 331 F.2d 1000, 1017 (D.C. Cir.) *cert. denied*, 337 U.S. 978 (1964) (Burger, W., dissenting) (emphasis in original).

26. Natanson v. Kline, 186 Kan. 393, 404, 350 P.2d 1093, 1104 (1960).

27. The attribution to Tertullian (?/160–c. 230) of the phrase, "Credo quia absurdum est," which is not found in any of his extant writings, is discussed by Etienne Gilson in *History of Christian Philosophy in the Middle Ages* (New York: Random House, 1955), p. 45. Similar passages can be found. Tertullian said with regard to the death of Christ, "Prorsus credibile est quia ineptum est" (It is straightforwardly believable because it is silly) and with regard to the Resurrection, "Certum est, quia impossibile est" (It is certain because it is impossible). *De carne Christi*, sec. 5. There are similarities with Augustine, who argued that one must believe in order to understand. *De Trinitate* 8.5.8 and 9.1.1. As St. Augustine stated in *In Ioannis evangelium tractatus* 40. 8.9, "Non quia cognoverunt crediderunt, sed ut cognoscerent crediderunt. Credimus enim ut cognoscamus, non cognoscimus ut credamus." (We have not known because we have believed, but so that we might know we have believed. For we believe in order to know, we do not know in order to believe.) These writings provide an example of the position that only through the special grace of belief is true knowledge of the important goals of life and the truths of existence available. Outside of such grace, belief often will seem to be folly in the eyes of the Greeks and scandal in the eyes of the Jews (I Corinthians 1:23).

28. Baruch A. Brody and H. Tristram Engelhardt, Jr. (eds.), *Mental Illness: Law and Public Policy* (Dordrecht: Reidel, 1980).

29. In re President & Directors of Georgetown College, Inc., 1008. The court held that the duty was not directly to the infant but to the community regarding the infant: "The patient had a responsibility to the community to care for her infant. Thus the people had an interest in preserving the life of this mother." The court was correct in holding that individuals ought not to create new burdens for the community. On the other hand, insofar as communities allow parents to place their children for adoption or as state wards, and one circumscribes that right created by civil beneficence simply because the individual wishes to exercise it so as to refuse lifesaving treatment, that circumscription may offend against important values of liberty and evenhandedness. In addition to the community's interest in the child and the society's interest in not being subjected to undue financial burden, there is also the question of the obligation of the parent to secure the well-being of the child.

30. In re Osborne, 294 A.2d 372, 374 (D.C. 1972).

31. Colin M. Turnbull, *The Mountain People* (New York: Simon and Schuster, 1972), p. 121.

32. The reader should note that this view of lying departs radically from the Kantian understanding. See, for example, Immanuel Kant, *The Metaphysics of Morals*, Akademie Textausgabe, vol. 6, pp. 429–31. Kant argues for the immorality of lying on the grounds that it violates a person's duty to himself considered as a moral being, as well as making that individual responsible for all of the unforeseen consequences of the lie. The significance of lying changes when one distinguishes between freedom as a value and freedom as a side constraint. If the freedom at stake in the morality of mutual respect is freedom as a side constraint, as I have argued in chapter 3, then individuals may free themselves of duties to themselves. In addition, the moral significance of lying changes when it is seen as a justified use of defensive force. The same arguments that Kant employs to justify defensive force (and for that matter retributive force) will justify defensive lying and deception as well. An individual who acts against the very possibility of mutual respect loses the grounds for consistently protesting against defensive force, including lying, and those who use defensive force cannot be held to have violated the notion of mutual respect, in that they have treated the violator in a way consistent with the violator's expressed moral principles. Not only does the individual using defensive force (including lying) have a warrant for its use, but the individual who occasions its use through imperiling an innocent individual is the one most reasonably to be held accountable for the consequences of the defense. Among other things, this argument shows that spies in a just war may not only kill the enemy but also deceive them.

33. William H. Masters and Virginia E. Johnson, *The Pleasure Bond* (Boston: Little, Brown, 1970). On this point, consider the poem of William Blake, "The Question Answer'd":

What is it men in women do require?
The lineaments of Gratified Desire.
What is it women do in men require?
The lineaments of Gratified Desire.

Insofar as relationships are based at least in part on the satisfactions of desires, not simply on rational considerations, they are open to being structured by peaceable manipulations of the sort, "I will do this for you if you do that for me."

34. If one agrees with Frankfurt, one might hold that a manipulation is peaceable, even if the person manipulated can no longer turn down the inducement offered as long as the manipulated individual rationally affirms the state of affairs. Even if the manipulation moves the individual who is being manipulated so that his first-order volitions compel him to agree, the action is still free if it is affirmed by second-order volitions. An example of this might be an experimenter offering a would-be research subject a million dollars to participate in a risky experiment. Even if the individual is so interested in the money that it would be impossible to decline the offer, the choice is still free, to develop Frankfurt's suggestions, if the individual affirms this state of affairs. Compare "I wish he hadn't offered me that money: I wish I could turn it down, but I just can't," and "I'm glad she offered me that money: I couldn't turn it down if I wanted to, but I would never want to turn down such an offer: I'm very glad it was made." H. Frankfurt, "Freedom of the Will and the Concept of a Person," *Journal of Philosophy* 68 (1971): 5–20; "Coercion and Moral Responsibility," in T. Honderich (ed.), *Essays on Freedom of Action* (London: Routledge, 1972), pp. 72–85; and H. Frankfurt and D. Locke, "Three Concepts of Free Action," *Proceedings of the Aristotelian Society*, supp. vol. 49 (1975): 95–125. See also Irving Thalberg, "Motivational Disturbances and Free Will," pp. 201–20, and Caroline Whitbeck, "Towards an Understanding of Motivational Disturbance and Freedom of Action," pp. 221–31, in H. T. Engelhardt, Jr., and S. F. Spicker (eds.), *Mental Health: Philosophical Perspectives* (Dordrecht: Reidel, 1978).

35. Robert Nozick, "Coercion," in S. Morgenbesser et al. (eds.), *Philosophy, Science, and Method* (New York: St. Martin's Press, 1969), pp. 440–72; Joel Rudinow, "Manipulation," *Ethics* 88 (1978): 338–47.

36. It should be evident to the reader that the term *force* in phrases such as "the use of unconsented-to force against the innocent" is employed in an extended sense to include all violations of the principle of mutual respect. Such violations will include not only the use of direct violence but also attempts to intervene in the lives of others by means of deceptions, threats, or duress. One should note also that failing to honor a contract is not simply an omission but a form of intervention in that it depends on the prior creation of a contract. Interventions will not include the failure to provide goods needed by another, but not due to another through prior contracts or just possession. Without the existence of a prior set of understandings, such an omission cannot be seen to be a form of intervention. The term force underscores the border crossing involved in the use of violence, the threat of violence, the breach of a contract, or the employment of deception. In such circumstances one uses a means to compel another individual so as to control or interfere with that individual in ways to which that individual has not consented.

There may be some circumstances in which unconsented-to force can be used against an individual who is in a strict sense innocent. Imagine that one is sitting at the bottom of a building with a shoulder-launchable surface-to-air missile. An innocent individual has just been pushed from the top of the building. One does not have enough time to run away so as to avoid being seriously injured if not killed by the impact of the falling individual. However, one has sufficient time to fire the surface-to-air missile. The firing is justified because the falling individual, innocent or not, willing or not, is in fact threatening the person at the bottom. The falling individual is about to engage in an unauthorized border crossing, willing or not. Were we dealing with cases such as this in some detail, we would be committed to a more ample analysis of "innocent person" and "proper defense against unjustified force." Here it is enough to suggest that in some circumstances compulsory vaccination may be like the use of a surface-to-air missile. If others are likely to contract a disease if left unvaccinated and spread it to innocent individuals who cannot vaccinate themselves or otherwise protect themselves, force may be justified to require vaccination in order to protect individuals who otherwise would be brought into contact with the disease without their consent, without an opportunity to avoid the contact, and without an opportunity to avoid contracting the disease. There will be the problem of how much energy innocent third persons must invest in avoiding the contact or in avoiding the development of the disease, before one may vaccinate others in order to protect the unvaccinated group. One must note that if the individuals who make contact with the disease do so in part of their own free choice, they may totally defeat their claim that others must vaccinate themselves or otherwise take precautions. As a consequence, this argument may support compulsory vaccinations against highly contagious diseases, such as smallpox (in order to protect those who cannot be vaccinated for medical reasons), but not against diseases such as AIDS, which can usually be contracted only through positive actions that are already generally known to carry certain risks, including that of AIDS. It is hard to step out of the way of highly contagious diseases such as smallpox, but easy to step out of the way of diseases such as AIDS. Hemophiliacs are in the unhappy position of needing a good from others (blood products) to which they have no prior rights. In the terms of chapter 8, if they contract AIDS in such circumstances, it is highly unfortunate, but not unfair.

37. An exception may be certain forms of psychoanalysis, which are focused on increasing the capacity to choose freely and/or responsibly. See, for example, Thomas Szasz, *The Ethics of Psychoanalysis* (New York: Basic Books, 1965). I have analyzed some of the issues raised by such approaches in H. T. Engelhardt, Jr., "Psychotherapy as Meta-ethics," *Psychiatry* 36 (Nov. 1973): 440–5.

38. Nishi v. Hartwell, 473 P 2d 116, 119 (Hawaii 1970), quoting Watson v. Clutts, 136 S.E. 2d 617, 621 (N.C. 1964).

39. Plato, *Laws*, trans. A. E. Taylor, in Hamilton and Cairns (eds.), *Collected Dialogues of Plato*, pp. 1310–11.

40. Alexander M. Capron, "Informed Consent in Catastrophic Disease Research and Treatment," *University of Pennsylvania Law Review* 123 (Dec. 1974): 364–76.

41. Natanson v. Kline, 186 Kan. 393, 404, 350 P.2d, 1093, 1106 (1960).

   For discussion of the strong support of the professional standard by British courts, see George J. Annas, "Why the British Courts Rejected the American Doctrine of Informed Consent," *American Journal of Public Health* 74 (November 1984): 1286–78.

42. Aiken v. Clary, 396 S.W.2d 668, 674-675 (Mo. Sup. Ct. 1965).

43. Sard v. Hardy, 397 A. 2d 1014, 1020 (Md. 1977).

44. Canterbury v. Spence, 464 F.2d 772, 797 (D.C. Cir. 1972).

45. Cobbs v. Grant, 8 Cal. 3.d 229, 245; 502 P.2d 1, 11; 104 Cal. Rptr. 505, 515 (Calif. 1972).

46. Canterbury v. Spence, 464 F.2d 772, 791 (D.C. Cir. 1972).
47. Cobbs v. Grant. Capron, "Informed Consent in Catastrophic Disease Research and Treatment," pp. 407, 416.
48· Cobbs v. Grant, 502 P.2d 1, 12 (Calif. 1972). Sard v. Hardy, 397 A.2d 1014, 1022 (Md. 1977).
49. Canterbury v. Spence, 464 F.2d 772, 789 (D.C. Cir. 1972).
50. Cobbs v. Grant, 8 Cal. 3.d 229, 246; 502 P.2d 1, 12; 104 Cal. Rptr. 505, 516 (Calif. 1972).
51. Hubert W. Smith, "Therapeutic Privilege to Withhold Specific Diagnosis from Patient Sick with Serious or Fatal Illness," *Tennessee Law Review* 19 (1946): 349–60.
52. Natanson v. Kline, 350 P.2d 1093, 1103 (1960).
53. In emergency circumstances, when physicians choose by their own lights, as well as in circumstances when the therapeutic privilege is invoked, one must presume that it is not feasible to consult with someone in authority over that patient or with someone who can accurately convey the wishes of the patient with respect to treatment. Such consultation would be morally required when feasible.
54. For an introduction to the literature concerning paternalism, see Joel Feinberg, "Legal Paternalism," *Canadian Journal of Philosophy* 105 (1971): 113–16; Allan Buchanan, "Medical Paternalism," *Philosophy and Public Affairs* 7 (1978): 370–90; Charles M. Culver and Bernard Gert, "The Morality of Involuntary Hospitalization," in S. F. Spicker et al. (eds.), *The Law-Medicine Relation*, pp. 159–75; and James F. Childress, *Who Should Decide? Paternalism in Health Care* (New York: Oxford University Press, 1982).
55. John Mill, *On Liberty*, ed. G. Himmelfarb (New York: Penguin, 1982): 165–6.
56. Calif. Welf. & Inst. Code, sec. 5150 (West 1972 & Supp. 1982).
57. Ibid., sec. 5260.
58. James F. Drane, "Competency to Give an Informed Consent," *Journal of the American Medical Association* 252 (Aug. 17, 1984): 925–7.
59. Gerald Dworkin, "Paternalism," *Monist* 56 (1972): 64–84.
60. Charles M. Culver and Bernard Gert, "Paternalistic Behavior," *Philosophy and Public Affairs* 6 (1976): 49–50.
61. Childress, *Who Should Decide?* pp. 237–41.
62. I borrow here, as elsewhere, from the distinctions between being in authority and being an authority, which are summarized by Richard E. Flathman, "Power, Authority, and Rights in the Practice of Medicine," in George Agich (ed.), *Responsibility in Health Care* (Dordrecht: Reidel, 1982), pp. 105–25.
63. Katherine-Marie Drews, "When Minors Seek Medical Treatment on Their Own Behalf," *Medicine and Law* 2 (1983): 209–20; and Susan L. Brackshaw, "Health Care of Children Over Objections of the Parents: Clash of Rights," *Medicine and Law* 2 (1983): 221–30.
64. An overview of the child–parent relation in modern Western thought is provided by Jeffrey Blustein, *Parents and Children* (New York: Oxford University Press, 1982).
65. Edward Wallerstein, *Circumcision: An American Health Fallacy* (New York: Springer, 1980).
66. Marie Bassill Assaad, "Female Circumcision in Egypt: Social Implications, Current Research, and Prospects for Change," *Studies in Family Planning* 11 (Jan. 1980): 3–16: Franziska P. Hosken, "The Epidemiology of Female Genital

Mutilations," *Tropical Doctor* 8 (1978): 150–6; Fran P. Hosken, "Women and Health: Genital and Sexual Mutilation of Females," *International Journal of Women's Studies* 3 (May 1980): 300–16; H. T. Laycock, "Surgical Aspects of Female Circumcision in Somaliland," *East African Medical Journal* 27 (1950): 445–50. One should note that great consternation has been caused by well-educated women from northern Africa requesting that their daughters receive radical circumcision in European hospitals and clinics.

67. Hoskin, "Women and Health: Genital and Sexual Mutilation of Females," p. 308. One should note that various forms of sexual mutilation were accepted in nineteenth- and early twentieth-century America. Ben Barker-Benfield, "Sexual Surgery in Late-Nineteenth-Century America," *International Journal of Health Services* 5 (1975): 279–98; Carroll Smith-Rosenberg and Charles Rosenberg, "The Female Animal: Medical and Biological Views of Woman and Her Role in Nineteenth-Century America," *Journal of American History* 60 (Sept. 1973): 332–56. For reference to current surgery aimed at enhancing female sexual response, see Wallerstein, *Circumcision: An American Health Fallacy*, pp. 182–90.

68. These views lead to an approval of the actions by the defenders of Masada, which included taking the lives of children, insofar as all participating who were competent agreed to the mutual suicide. One might note that there is some evidence of compulsion, Flavius Josephus, *Wars of the Jews*, book VII, chap. IX.

   One might note how difficult it is to decide whether parental decisions show reckless disregard of the welfare of a child. Individuals are generally ready to intervene to provide treatment for the children of parents who refuse treatment due to religious commitments to a nonmainline religion. Consider the report of an Italian couple who declined surgery and radiotherapy for their child diagnosed as having Ewing's sarcoma, and instead took the child to Lourdes. The child experienced a spontaneous remission. Eugene F. Diamond, "Miraculous Cures," *Linacre Quarterly* 51 (August 1984): 224–32.

   The view of toleration to which the arguments in this volume lead (no matter how unpleasant such conclusions may be) are similar to the position of Ohio, at least through 1983, regarding the right of parents to forego standard medical care for their children and to rely instead on prayer. "Nothing in this section shall be construed to define as an abused or neglected child any child who is under spiritual treatment through prayer in accordance with the tenets and practice of a well-recognized religion in lieu of medical treatment, and no report shall be required as to such child." Ohio's Juvenile Code 2151.421. The conclusions may not be as radical as they appear at first blush.

69. Darrel Amundsen, "Casuistry and Professional Obligations: The Regulation of Physicians by the Court of Conscience in the Late Middle Ages" (Part I), *Transactions and Studies of the College of Physicians of Philadelphia* 3 (1981): 22–39; "Casuistry and Professional Obligations: The Regulation of Physicians by the Court of Conscience in the Late Middle Ages" (Part II), *Transactions and Studies of the College of Physicians of Philadelphia* 3 (1981): 93–112.

70. Amundsen, Part I, p. 35.

71. Brown v. Hughes, 94 Colo. 295, 30 P. 2d 259 (1934); Carpenter v. Blake, 60 Barb., 488 (N.Y., 1871).

72. Hans Jonas, "Philosophical Reflections on Experimenting with Human Subjects," in P. A. Freund (ed.), *Experimentation with Human Subjects* (New York: Braziller, 1969), pp. 3–4.

73. Ibid., pp. 16–17.
74. Hans Jonas, "Philosophical Reflections on Experimenting with Human Subjects," *Daedalus* 98 (1969): 235.
75. Jay Katz, "Prologue—Experiments Prior to 1939," in Jay Katz, *Experimentation with Human Beings* (New York: Russell Sage Foundation, 1972), pp. 284–92.
76. J. H. Jones, *Bad Blood: The Tuskegee Syphilis Experiment* (New York: Free Press, 1981).
77. Hans-Martin Sass, "Reichsrundschreiben 1931: Pre-Nuremberg German Regulations Concerning New Therapy and Human Experimentation," *Journal of Medicine and Philosophy* 8 (1983): 99–111.
78. See, for example, William Cullen, *Treatise of the Materia Medica* (Philadelphia: Mathew Carey, 1808).
79. Thomas Sydenham, preface to "The History of Acute and Chronic Disease," in *The Entire Works of Dr. Thomas Sydenham*, ed. and trans. John Swan. 3d ed. (London: E. Cave, 1753), p. xiii.
80. P. C. A. Louis, *Recherches sur les effets de la saignée dans quelques maladies inflammatoires* (Paris: Baillière, 1835). See also the first treatise on the use of confidence levels in medical statistics, J. Gavaret, *Principles généraux de statistique médicale* (Paris: Bechet jeune et Labe, 1840).
81. *Protection of Human Subjects*, 45 Code of Federal Regulations, 46.116(a).
82. Ibid., 46.111(a) 2.
83. I am indebted to Hans-Martin Sass for his discussions of this issue with me.
84. For an attempt to set out general moral principles for research, see the National Commission for the Protection of Human Subjects of Biomedical and Behavioral Research, *The Belmont Report* (Washington, D.C.: U.S. Government Printing Office, 1978, DHEW [OS] 78-0012). As the reader will notice, this report defends a principle of justice, in addition to principles of autonomy and beneficence. The analyses in this volume indicate that the principle of justice can in fact be reduced to the principles of autonomy and beneficence. The two appendices to this report offer an introduction to the philosophical issues bearing on the use of human research subjects.
85. *Nobel Lectures, Physiology or Medicine, 1942–1962* (Amsterdam: Elsevier, 1964), p. 511.
86. One should note that the appeal to future agreement by the ward in the principle of proxy consent as I have outlined it has a similarity with Richard McCormick's view of what a responsible ward would have acknowledged as his duty to participate in research. A difference between our positions lies in my acknowledgment of the heterogeneity of the views of the good life and therefore of moral duty. As a consequence, my view does not depend on the notion of the ward having a general moral duty, but rather (at least in part) on what is likely to be the judgment of an individual when competent. Richard A. McCormick, "Proxy Consent in the Experimental Situation," *Perspectives in Biology and Medicine* 18 (Autumn 1974): 2–21.
87. *Protection of Human Subjects*, 45 Code of Federal Regulations, 46.406.
88. Ibid., 46.407.
89. Ibid., 46.102(g).
90. Ibid., 46.301–6.
91. Hans Jonas, "Philosophical Reflections on Experimenting with Human Subjects," p. 246fn.
92. Arthur Elstein, "Human Factors in Clinical Judgment," in H. T. Engelhardt,

Jr., et al. (eds.), *Clinical Judgment* (Dordrecht: Reidel, 1979), pp. 17–28. Michael Scriven, "Clinical Judgment," in *Clinical Judgment*, pp. 3–16.

93. Norwood Hanson, *Patterns of Discovery* (Cambridge: Cambridge University Press, 1961).

94. See, for example, J. S. Carey, "Veterans Administration Coronary Cooperative Study," *Journal of the American Medical Association* 24 (1979): 2791–2; R. G. Hoffman et al., "The Probability of Surviving Coronary Study," *Journal of the American Medical Association* 241 (1980): 621–7; M. L. Murphy et al., "Treatment of Chronic Stable Angina," *New England Journal of Medicine* 297 (1977): 621–7.

95. See, for example, G. Crile, Jr., "The Breast Cancer Controversy," *Transactions and Studies of the College of Physicians of Philadelphia* 41 (1974): 243–53; J. A. Urban, "Treatment of Primary Breast Cancer," *Journal of American Medical Association* 244 (1980): 800–3; and U.S. Department of Health, Education, and Welfare, *The Breast Cancer Digest* (Bethesda, Md.: NIH Pub. 80-1691, 1979), pp. 26–35.

96. A random clinical trial is usually halted when the data show that there is only a very small likelihood, say five times out of a hundred, or one time out of a hundred that the results are likely to be due to chance rather than to a true relation. How certain ought one to be before one stops a trial? The sooner one stops, the likelier it is that the findings were due only to chance. The longer one continues the trial, the longer individuals who would benefit from the new treatment must wait for a final decision to be made. There are no answers that can be discovered for such questions, since they represent a balance among various possible harms and benefits. One must create a balance in terms of a general view of the need to protect patients over the long run from physicians prematurely establishing treatments as "accepted treatments."

97. The reader should recognize that deception plays a major role in psychological studies. Here the same moral principle should apply as I have outlined in the body of the chapter. Individuals should be warned that they will be subjected to deceptions. Where the risks from the deception are minor, it can usually be presumed that a general disclosure with few details will adequately serve the purpose of respecting the freedom of the would-be subject (e.g., "Over the next few weeks you will be subjected to certain minor deceptions in order to study the process of learning"). Finally, researchers need not provide more information than is ordinarily provided in everyday life. Thus, participant researchers who actually take on a bona fide role need not disclose that they are also psychologists. Here as elsewhere there may be a divergence of law and morals.

98. Hippocrates, "Oath," in *Hippocrates*, vol. 1. p. 301.

99. One should note that it is highly unlikely that courts would attempt to break priest–penitent confidentiality, even in jurisdictions where there is no legally recognized privilege.

100. For an analysis of the development of the legal duty to disclose to third parties the dangerousness of the patient, see William J. Winslade, "Psychotherapeutic Discretion and Judicial Decision: A Case of Enigmatic Justice," in Spicker *et al.* (eds.), *The Law-Medicine Relation*, pp. 139–57.

101. Monroe H. Freedman, *Lawyers. Ethics in an Adversary System* (Indianapolis: Bobbs-Merrill, 1975). See also Stephen Toulmin, "The Meaning of Professionalism: Doctors' Ethics and Biomedical Science," in H. T. Engelhardt, Jr., and D. Callahan (eds.), *Knowledge, Value, and Belief* (Hastings-on-Hudson: Institute of Society, Ethics and the Life Sciences, 1977), pp. 254–78.

102. Henry Charles Lea, *A History of Auricular Confession and Indulgences in the Latin Church* (New York: Greenwood Press, 1968), vol. 1, p. 444.
103. Ibid., p. 445.
104. Nancy Lee Beaty, *The Craft of Dying* (New Haven, Conn.: Yale University Press, 1970).
105. A very useful review of recent law and public policy regarding both treatment refusal and the use of advance directives is provided in President's Commission for the Study of Ethical Problems in Medicine and Biomedical and Behavioral Research, *Deciding to Forego Life-Sustaining Treatment* (Washington, D.C.: U.S. Government Printing Office, 1983).
106. *Rituale Romanum* (Tours: Typis Mame, 1952), pp. 233–57.
107. Darrel W. Amundsen, "Prolonging Life: A Duty without Classical Roots," *Hastings Center Report* 8 (Aug. 1978): 23–30.
108. Seneca, "On the Sadness of Life," in *The Stoic Philosophy of Seneca*, trans. Moses Hadas (New York: Norton, 1958), p. 205.
109. Natanson v. Kline, 186 Kan. 393, 404, 350 P.2d 1093, 1104 (1960).
110. For instances of Jehovah's Witnesses being allowed to refuse lifesaving treatment, see, for example, In re Estate of Brooks 205 N.E.2d 435 (Ill. 1965); In re Milideo 390 N.Y.S.2d 523 (Sup. Ct. 1976); for a case where the right to refuse treatment was upheld, even if it were tantamount to suicide and suicide were a crime, see, Erikson v. Dilgard, 252 N.Y.S.2d 705, 706 (Sup. Ct. 1962).
111. Contra, J.F.K. Mem. Hosp. v. Heston, 279 A.2d 670, 672–673 (N.J. 1971).
112. Satz v. Perlmutter, Fla. Sup. Ct. 379 So.2d 359 (1980).
113. William Blackstone, *Commentaries on the Laws of England in Four Books*, Book 4, p. 189.
114. H. T. Engelhardt, Jr., and Michele Malloy, "Suicide and Assisting Suicide: A Critique of Legal Sanctions," *Southwestern Law Journal* 36 (Nov. 1982): 1003–37. For a general review of some of the philosophical issues raised by suicide, see M. Pabst Battin, *Ethical Issues in Suicide* (Englewood Cliffs, N.J.: Prentice-Hall, 1982) and M. Pabst Battin and David J. Mayo (eds.), *Suicide: The Philosophical Issues* (New York: St. Martin's Press, 1980).
115. 415 N.E.2d at 940 n.3, 434 N.Y.S.2d at 951 N.3 (citations omitted from the text).
116. Alaska Stat. § 11.41.120 (1978): Ariz. Rev. Stat. Ann. § 13-1103 (1978); Ark. Stat. Ann. § 41-1504 (1977); Calif. Penal Code § 401 (West 1970); Colo. Rev. Stat. § 18-3-104 (1978); Conn. Gen. Stat. § 53a-56 (1981); Del. Code Ann. tit. 11, § 645 (1979); Fla. Stat. Ann. § 782. 08 (West 1976); Hawaii Rev. Stat. § 701-702 (1976); Kans. Stat. Ann. § 21-3406 (1981); Commonwealth v. Hicks, 118 Ky. 637, 82 S.W. 265 (1904); Maine Rev. Stat. Ann. tit. 17-A, § 204 (1982); Commonwealth v. Mink, 123 Mass. 422 (1877); Minn. Stat. Ann. § 609.215 (West 1964); Miss. Code Ann. § 979-3-49 (1972); Mo. Ann. Stat. § 565.021 (Vernon 1979); Mont. Code Ann. § 45-5-105 (1981); Nebr. Rev. Stat. § 28-307 (1979); N.J. Stat. Ann. § 2C:11-6 (West 1981); N.Mex. Stat. Ann. § 30-2-4 (1978); N.Y. Penal Law § 120.30 (McKinney 1975); Blackburn v. State, 23 Ohio St. 146 (1872); Okla. Stat. Ann. tit. 21, § 813-818 (West 1958 & Supp. 1981–2); Oreg. Rev. Stat. § 163.125 (1981); 18 Pa. Cons. Stat. Ann. § 2505 (Purdon 1973); P.R. Laws Ann. tit. 33, § 1385 (1969); State v. Jones, 86 S.C. 17, 67 S.E. 160 (1910); S.Dak. Codified Laws Ann. § 22-16-37 (1979); Turner v. State, 119 Tenn. 663, 108 S.W. 1139 (1908); Tex. Penal Code Ann. § 22.08 (Vernon 1974); Wash. Rev. Code Ann. 9A.36.060 (1977); Wis. Stat. Ann. § 940.12 (West 1982). The list reflects the law circa 1981.

There is apparently no treatment of either suicide or assisting or aiding and abetting suicide in either statutory or case law in some states. These states could rely on the theory that assisting suicide is the same as acting as a principal to the crime of self-murder. See, e.g., McMahan v. State, 168 Ala. 70, 63 So. 89 (1910).

117. Sanders v. State, 54 Tex. Crim. 101, 105, 112 S.W. 68, 70 (1908).

118. The Texas Court of Criminal Appeals held that suicide had never been a crime in Texas and that aiding and abetting suicide also was not. The case involved a physician, Dr. Grace, who retired one evening, sleeping in one bed, his wife in the other, and his mistress on the floor between the two beds. The mistress, who was despondent, took her own life with a pistol that Dr. Grace had placed on a nightstand. Grace v. State, 44 Tex. Crim. 193, 69 S.W. 529 (1902). Dueling was first criminalized in Texas on Dec. 21, 1836. See Oliver C. Hartley, *A Digest of the Laws of Texas* (Philadelphia: Thomas, Cowperthwait, 1850), p. 288.

119. Common law did not generally excuse individuals from mayhem or murder on the basis of the defense of consent. See, for example, Matthew v. Ollerton (1693), Comberbach 218, where the court held that "if I licence a Man to beat me, such Licence is void . . . because 'tis against the Peace."

120. Joseph T. Mangan, "An Historical Analysis of the Principle of Double Effect," *Theological Studies* 10 (March 1949): 41–61. See also Richard McCormick, *Ambiguity in Moral Choice* (Milwaukee: Marquette University Press, 1973).

121. For a review of issues raised by the principle of double effect, see Richard McCormick and Paul Ramsey (eds.), *Doing Evil to Achieve Good* (Chicago: Loyola University Press, 1978).

122. Gerald Kelly, *Medico-Moral Problems* (St. Louis, Mo.: Catholic Hospital Association, 1958), p. 129.

The tradition required treatment only if there was hope of health (*si sit spes salutis*) or where hope of recovery appeared (*ubi spes affulget convalescendi*). Also, one was never required to engage in futile treatment (*nemo ad inutile tenetur*) or even treatment when it could only postpone death or briefly blunt the illness (*parum pro nihilo reputatur moraliter*). In addition, the very aversion to a form of treatment (*horror magnus*) could defeat the obligation to accept treatment by constituting an undue burden. It is worth noting that one Jesuit theologian determined in the 1940s that the maximum amount of money that even a rich individual was obliged to invest in his own treatment was two thousand dollars. Gerald Kelly, "The Duty of Using Artificial Means of Preserving Life," *Theological Studies* 11 (1950): 203–20.

One should note that similar constraints on the obligation to treat were recognised by Jewish scholars. One of the most interesting analyses comes from the Talmud account of the death of Judah the Prince. "Rabbi's handmaid ascended the roof and prayed: 'The immortals desire Rabbi [to join them] and the mortals desire Rabbi [to remain with them]; may it be the will [of God] that the mortals may overpower the immortals.' When, however, she saw how often he resorted to the privy, painfully taking off his tefillin and putting them on again, she prayed: 'May it be the will [of the Almighty] that the immortals may overpower the mortals.' As the Rabbis incessantly continued their prayers for [heavenly] mercy she took up a jar and threw it down from the roof to the ground. [For a moment] they ceased praying and the soul of Rabbi departed to its eternal rest." *Kethuboth* 104a (Soncino edition).

123. Kelly, *Medico-Moral Problems,* p. 130.

124. Ibid., p. 132.

125. Susanna E. Bedell and Thomas L. Delbanco, "Choices about Cardiopulmonary Resuscitation in the Hospital," *New England Journal of Medicine* 310 (April 26, 1984): 1089–93.
126. Ibid., p. 1091. See also Stuart J. Youngner et al., " 'Do Not Resuscitate' Orders: Incidence and Implications in a Medical Intensive Care Unit," *Journal of the American Medical Association* 253 (Jan. 4, 1985): 54–61.
127. Marcia Angell, "Respecting the Autonomy of Competent Patients," *New England Journal of Medicine* 310 (April 26, 1984): 1115–16; Sidney H. Wanzer et al., "The Physician's Responsibility toward Hopelessly Ill Patients," *New England Journal of Medicine* 310 (April 12, 1984): 955–9.
128. Bernard Lo and Laurie Dornbrand, "Guiding the Hand that Feeds," *New England Journal of Medicine* 311 (Aug. 9, 1984): 402–4.

The arguments in this volume support the general conclusion that there is nothing special about expediting death through the cessation of feeding or hydration. The morality of such decisions must be judged in terms of the principles of autonomy and beneficence, not in terms of some special obligation to feed or provide fluids. The law is now struggling with these issues.
129. Information on natural death acts and living wills is available in Society for the Right to Die, *Handbook of Enacted Laws* (New York: Society for the Right to Die, 1984). See also for a review of background issues, Alexander Capron, "Death and the Law: A Decade of Change," *Soundings* 63 (Fall 1980): 290–320.
130. Cal. Stat. Chapter 1439, Code § Health and Safety, §–§ 7185 through 7195 (Sept. 30, 1976).
131. For a review of durable power of attorney and natural death statutes up until March 1983, see President's Commission for the Study of Ethical Problems in Medicine and Biomedical and Behavioral Research, *Deciding to Forego Life-Sustaining Treatment*, pp. 318–437.
132. Legal Advisors Committee of Concern for Dying, "The Right to Refuse Treatment: A Model Act," *American Journal of Public Health* 73 (Aug. 1983), 918–21.
133. Eichner v. Dillon, 420 N.E. 2d 64 (N.Y. Ct. App. 1981).
134. Superintendent of Belchertown State School v. Saikewicz, Mass. 370 N.E. 2d 417 (1977).
135. Ernest Jones, *The Life and Work of Sigmund Freud* (New York: Basic Books, 1957), vol. 3, p. 246.
136. Ibid.
137. Ibid., pp. 144–5.
138. Percy W. Bridgman, "The Struggle for Intellectual Integrity," *Harpers Magazine* 168 (Dec. 1933): 18–25.
139. Gerald Holton, "Percy Williams Bridgman," *Bulletin of the Atomic Scientists* 18 (Feb. 1962): 23.
140. Ibid.
141. Seneca, *Stoic Philosophy of Seneca*, p. 202.
142. Ibid., pp. 204–5.
143. Tacitus records how Seneca committed suicide with his wife when faced with the alternative of suicide or an execution by Nero. "Then by one and the same stroke they sundered with the dagger the arteries of their arms. Seneca, as his aged frame attenuated by frugal diet, allowed the blood to escape but slowly, severed also the veins of his legs and knees. Worn out by cruel anguish, afraid too that his sufferings might break his wife's spirit, and that, as he looked on her

tortures he might himself sink into irresolution, he persuaded her to retire into another chamber. Even at the last moment his eloquence failed him not; he summoned his secretaries and dictated much to them which, as it has been published for all readers in his own words, I forbear to paraphrase." Moses Hadas (ed.), *The Complete Works of Tacitus* (New York: Random House, 1942), pp. 391–2.

144. David Hume, "Of Suicide," in T. H. Green and T. H. Grose (eds.), *Essays Moral, Political, and Literary* (London: Scientia Verlag Aalen, 1964), p. 414.
145. Immanuel Kant, *The Metaphysical Principles of Virtue: Part II of The Metaphysics of Morals*, trans. James Ellington (Indianapolis: Bobbs-Merrill, 1964), pp. 83–4; Akademie Textausgabe, vol. 6, 423–4.
146. "He who contemplates suicide should ask himself whether his action can be consistent with the idea of humanity *as an end in itself.* If he destroys himself in order to escape from painful circumstances, he uses a person merely as *a means* to maintain a tolerable condition up to the end of life." Kant, *Fundamental Principles of the Metaphysic of Morals*, in *Critique of Practical Reason and Other Works on the Theory of Ethics*, trans. Thomas K. Abbott. 6th ed. (London: Longmans, Green, 1909), p. 47; Akademie Textausgabe, vol. 4, p. 429.
147. Kant in fact argues that masturbation is a violation of one's duty to oneself, which is more heinous than suicide. *The Metaphysical Principles of Virtue*, Akademie Textausgabe, vol. 6, p. 425.
148. Ellington, p. 84; Akademie Textausgabe, vol. 6, p. 423.
149. David Hume, "Of Suicide," p. 413.
150. H. T. Engelhardt, Jr., and Michele Malloy, "Suicide and Assisting Suicide: A Critique of Legal Sanctions," esp. pp. 1022–7.
151. Norman Cantor, "A Patient's Decision to Decline Life-Saving Medical Treatment: Bodily Integrity Versus the Preservation of Life," *Rutgers Law Review* 26 (1973): 228–64.
152. Ludwig Edelstein, *The Hippocratic Oath: Text, Translation and Interpretation*, supp. no. 1 to *Bulletin of the History of Medicine* (Baltimore: Johns Hopkins University Press, 1943), pp. 10–15.
153. Suicide would appear still to be a crime in Alabama, Oregon, and South Carolina. See Southern Life & Health Ins. Co. v. Wynn, 29 Ala. App. 209, 194 So. 421 (1940); Wyckoff v. Mutual Life Ins. Co., 173 Or. 592, 147 P.2d 227 (1944); State v. Levell, 13 S.E. 319 (S.C. 1891).
154. Attempted suicide would seem still to be a crime in Illinois and Indiana. See Royal Circle v. Achterrach, 204 Ill. 549, 68 N.E. 492 (1903); and Wallace v. State, 232 Ind. 700, 116 N.E.2d 100 (1953). In New Jersey suicide, if not a misdemeanor, is at least against public policy. See State v. Carney, 69 N.J.L. 478, 55 A. 44, 45 (1903), and John F. Kennedy Memorial Hospital v. Heston, 58 N.J. 476, 279 A.2d 670, 672–673 (1971). For a general review of the legal issues raised by critically and terminally ill patients, see A. Edward Doudera and J. Douglas Peters (eds.), *Legal and Ethical Aspects of Treating Critically and Terminally Ill Patients* (Ann Arbor, Mich.: AUPHA Press, 1982).
155. Tex. Penal Code Ann. § 22.08 (Vernon 1974).
156. Uruguay Penal Code art. 37, at 367 n.74. Jo Thomas, "Dutch High Court Acts in 'Right to Die' Case," *New York Times* (Nov. 28, 1984), p. 4.
157. For a review of some of the issues concerning civil and criminal liability of physicians who aid and abet suicide, see H. T. Engelhardt, Jr., and Michele

Malloy, "Suicide and Assisting Suicide: A Critique of Legal Sanctions," pp. 1029–32.
158. The phrase *captain of the ship* was introduced in the context of medical malpractice in the case of McConnell v. Williams, 361 Pa. 355, 65 A.2d 243 (1959). This doctrine made nurses and others the borrowed servants of the physician performing surgery. As such, these other individuals were not regarded as independent agents or as employees of the hospital. The history of this doctrine, which is varied, does raise the question of the lines of responsibil·ity and authority in health care generally.
159. S. J. Eisendrath and Albert R. Jonsen, "The Living Will: Help or Hindrance?" *Journal of the American Medical Association* 249 (April 15, 1983): 2054–8.
160. A. M. Sadler, B. L. Sadler, and A. A. Bliss, *The Physician's Assistant—Today and Tomorrow* (New Haven, Conn.: Yale University Press, 1972).
161. For a comprehensive review of the lines of responsibility in health care, including the position of nurses, see George J. Agich (ed.), *Responsibility in Health Care*.

8

Rights to Health Care

A basic human right to the delivery of health care, even to the delivery of a decent minimum of health care, does not exist. The difficulty with talking of such rights should be apparent. It is difficult if not impossible both to respect the freedom of all and to achieve their long-range best interests. Rights to health care constitute claims against others for either their services or their goods. Unlike rights to forbearance, which require others to refrain from interfering, rights to beneficence require others to participate actively in a particular understanding of the good life. Rights to health care, unless they are derived from special contractual agreements, depend on the principle of beneficence rather than that of autonomy, and therefore may conflict with the decisions of individuals who may not wish to participate in realizing a particular system of health care. If the resources involved in the provision of health care are not fully communal, private owners of resources may rightly have other uses in mind for their property than public health care. As chapters 3 and 4 have already suggested, the principles of autonomy and beneficence that lie at the foundations of justice will spawn conflicts within any portrayal of a just allocation of health care resources.

The limits to justice as beneficence

These fundamental conflicts between respecting the freedom and achieving the best interests of persons are made worse by commitments to goals that, if

336

pursued without qualification, lead to even more elaborate tensions within any concrete vision of a just health care system. Consider the following four goals that are at loggerheads.

1. The provision of the best possible care for all
2. The provision of equal care for all
3. Freedom of choice on the part of health care provider and consumer
4. Containment of health care costs

One cannot provide the best possible health care for all and contain the cost of health care. One cannot provide equal health care for all and maintain freedom in the choice of health care provider and consumer. For that matter, one cannot maintain freedom in the choice of health care services while containing the costs of health care. One also may not be able to provide all with equal health care that is at the same time the very best care because of limits on the resources themselves. These tensions spring not only from a conflict between freedom and beneficence, but from competing views of what it means to pursue and achieve the good in health care (e.g., is it more important to provide equal care to all or the best possible care to the least well-off class?).

Reflections concerning the proper provision of health care have an ancient lineage. Plato in Book III of the *Republic* explores what resources ought to be devoted to health care. He concludes that the protracted treatment of chronic illnesses is boonless when medicine cannot restore an individual to his occupation and his duties. Such an individual should instead accept death.[1] The *Republic* endorses acute health care if it promises to restore individuals to a useful life, but very little if any chronic health care. Preventive health care would be provided in the form of gymnastics. Plato's reflections suggest the following general points: (1) limits should be set to the amount of resources invested in health care, (2) the resources invested in health care often do not secure a high quality of life for those treated, and (3) such investments often constitute a major drain on common resources with very little return. The notion of rights to health care for Plato was understood in terms of the goal of maintaining the republic, not in terms of individual rights to health services. Though Plato gives little place for free choice and sees the individual living in and through the polis, he recognizes a tension between an individual's desire to pursue life at all costs, even if that life is often of marginal quality, and the fact that there are numerous other goals besides health care in which one might better invest resources than in the marginal extension of life at minimal quality. Plato recognizes the quandary of infinite expectations and finite resources that characterizes the predicament of health care allocations. He also implicitly acknowledges the conflict between attempts to discover the proper pattern for the allocation of health care resources and the role of free choice in their allocation. He recognizes as well how private property may undermine societal efficiency as individuals attempt to extend their lives in a protracted struggle with death, as in the case of Herodicus, of whom Plato speaks with disapproval.[2] He anticipates in an embryonic fashion the conflict between claims that the proper pattern for allocating resources can be discovered and claims that the proper pattern is that created by the free choice of innumerable men and women. He sees the tension between individual and societal concerns.

In order to understand what amount of health care ought to be provided for the indigent and why, one will need to come to terms with these tensions and the moral confusions they engender. They must be surmounted in order to answer whether, for example, funds for liver and heart transplantation ought to be provided to those in need who cannot pay.[3] They must be overcome in order to answer whether one's duties to provide health care stop at national boundaries or reach out so as to oblige one to provide health care to those in need throughout the world. This chapter will explore the prospects for surmounting these difficulties, while recognizing the various limitations to the possibility of achieving the most beneficent pattern for the distribution of health care resources:

1. Individual rights to free choice, which will limit the authority of societies and states to appropriate the services of persons (e.g., there will be limits on the authority of societies to forbid particular forms of health care provider–patient relationships or to draft health care workers to provide services);
2. Private property, which will limit the authority of societies and states to appropriate and redistribute resources (e.g., there will be limits to the authority of the state to tax away private resources in order to provide medical care to preserve the health and save the life of needy indigents);
3. The limited authority of the state, which, being drawn from the society's free participants, is limited by the wishes of its participants (e.g., a society will need to have legitimately acquired resources in order to establish a communal health system). As chapter 4 has shown, these first three points spring from a weakening of the myth of the sovereign state;
4. Societal or communal free choice, which will direct the resources of a group to endeavors other groups may find frivolous or ill considered (e.g., a community may decide to invest its resources in a new sports stadium rather than a badly needed well-baby clinic);
5. The finitude of all resources, which will limit the capacities of both individuals and groups to pursue health care goals or the allocation of resources to health care (e.g., one will not be able to invest all available

resources in the maximum extension of life for all at all costs without draining resources from other major societal endeavors, if not theoretically consuming all available resources);

6. The limits of reason, which make it difficult to establish a particular allocation of resources as obligatory (e.g., is it more important to invest communal resources in programs that extend the lives of the young by treating pediatric leukemia, or to invest those resources in treating the pains of the elderly who have degenerative osteoarthritis?).

These limitations define attempts to frame an ideal system for allocating resources to health care.

Justice and inequality

Interests in justice as beneficence are sustained in part because of inequalities among persons. That some have so little while others have so much properly evokes moral concerns of beneficence to provide help for those in need. As the previous section as well as chapters 3 and 4 show, the moral authority to use force to set such inequalities aside is limited. These limitations are in part due to the fact that the resources one could use to aid those in need are often already owned by other people. One is forced to examine the very roots of inequality to determine whether such inequality and need constitute a claim against those in a position to aid.

The natural lottery

Natural lottery is used here to identify changes in individual fortune that are the result of natural forces, not the actions of persons. It is not used to identify the distribution of natural assets. The natural lottery contrasts with the social lottery, which is used here to identify changes in individual fortune that are not the result of natural forces but the actions of persons. The social lottery is not used to identify the distribution of social assets. The natural and social lotteries together determine the distribution of natural and social assets. The social lottery is termed a lottery, though it is the outcome of personal actions, because of the complex interplay of personal choices. They are both aptly termed lotteries because of the unpredictable character of their outcomes, which do not conform to an ideal pattern.

All individuals are exposed to the brutal vicissitudes of nature. Some are born healthy and by chance remain so for a long life, free of disease and major suffering. Others are born with serious congenital or genetic diseases, others contract serious crippling fatal illnesses early in life, and yet others are injured and maimed. These natural forces, insofar as they occur outside of human responsibility, can be termed the natural lottery. They bring individuals to good health or disease through no merit or fault of their own or others. Those who win the natural lottery will not be in need of medical care. They will live extraordinarily full lives and die painless and peaceful deaths. Those who lose the natural lottery will be in need of health care to blunt their sufferings and, where possible, to cure their diseases and to restore function. There will be a spectrum of losses, ranging from minor problems such as having bad teeth to major tragedies such as developing childhood leukemia, inheriting Huntington's chorea, or developing amyelotrophic lateral sclerosis.

These tragic outcomes, as the blind deliverances of nature, are acts of God for which no one is responsible (unless, that is, one wishes to impeach divine providence). The fact that individuals are injured by hurricanes, storms, and earthquakes is often simply no one's fault. Since no one is to blame, no one can be charged with the responsibility of making those whole who lose the natural lottery on the ground that they are accountable for the harm. One will need a special argument to show that the readers of this volume should submit to the forcible distribution of their resources in order to provide health care for the individuals injured. It may very well be unfeeling or unsympathetic not to provide such help, but it is another thing to show that one owes others such help in a way that would morally authorize state force to redistribute resources, as one would collect funds owed in a debt. The natural lottery creates inequalities and places individuals at disadvantage without creating a straightforward obligation on the part of others to aid those in need.

The social lottery

Individuals differ in their resources not simply because of outcomes of the natural lottery, but also due to the actions of others. Some deny themselves immediate pleasures in order to accumulate wealth or to leave inheritances to others. Through a complex web of love, affection, and mutual interest, individuals convey resources, one to another, so that those who are favored prosper, and those who are ignored languish. Some will grow wealthy and others will grow poor, not through anyone's maleficent actions or omissions, but simply because they were not favored by the love, friendship, collegiality, and associations through which fortunes develop and individuals prosper. In such cases there will be no fairness or unfairness, but simply good and bad fortune. In addition, some will be advantaged, disadvantaged, rich, poor, ill, diseased, deformed, or disabled because of the malevolent actions of others. Such will be unfair circumstances, which just and beneficent states should try to prevent and to rectify through retributive justice and forced restitution.

Insofar as the injured party has a claim against the injurer to be made whole, not against society, the outcome is unfortunate from the perspective of society's obligations to make the actual restitution. Restitution is owed by the injurer.

When individuals come to purchase health care, some who lose the natural lottery will be able in part at least to compensate for that loss through their winnings at the social lottery. They will be able to afford expensive health care needed to restore health and to regain function. On the other hand, those who lose in both the natural and the social lottery will be in need of health care and without the resources to acquire it.

The rich and the poor: differences in entitlements

If one owns property by virtue of just acquisition or just transfer, then one's title to that property will not be undercut by the needs of others. One will simply own it. On the other hand, if one owns property because such ownership is part of a system that ensures a beneficent distribution of goods (e.g., the greatest balance of benefits over harms for the greatest number, the greatest advantage for the least-well-off class), one's ownership will be affected by the needs of others. In chapter 4, we saw reasons why one should suspect that property is in part privately owned in a strong sense that cannot be undercut by the needs of others. In addition, it would appear that all have a general right to access to the fruits of the earth, if not the universe, which would constitute the basis for a form of taxation as rent in order to provide for fungible payments to individuals, whether or not they are in need. Finally, there are likely to be resources held in common by groups that will need to find reasonable and equitable means for their distribution. The first two forms of entitlements will exist independently of medical or other needs; the last form of entitlement, through the decision of a community, may be conditioned by need.

The existence of any amount of private resources is the basis of an inequality among persons. Insofar as one owns things, one will have a right to them, even if others are in need, and even if the taxation as rent on one's resources is far from excessive or onerous. The test of whether one should transfer one's goods to others will not be whether such a redistribution will prove onerous or excessive for the person subjected to the distribution, but whether the resources belong to that individual. Goal-oriented approaches to the just distribution of resources will need to be restricted to commonly produced and commonly owned goods. Therefore, one must qualify the conclusions of the President's Commission that suggest that excessive burdens should determine the amount of tax persons should pay to sustain an adequate level of health care for those in need.[4] One will need to face a more complicated moral world with three sources of goods for the support of health care.

Drawing the line between the unfortunate and the unfair

How one regards the moral significance of the natural and social lotteries and the moral force of private ownership will determine how one draws the line between circumstances that are simply unfortunate and those that are unfortunate and in addition unfair in the sense of constituting a claim on the resources of others. Life in general and health care in particular reveal circumstances of enormous tragedy, suffering, and deprivation. The pains of illness and disease and the despair of deformity call upon the sympathy of all to provide aid and give comfort. Injuries and diseases due to the unconsented-to actions of others are unfair. Injuries and diseases due to the forces of nature are unfortunate. As noted, unfortunate outcomes of the unfair actions of others are not necessarily society's fault. The horrible injuries that come every night to the emergency rooms of major hospitals may be someone's fault, even if they are not society's. Such outcomes, though unfair with regard to the relationship of the injured with the injurer, may be simply unfortunate with respect to society. One is thus faced with drawing the difficult line between acts of God and acts of malicious individuals that do not constitute a basis for societal retribution and injuries that provide such a basis. Such a line was drawn by Patricia Harris, the former secretary of the Department of Health, Education, and Welfare, when she ruled that heart transplantations should be considered experimental and therefore not reimbursable through Medicaid.[5] To be in need of a heart transplant and not have the funds available would be an unfortunate circumstance but not unfair. One was not eligible for a heart transplant even if another person had intentionally damaged one's heart. From a moral point of view, things could change if the federal government had in some culpable fashion injured one's heart. So, too, if promises of treatment had been made. For example, to suffer from appendicitis or pneumonia and not receive treatment reimbursable through Medicaid would be unfair, not simply unfortunate.

The line between the unfair and the unfortunate can be drawn because it is difficult if not impossible to translate all needs into claims against the resources of others. First it is hard to distinguish needs from mere desires. Is the request of an individual to have his life extended through a heart transplant at great cost and perhaps only for a few years a desire for an inordinate extension of life, or is it a need to be secure against a premature death? The difficulty of discovering such rankings has already been explored in chapters 2 and 3. Outside a particular view of the good life, needs do not create rights to the services or goods of others. Finally, there is a certain impracticality in seeing such circumstances as needs that generate claims. Attempts to restore health could indefinitely deplete societal resources in the pursuit of ever-more incremental extensions of life of marginal quality. A relatively limited amount of food and shelter is required to preserve the lives of individuals. But an indefinite amount of resources can be committed to the further preservation of human life. One is forced to draw a line between those needs that constitute claims on the aid of others and those that do not.

Beyond equality

The line between the unfortunate and the unfair justifies certain social and economic inequalities. In particular, it justifies inequalities in the distribution of health care resources that are the result of differences in justly acquired resources and privileges. To this one must add that the very notion of equal distribution of health care is itself problematic, a point recognized in *Securing Access to Health Care*, the report of the President's Commission.[6]

1. Though in theory at least one can envisage providing all with equal levels of decent shelter and nutrition, one cannot restore all to or preserve all in an equal state of health. Health needs cannot be satisfied in the same way in which one can address needs for food and shelter.
2. If one provided all with the same amount of funds to purchase health care or the same amount of services, the amount provided would be far too much for many and still insufficient for some who could have always used more investment in treatment and research in the attempt to restore them to a level of function that would ensure equal opportunity.
3. If one attempts to provide equal health care in the sense of allowing individuals to select health care only from a predetermined list of available therapy, which would be provided to all so as to prevent the rich from having access to better health care than the poor, one would have confiscated a portion of the private property of individuals and have restricted the freedom of individuals to join in voluntary relationships. That some are fortunate in having more resources is neither more nor less arbitrary or unfair than some having better health, better looks, or more talents. If significant restrictions were placed on the ability to purchase special treatment with one's resources, one would need not only to anticipate that a black market in health care services would inevitably develop, but also to acknowledge it as a special bastion of liberty and freedom of association. As chapters 3 and 4 have shown, there would be no moral authority to interfere in that market.

Living with inequalities and tragedy

The health care arts and sciences are undertakings of finite men and women with finite resources, living and practicing their professions under moral limitations that do not allow them to attempt all they would to achieve the good. All human undertakings are characterized by limitation. This is most painfully the case in medicine, which must live with and attempt to comfort, care for, and where possible cure the sufferings of helpless and innocent individuals. The natural and social lotteries, the existence of private entitlements, and the outcomes of free choice, both individually and communally, destine individuals to living lives of unequal scope and fulfilment. Up to a point, it will be proper to attempt to set these inequalities aside. There will be limits on what attempts are morally permissible. These limits will define where inequalities are not inequities, and where unfortunate outcomes are not unfair. There will still be the possibility of blunting many of the unfortunate outcomes of natural forces and social undertakings. As we will see, though we possess neither the insight nor the resources of gods and goddesses, we can still come to understand the lineaments of a just health care system.

From macroallocations to microallocations and back

Decisions about who should receive health care and in what amount must be made in terms of what funds are available for health care in general, and for specific forms of health care in particular. In addition, choices by particular health care professionals regarding who receives what level of care are made against a background of views about the proper patterning of such allocations. The different levels of health care choices interact systematically. Each level brings with it its own set of moral concerns and problems. Yet each level influences the other and shapes the character of its quandaries. Somewhat procrusteanly, these can be viewed as four levels of concerns.[7]

Higher-level macroallocational choices

One must determine what portion of total available resources should be given to health care. Even if one supports a general market solution for most problems of distribution, there still will be common funds in the hands of societies and states, which will be the subject of explicit allocational choices. One will need, for example, to decide what portion of a society's budget should be invested in defense, education, the construction of museums, in health care, and so on. Here the question will arise whether one can in general hold that health care expenditures have a more pressing claim on a society's attention and resources than, for example, the construction of museums. To some extent, one will be forced to make decisions globally, that is, in terms of general categories such as defense versus education versus health care, because it will be difficult for legislators and higher-level administrators to grasp in detail how the particular components of the defense, education, or health care budget strengthen the general importance of that budget category. However, it will always be best, insofar as it is possible, to analyze the components of each budget category.

Lower-level macroallocational choices

To appreciate adequately the importance of allocations to the category of health care, one will need to examine what is encompassed by that term. Health care, after all, includes not only the treatment of coronary artery disease, cancer, pneumonia, and tuberculosis, but arthritis, headaches, athlete's foot, and acne. Health care includes as well the psychiatric treatment of neuroses and the general support given by physicians to the worried well and vexed ill. It encompasses genetic counseling, the provision of contraceptives, and abortion. Cosmetic surgery to raise sagging breasts and buttocks and to make noses better conform to particular cultural aesthetic norms also falls within its purview. In order to decide which of these elements of health care are more or less worthy of urgent support, one must decide which count as true needs, and which are mere desires. In addition, one must fashion a hierarchy of needs and desires in order to rank coherently the claims made by different areas of health care for support. We have already seen in chapter 2 why it will be difficult to discover a single and univocal normative hierarchy that will determine how much of a communal budget should be allocated to the cure and treatment of pediatric leukemia versus cataracts of the elderly. Such a discovery would require an authoritative evaluative sense. If such a hierarchy cannot be discovered, one will need to determine how one is fairly to create such a hierarchy for a community's use.

The amount of funds one provides for any health care category will be determined by the legitimate demand for such care, whether or not the normative hierarchy is acquired by discovery or creation. That is, one will need to know how great the legitimate demand is for treatment of pediatric leukemia, pneumonia, acne, or sagging buttocks. One has to add *legitimate* to underscore that theories have been advanced regarding the proper ways in which one ought to select particular patients for particular forms of treatment[8] and with regard to what forms of treatment are truly medical.[9] In order to determine the proper allocations to particular areas of health care, one will need to understand how one determines that particular patients have a claim on a particular form of care. To determine the pattern of lower-level macroallocational distributions, one will have to decide on the proper pattern for microallocational decisions.

Higher-level microallocational choices

In deciding which patients should receive what form of treatment, one makes choices against background assumptions about the ways in which resources ought to be allocated to particular patients. Though the focus is on particular patients, they are seen through presumptions regarding the proper patterns within which such choices should be made. If the question is the provision of a liver transplant to a patient with liver failure, one will need to decide how one ought to select candidates for the procedure if there is an insufficient number of livers available for transplantation or insufficient funds to provide for the care of all. George Deukmejian, governor of California, ordered that a liver transplantation be paid for out of state funds for Koren Crosland, whereas friends and strangers raised $265,000 to cover the cost of a liver transplant for Amy Hardin of Cahokia, Illinois.[10] The action of Governor Deukmejian can be seen as a recognition of the state's obligation to provide lifesaving health care for those in need. The events in Illinois can be interpreted as the free actions of numerous men and women to provide care for an individual who, though in unfortunate circumstances, had no claim on state funds. In deciding how particular patients ought to be selected, one must determine whether such health care should be provided (1) equally to all in need (and, if resources are not sufficient, to those chosen by a lottery), (2) to all who can pay or who have friends and acquaintances who will pay for the treatment, (3) to those individuals who are most likely to return to a productive life and thus maximally benefit society, or (4) in terms of some other set of considerations, such as providing treatment to those who merit it through special services to society. The choice of a vision for proper microallocational decisions sets the stage but does not absolutely determine those decisions. One may still argue that in particular cases particular forms of exceptions should be allowed.

Lower-level microallocational choices

Charles Fried has argued that physicians and other health care providers should not be put in the place of making allocational decisions.[11] Government bureaucrats and other administrators may properly set limits to the availability of communal resources. It is their function to make both higher-level and lower-level macroallocations. Hospital administrators, for example, may decide what portion of the hospital budget will be allocated to particular hospital services. In addition, they may establish patterns for the allocation of resources for a particular service to particular kinds of patients. They may set the pattern for microallocations. In contrast, individual physicians and other health care professionals may properly see their role as securing the best care for their patients, even if the pursuit of such care conflicts with the ideal pattern for microallocations. Fried can be understood as holding that the tension between physicians and bureaucrats is wholesome. This tension is analogous to that between an attorney for the defense and an attorney for the prosecution. The counsel for the defense attempts to establish the defendant's innocence with all available energies, even if that attorney believes the defendant is in fact guilty, while the prosecutor attempts to establish the guilt of the defendant, even in the face of doubts regarding the guilt of the defendant. The Anglo-American adversary system of law presumes that this conflict of interests will optimally direct energies to the disclosure of the truth and the service of justice. So, too, one might hold that from the conflict between the hospital administration seeking to impose a particular efficient or just system of health care and the physician seeking to acquire for a patient the very best health care regardless of the system, there will develop the best balancing of forces needed to secure a health care system that is attentive to general goals of efficiency and social justice, while at the same time having concern for the particular interests of particular patients.

The more the ideal pattern or rule for microallocational choices functions as a rule of thumb, a guiding principle, or a regulative ideal, the more there will be a distance between higher-level microallocational choices regarding what pattern of choosing particular levels of treatment for particular patients is proper, and lower-level microallocational decisions about the proper level of treatment for a particular patient. As this distance increases, the lower-level microallocational choices will put pressures on the system, which may lead to recasting the rules of thumb, and consequently reshaping lower-level macroallocational choices, and then in the end revising the higher-level microallocational pattern. If, out of consideration for particular patients, physicians continually secure funds for expensive lifesaving treatment such as liver and heart transplant, this will force a reconsideration of the policies for macroallocational choices, given this de facto major focus in the investment of resources. In great measure this occurred in the case of liver transplantation. Individuals such as Charles and Marilyn Fiske, who secured payment for a liver transplantation for their daughter Jamie, influenced not only changes in rules for the selection of recipients (i.e., from only those who could pay to those in need), but occasioned congressional hearings regarding organ transplantation in general. In the end, microallocational choices raise the issue of rethinking macroallocational decisions.[12] There is, in short, a dialectic among these four levels through which one seeks a balancing of these levels of moral concern.

The British investment of 6.3 percent of their gross national product in the
National Health Service, versus the 10.5 percent expenditure of the United
States in the same year (1982), reflects in part the cost savings due to long
queues or waits for elective treatment in the United Kingdom and the
restriction on the provision of expensive therapeutic measures such as
coronary bypass surgery and hemodialysis.[13] The United Kingdom would
appear not to provide hemodialysis routinely for individuals in end-stage
renal failure over the age of fifty-five.[14] The smaller allocation of resources to
health care in the United Kingdom is thus tied to an acceptance of the
propriety of certain microallocational choices. On the other hand, recent
interest in the United Kingdom in the purchase of private medical insurance
(now covering one out of every fourteen Britons) is likely to lead to an
increase in the proportion of the gross national product devoted to medical
care.[15] If such interest were to continue to grow, and the number of private
beds were to increase, the proportion of resources devoted to health care in
the United Kingdom might indeed approach that of the United States.
Though the interplay among various forces in such cases is very complex,[16]
here it is enough to indicate that the notion of what will count as proper
microallocational choices is closely tied to what will count as proper
macroallocational choices, and vice versa. Each level influences the other,
whether directly or indirectly.

Such happens automatically if the pattern of distribution of resources is
controlled by the market. Free individuals, using their private property, trade
for the services of others and fashion patterns of allocation even without any
explicit choice of a pattern. In part, one must presume an element of all
allocations in health care will be determined in this fashion. Matters are
complicated as one turns to the communal support of health care. There one
is committed to establishing explicitly a pattern of allocation, as long as one
does not simply provide in-cash support. One is thus returned to the
fundamental issue of whether just patterns for the distribution of resources to
and in health care can be discovered or whether they must be created through
some form of common and fair negotiation or agreement. The issue of
whether one can know truly what a just pattern of health care distribution is,
or whether one must instead in some fair, and in that sense just, fashion
create a pattern of health care distribution, lies at the very heart of the
question of justice in heath care. One must decide to what extent justice in
health care distributions at the macro- and microlevels can be discovered and
the extent to which it is the product of a fair procedure of negotiation and
agreement among the individuals involved.

Conflicting models of justice

We will therefore turn to a comparison of two radically different understandings of what counts as justice in general and what should count as justice in health care in particular: justice as primarily procedural, a matter of fair negotiation, and justice as primarily structural, a pattern of distributions that is amenable to rational disclosure. As examples of these two contrasting approaches, John Rawls's *A Theory of Justice* and Robert Nozick's *Anarchy, State, and Utopia*, will be briefly examined.[17] Rawls presumes that there is an ahistorical way to discover the proper pattern for the distribution of resources, and therefore presumably for the distribution of health care resources. Moreover, he presumes that societally based entitlements are morally prior to privately based entitlements. Nozick, in contrast, provides a historical account of just distributions. Justice in patterns for the allocation of goods, including health care services, depends on what individual men and women have agreed to do with and for each other. Nozick holds that privately based entitlements are morally prior to societally based entitlements. In contrast with Rawls, who argues that one can discover a proper pattern for the allocation of societal resources, Nozick argues that such a pattern cannot be discovered and that instead one can only identify the characteristics of a just process for fashioning rights to health care.

Rawls is of interest to us because of this claim to be able to discover a proper pattern for distributing the primary social goods. Though he avoids the issues of allocating health care resources, his theory is often invoked in the discussion of the distribution of health care resources.[18] To appreciate Rawls, one might approach the problem of distributive justice through imagining how one might divide plots of land on an unowned island.[19] Let us imagine that some readers of this book are adrift in a powerless boat approaching an uninhabited and unowned island. Let us also imagine that all have an equal interest in owning land on the island. We might assign one individual the task of managing the distribution. That individual would need to survey the island and divide it equally. To ensure fairness, we might give to that individual the destiny of taking that parcel of land that no one else wanted, the last parcel after all other persons had selected a tract. That individual would wish to lay out tracts with great care, to ensure that each tract would be equal. Or if the tracts were unequal, the inequality would need to produce an advantage for the person receiving the tract, so that it would be as desirable as the rest. In this way we could establish a procedure for the just distribution of land on the island. The procedure would presuppose that we all had equal rights to the land and equal concerns not to be harmed by receiving a tract of land with a value less than the tracts received by others.

The procedure presumes as well that prior to the distribution the land is commonly owned. With these presumptions, self-interest combined with a veil of ignorance to prevent actions against the interests of others produces a just outcome in the sense that all secure their share.

Rawls has developed this procedure on a grand scale. He introduces it by asking us to imagine what would count as a just distribution of the primary social goods. In doing so, he presumes that the things in the world are not already owned. He presumes as well that all would want an equal distribution unless an unequal distribution would be to the advantage of the person receiving the smallest allocation. Rawls develops the conceptual machinery for this procedure around three key notions: (1) that there is a single, normative view of what should characterize a rational individual, namely, someone who is risk aversive and therefore unwilling to take the risk to be a member of an exploited class (e.g., as might occur in a utilitarian scheme, which would distribute the primary social goods so as to create the greatest good for the greatest number, but with the possibility of some harm to a small minority) but who also lacks envy and is therefore willing to accept unequal distributions if they redound to the benefit of the least-advantaged class in that society (i.e., thereby ensuring all who risk an unequal distribution against receiving less than they would have through an equal distribution); (2) that these rational contractors have certain interests expressed in a minimal or thin theory of the good that supports a lexical ordering of the primary social goods, which ranks liberty higher than the other primary social goods; and (3) that these rational contractors can be envisioned as deciding on their future circumstances in an original contracting position within which they are ignorant of circumstances that would otherwise bring them to be biased contractors, such as (a) their position in society, (b) their natural assets and abilities, (c) their conception of the good, including their rational plan of life, (d) special features of their psychology, (e) the particular circumstances of their society, and (f) the generation to which they belong.[20] By placing the distribution of natural assets and abilities behind the veil of ignorance, as well as one's position in society, which may result from the free choice of others, Rawls erases many of the usual lines between what is unfair and what is simply unfortunate. This is the basis of his seeing a moral obligation to compensate others for the unfortunate results of the natural lottery (i.e., the outcomes of natural forces) and the social lottery (i.e., the outcomes of the choices of individuals and society). If one does not yet know whether one will be favored by the natural or social lottery, and if all things are still unowned, one will wish to distribute resources so as to ensure against one's possible losses in either of these lotteries. Unfortunate outcomes therefore become unfair outcomes, outcomes that individuals in the original position would have seen as requiring compensation as an element of an acceptable social structure. In this fashion, one could presumably argue for health care insurance as a basic right.

In terms of these presuppositions John Rawls is able to fashion what he offers as his two principles of justice.

First Principle

Each person is to have an equal right to the most extensive total system of equal basic liberties compatible with a similar system of liberty for all.

Second Principle

Social and economic inequalities are to be arranged so that they are both:

(a)   to the greatest benefit of the least advantaged, consistent with the just savings principle, and

(b)   attached to offices and positions open to all under conditions of fair equality of opportunity.[21]

With respect to issues of health care, one will have to decide whether it is governed under the first or the second half of the second principle.

If the allocation of health care resources is like the allocation of other primary social goods, differences in allocation will be justifiable as long as these differences redound to the benefit of the least-well-off class. There will then be a problem of defining the least-well-off class with regard to either economic characteristics or economic plus health status characteristics.[22] If the allocation of health care resources is integral to assuring fair equality of opportunity, one will need to allocate funds for health care prior to allocations for other primary social goods such as income support or the achievement of an attractive standard of living. If this is the case, one will face the problem of the very ill and incapacitated draining a great deal of resources in the pursuit of only a modest gain in health status in order to achieve a modicum of greater equality of opportunity.

One must remember that Rawls is offering an ahistorical foundation for the allocation of resources, what one can term, following Nozick, an end-state view of distributive justice. It is just in aiming toward a particular condition, pattern, or end state that individuals would find acceptable as a condition for the distribution of commonly owned resources. Nozick, in contrast, gives a historical account. He assumes that (1) the condition for morality is mutual respect, and (2) people actually already own things prior to any particular society. Therefore, the principles of justice are those of just acquisition, just transfer, and retribution for past injustices in acquisition or transfer under the general formal principle of justice, "*From each as they choose, to each as they are chosen.*"[23] As a result, for Nozick the results of the natural and social lotteries are unfortunate, though not unfair, insofar as they have not been influenced by unjustified force, coercion, or overreaching. Unfortunate outcomes do not of themselves create obligations in justice. For Nozick, moral agents are not obliged out of considerations of fairness to attempt to blunt the consequences of the natural lottery through which some are born healthy and others with serious diseases. In addition, for Nozick the adverse outcomes of the social lottery, through which some are wealthy through gifts, inheritances, or the cooperation of others, and others impoverished, are also simply unfortunate if unjustified societal force, coercion, or overreaching has not been involved (individuals may have acted unfairly, for which compensation will be due from those individuals). That some do not have funds to pay for health care does not of itself create a societal obligation of redress.

This difference between Nozick and Rawls derives as well from their different theories of entitlements and ownership. For Rawls, one has a justifiable title to goods if such a title is part of a system that ensures the greatest benefit to the least advantaged, consistent with a just savings principle, and with offices and positions open to all under conditions of fair equality and opportunity, and where each person is to have an equal right to the most extensive total system of equal basic liberties compatible with a similar system of liberty for all. In contrast, for Nozick, one simply owns things: "Things come into the world already attached to people having entitlements over them."[24] If one really owns things, there will be freedom-based limitations on principles of distributive justice. The needs of others will not erase one's ownership in one's property. The readers of this book should consider that they may be wearing wedding rings or other jewelry not essential to their lives, which they could sell in order to give money to Mother Teresa to buy antibiotics that would save identifiable lives in Calcutta. Those who keep such baubles may in part be acting in agreement with Nozick's account and claiming that "it is my right to keep my wedding ring for myself, even though the sale of it could save the lives of individuals in dire need."

Nozick's account requires a distinction between someone's rights and what is right to do. At times, selling some of one's property in order to support the health care of those in need will be the right thing to do, even though one has a right to refuse to sell. This contrast derives from the distinction Nozick makes between *freedom as a side constraint*, as the very condition for the possibility of a moral community, and *freedom as one value among others*. The contrast leads to a distinction between those claims of justice, which are based on the very possibility of a moral community, and those claims of justice that turn on interests in particular goods and values. For Nozick, one cannot do things to innocent free persons without their consent, even if that intervention will save the lives of others by providing needed health care or preserve their liberty by securing equality of opportunity—even if such would be a good thing to do (and in this sense the right thing to do). Because for Nozick one needs the *actual* consent of *actual* persons in order to respect them as free persons, their rights can morally foreclose the pursuit of many morally worthy goals. In contrast, Rawls treats freedom only as a value. As a consequence, in developing just institutions, Rawls does not require them to have the actual consent of all those involved with the consequence that claims to self-determination can be limited by important social goals.

In summary, the difference between Rawls's and Nozick's accounts in great measure derives from the fact that Rawls's theory of justice turns on an invitation to imagine what it would be like to sketch the principles of justice as fairness, so that no matter what class one is born into, one would not have grounds for saying that one's position as a result of being a member of that class was not rationally unacceptable. Nozick challenges why one should assume such a viewpoint, if indeed people actually own things. His retort is that a position such as Rawls would deliver principles of distributive justice that rational individuals should take to be normative at best, only if people do not already own things privately. However, people do already own things privately, as Nozick and this book in chapter 4 have argued. Freedom is not simply one value among others, but respect of self-determination is, to put Nozick in the somewhat Kantian terms of chapters 2 and 3, the condition for the possibility of a moral community. As a consequence, even if a just distribution could be effected in Rawls's sense, free individuals would be at liberty to decide through their own free transactions to erase that state of affairs.

This contrast between Rawls and Nozick can be appreciated more generally as a contrast between two quite different principles of justice, each of which would have remarkably different implications for the allocation of health care resources.

1. Freedom-based justice is concerned with those distributions of goods made in accord with the notion of the moral community as a peaceable community. It will therefore require the consent of the individuals involved in a historical, cultural nexus of justice-regarding institutions in conformity with the principle of autonomy. The principle of beneficence is pursued within constraints set by the principle of autonomy.

2. Goals-based justice is concerned with the achievement of the good of individuals in society, and where the pursuit of beneficence is not constrained by a strong principle of autonomy. Such justice will vary as one attempts to (a) give each person an equal share; (b) give each person what that person needs; (c) give each person a distribution as a part of a system designed to achieve the greatest balance of benefits over harms for the greatest number of persons; and (d) give each person a distribution as a part of a system designed to maximize the advantage of the least-well-off class within conditions of equal liberty for all and of fair opportunity.

Allocations of health care in accord with freedom-based justice will occur within major constraints to respect the free wishes of persons and their property rights. Allocations of health care in accord with goals-based justice will need to indicate what it means to provide a just pattern of health care, and what constitutes true needs, not mere desires, and how to rank the various health goals among themselves in comparison with nonhealth goals. Such approaches to justice in health care will require a way of ahistorically discovering the proper pattern for the distribution of resources.

Freedom-based and goals-based approaches to justice in health care contrast because they offer competing interpretations of Justinian's maxim, "Justitia est constans et perpetua voluntas jus suum cuique tribuens" (Justice is the constant and perpetual will to render everyone his due).[25] A freedom-based approach holds that justice is first and foremost giving to each the right to be respected as a free individual in the disposition of personal services and private goods: that is, what is due (*jus*) each individual. In contrast, a goals-based approach holds that justice is receiving a share of the goods, which is fair by an appeal to a set of ahistorical criteria specifying what a fair share should be, that is, what is due to each individual. Since there are likely to be various senses of a fair share of what is just (e.g., an equal share, a share in accordance with the system that maximizes the balance of benefits over harms), there will be various competing senses of justice in health care under the rubric of goals-based justice.

Health care systems

One's view of justice in health care will determine what system of delivery of health care will be acceptable. One's understanding of justice will indicate how one is to strike a balance among the four goals of a health care system mentioned in the first section of this chapter:

1. The provision of the best possible care for all
2. The provision of equal care for all
3. Freedom of choice on the part of health care provider and consumer
4. Containment of health care costs

The more one endorses a freedom-based view of justice, the more one will be committed to support freedom in the choice of health care provider, consumer, and services. The more one endorses a goals-based view of justice, the more one will be committed to achieving such goals as the best care for all.

Commitment to a freedom-based view of justice will set limits to the goals usually sought through a health care system. Health care systems are fashioned by societies to blunt the outcomes of the blind forces of nature through the rational planning of human beneficence. They are attempts to insure against losses in the natural lottery. They are social constructs established to relieve individuals of some of the anxieties associated with fear of disease, death, and deformity.[26] They are one of many human attempts to render nature congenial to persons. In addition, they are responses to the social lottery, for they function to blunt the uncaring choices by others, who will not respond with sympathy to those in need. Health care systems function as a societally fashioned web of caring, support, and aid.

In order to underscore the roles played by societal versus individual choice, one can classify systems of health care under three rubrics: (1) those that rely on the market alone and provide no special social safety net for those who lose in the natural and social lotteries; (2) those that attempt to provide an equal level of health care for all; and (3) those that allow for two tiers of health care, one provided through a social safety net, which affords all a decent minimum of health care, and a second tier that can be purchased by private resources and that encompasses care not included in the first tier. Each of these three general modes of health care distribution, as we shall see, can be grounded in more than one account of justice in health care.

Key terms will have different meanings in each of these three general systems. For example, *access to health care* in a free market system will mean only that individuals who wish to participate in the market will not be obstructed. A right of access to health care has only a negative meaning in this context. It indicates an obligation of forbearance, not of beneficence, on the part of others. No one is obliged to provide either services or resources. Any further sense of access to health care will depend on the charitable vision of the particular society that offers care to those in need and unable to pay. In contrast, systems attempting to provide equal care for all or a decent minimum of health care for all will construe access to health care in a positive sense, as an entitlement to particular services, given particular needs. In such systems, the notion of health care delivery takes on a new force, in that private or governmental insurance programs create (or discover?) entitlements to health care, which should then be efficiently delivered. Efficiency will mean not only cost effectiveness but also presumably responsiveness to patient needs, leading to the task of ranking patient needs. The right of access to health care when it takes on such a positive meaning is tied to positive obligations on the part of society or others to provide services and resources. Through the redistribution of resources such systems attempt to erase or ameliorate the cash barrier between those in need of health care (or who desire health care) and health care providers.[27]

Free market distribution of health care

In a market distribution of health care, only those who can afford health care or who are the objects of charity receive treatment. This general approach prevailed in much of early nineteenth-century America.[28] Though there was some support on the county and state level for the care of the indigent, the major burden of care for those who lost in the natural and social lotteries was borne by philanthropic individuals and institutions. Most health care was provided on the basis of a fee for service, and the existence of charitable institutions did not set aside the free choices of providers who received fees for care and patients who paid for care. Such charitable and fee-for-service care were in accord with Nozick's maxim, "*From each as they choose, to each as they are chosen.*"[29]

This approach to health care need not be justified on a libertarian or Nozickian basis. One might imagine a utilitarian or Rawlsian arguing that the efficiency of the market, when combined with charity, will secure the greatest good for the greatest number, or the greatest advantage for the least-well-off class. One would thus find a proponent of a goals-based account of justice in health care agreeing with the market distribution, not because the market essentially possessed especially endorsable moral properties, but because in empirical and contingent fact the market achieves the goals sought.

Many will suppose that the outcomes of the market and of charity will not be sufficient and will wish to provide at least a modest social safety net for certain severe losses in the natural and social lotteries. Still, given the arguments in chapters 2 and 3, this need not be the case. One could imagine individuals deciding that it would be best to avoid all formal systems of health care, as do the BaMbuti of Zaire discussed in chapter 6. They may value the opportunity to live their traditional way of life in the tropical rain forest undisturbed by modern science and technology more highly than the promise of protection against the outcomes of the natural and the social lotteries through participation in a health care system. But most will not. Most societies will make some provision for a formal system of health care, which includes at least the charitable underwriting of some modern health care services for those in need. In order to determine how much health care to provide, one will need to confront the issues raised in macroallocational decisions. One will need to decide in general how important health care is in relation to other undertakings. To make that judgment, one will need to decide which elements of health care are more important and in what order. One may in addition be committed to distinguishing between true needs and mere desires. Such explicit macroallocational choices are in great measure avoided by the market approach. The market approach avoids drawing the philosophical distinction between needs and desires. Each person can create a ranking of needs and desires in deciding what to purchase or not to purchase. The pattern of macroallocations will then be determined through innumerable free choices by individual men and women. The only exception will be charitable gifts to support health care for the indigent that do not come with explicit instructions for their use. The institutions receiving such gifts will need to make lower-level macroallocational choices regarding their use.

In summary, a market approach maximizes free choice in the sense of minimizing interventions in the free associations of individuals and in the disposition of private property. In not intervening, it allows individuals to choose as they wish and as they are able what they hold to be best for their health care. It makes no pretense at cost containment. Health care will cost as much and will receive as much commitment of resources as individuals choose. The percentage of the gross national product devoted to health care will rise to a level determined by the free choices of health care providers and consumers. If some element of health care becomes too expensive or not worth as much as a competing possible expenditure, individuals will engage in cost containment through not purchasing such health care, and its price will tend to fall. Finally, there will be no attempt to achieve equality, though there will be considerable room for sympathy and for the loving care of those in need. A free market economy, through maximizing the freedom of those willing and able to participate, may create more resources than any other system and thus in the long run best advantage those most harmed through the natural lottery. By creating a larger middle class, the market may tend to create greater equality at a higher standard of living and of health care than would alternative systems. Further, charity can at least blunt severe losses at the natural and social lotteries.

Whether one accepts a free market approach will depend on one's moral views regarding (1) the rights of individuals to create free associations, as occur in the market with physician–patient contracts; (2) the moral significance of the natural and social lotteries; and (3) the character and scope of private and communal ownership, as well as one's understanding of (4) the factual circumstances, that is, if and to what extent the market is in the long run the best provider of a high standard of living and of health care. If one holds that individuals and society have an obligation to provide a certain level of health care, which conforms to a particular pattern of distribution not achievable through the market and that the obligation overrides rights to free choice and the use of one's property, one will need to abandon market mechanisms either in whole or in part.

Equal health care for all

Many find it abhorrent that the rich should be able to purchase health care not available to the poor. Robert Evans, in defending the Canadian government's monopolization of health care insurance so as to provide an encompassing health care system for all, remarks, "The idea that one person's life and limb is more valuable than another's, more worth saving on the basis of his/her ability to pay, comes rather close to denying a fundamental 'cherished illusion' of equality which underlies our political and judicial system."[30] If one regards this abhorrence as having the moral significance of creating (or acknowledging) an obligation to avoid such conditions, one will have committed oneself to a health system that aims at equal care for all. Such a commitment to equality in care is not necessarily an element of all goals-based theories of justice. A utilitarian, for instance, would not endorse such an approach unless it in fact led to the greatest balance of benefits over harms for the greatest number. If permitting the rich to purchase care not available to the poor allows for the initial introduction and development of new health care technologies, which would otherwise not be undertaken or developed as quickly, and which when fully developed are at a price that allows for wide use, then a utilitarian may need to endorse such a trickle-down approach to medical technologies.[31] So, too, depending on how one applied Rawls, one could have a Rawlsian approach to health care distribution that allowed inequalities as long as these in fact either secured conditions of fair equality of opportunity or redounded to the greatest advantage of the least-well-off class.

The same genre of arguments, depending on the factual assumptions, can support an egalitarian system of health care. As an example, one might take Peter Singer's utilitarian argument that the only way to secure the best health care for the greatest number is to make sure that all, including the upper socioeconomic classes, participate in the general health care system. Only then, so arguments such as Singer's contend, will the privileged classes have a lively interest in achieving and preserving the highest quality of health care in the general health care system.[32] Others might argue within Rawlsian moral assumptions and on the basis of empirical findings that anything less than an all-encompassing health care system will undercut the conditions of equal opportunity required for Rawlsian fairness. One will then need to determine how encompassing an egalitarian system must be. Should it embrace all health care, including psychoanalysis and cosmetic surgery, or only health care that offers a significant extension of life, or the prevention or treatment of serious physical and mental diseases? One must then decide how to discover or agree on what will count as a *significant* extension of life or a *serious* physical or mental disease.[33]

The attempt to secure equality in health care faces the difficulties we have already seen with regard to the definition of equality. The most feasible interpretation will likely be the provision of health care only from a list of services underwritten through some national health care system and supplied to all. One would need to forbid individuals to contract with physicians for services outside the communal health care system. Such an approach to health care would presume that the interest in providing *equal* health care is sufficiently compelling as to override rights of free association and of the free disposition of private property. Where as a matter of fact such an egalitarian system would not provide the same minimal level of health care for all as would a free market system or a two-tiered system of health care, one would need to show that such a commitment to equality in principle is more important than the quality of health care itself. That is, one would need to show why it would be morally obligatory to have equality even at the price of the greatest number (or the least advantaged) receiving inferior care.

Such an approach to health care requires suppressing: (1) the drive to purchase additional or better health care for oneself and one's loved ones, and (2) the interest of health care providers in providing additional services or working harder if paid more. Such suppression can be only partially successful, and only at a price. This difficulty can be better appreciated if one considers systems of health care that at least in principle are committed to providing health care to all in need. One might consider as an example the Soviet Union, which, like the United States, encompasses a large territory with diverse ethnic populations. There is evidence that the Soviet health care system, though undirected by the open and explicit concerns for profit (one might even occasionally say greed) that move the American health care system, is encumbered by systemic inefficiency. Though officially dedicated to high-minded humanitarian goals, the system fails to function as well as those health care systems that provide at least some openly acknowledged place for private gain (and the privileges of private property).[34]

Not only does it become difficult to motivate efficient action in an egalitarian system, but corruption of the system produces a clandestine privileged tier. It would appear to be quite difficult, if not impossible, to create an egalitarian health care system. Those with political power and privilege will tend to be able directly or indirectly to acquire better health care for themselves and their families. When the law prohibits the satisfaction of any strong, important set of human concerns and desires, a black market inevitably develops. For this reason it is difficult to identify truly egalitarian systems anywhere in the world. Even in the People's Republic of China, the quality of health care may differ from commune to commune, depending on how much each commune invests in its own health care. In addition, private individuals can accumulate savings, which they may invest in special health care available elsewhere. In the Soviet Union, at least unofficially, health care is provided after hours on a fee-for-service basis. A significant proportion of health care in Poland is provided through private transactions.[35] Whether one sees such black markets as brave testimonies to the dedication of individuals to their personal liberties or as a moral weakness blocking the realization of important moral goods (it should be clear to the reader that this author sides with the former, not the latter, interpretation), the existence of such markets is a problem for all egalitarian undertakings.

In summary, the extent to which one judges that an egalitarian approach meets the four desiderata of a health care system will depend on one's view of individual rights and the character of the good life. The achievement of an egalitarian health care system can be purchased only at the price of dramatically curtailing individual rights to free association and the use of private property. There may in addition be costs to the vitality of the system as one attempts to suppress drives for profit and the incentives tied to success in accumulating privately owned goods. On the other hand, an egalitarianly oriented system can contain costs by restricting the kinds of treatment available to individuals seeking care. Whether the treatment received is the best will depend on how important equal treatment is for the ideal of best care and on one's judgments regarding the importance of the market for creating wealth. If one is egalitarian in principle, the second condition will be superfluous. One would be committed to pursuing equal health care, even if an egalitarian system does not provide the best of health care (i.e., in terms of morbidity and mortality statistics) for the greatest number or for the least-well-off class. Equality would function as an overriding moral ideal.

Even if the difficulties with an egalitarian system defeat its moral and economic feasibility, the system provides an example of an encompassing attempt to structure health care allocations according to a pattern that is independent of the individual choices of men and women and that contrasts sharply with free market distributions. Ideally, one would wish to combine in one system both respect for the free choices of providers and receivers of care and that element of the egalitarian approach that secures protection for the unfortunate.

Two classes of health care

It is better to harness human passions than to suppress them. This is one of the features of Rawls's theory of justice: it does not deny a place for greed, for acquisitiveness, for a desire to acquire more property than others. It offers rather a scheme for harnessing that passion within a taxation system that will distribute as much of those goods as possible to the least-well-off class without discouraging those who produce resources (as long as all of this

occurs within conditions of fair opportunity and of equal basic liberties).
Egalitarian schemes share a difficulty with all austere attempts to secure
virtue, which aspire to suppress fundamental human drives and needs. One
might think of the medieval ideal of purity in love, which led to the
condemnation of sexual intercourse for pleasure even in marriage.[36] Such
condemnations surely did not succeed in eradicating concupiscence,[37] though
they did undoubtedly lead to special burdens of guilt.[38] So, too, as we have
noted, an egalitarian system must suppress the normal human inclination
to devote one's private resources to the purchase of the best care for
those whom one loves. This desire to have more than equal treatment for
oneself or those one loves is made into a vice in an egalitarian system. A
two-tiered system allows for expression of such desires for individual love
and private gain, while supporting a general social sympathy for those in
need.

A two-tiered system of health care is in many respects a compromise. On
the one hand, it provides at least some amount of health care for all, while on
the other hand allowing those with resources to purchase additional health
care. It can endorse the provision of communal resources for the provision of
a decent minimal amount of health care for all, while acknowledging the
existence of private resources at the disposal of some individuals to purchase
better care. This compromise character of a two-tiered system can find a
number of justifications. The utilitarian may in fact find that this approach
maximizes the greatest good for the greatest number because it is a
compromise. In allowing free choice while providing some health care for all,
the system supports two important human goals and sources of satisfaction
(i.e., liberty and well-being). A two-tiered system can also be justified in
Rawlsian terms insofar as health care is to be treated under the difference
principle, that is, to the extent it is to be regarded as justly distributed if the
distribution redounds to the benefit of the least-well-off class. One would
then allow that amount of additional health care to be purchased by the
affluent, which would maximize the quality of care for the least-well-off, or
the general status of the least-well-off class.

This volume's analyses of the principles of autonomy and beneficence and
of entitlements to property support a two-tiered system of health care. Not
all property is privately owned. Nations and other social organizations may
invest their common resources in insuring their members against losses in the
natural and social lotteries. On the other hand, as we have seen in chapter 4,
not all property is communal. There are private entitlements, which individuals may freely exchange for the services of others. The existence of a two-
tiered system (whether officially or unofficially) in nearly all nations and
societies reflects the existence of both communal and private entitlements, of
social choice and individual aspiration. A two-tiered system with inequality

in health care distribution would appear to be both morally and factually inevitable.

The serious task will be to decide how to create a decent minimum as a floor of support for all members of a society, while allowing money and free choice to fashion a special tier of services for the advantaged members of society. The problem will be to define what will be meant by a "decent minimum" or "minimum adequate amount" of health care. In addressing this general issue, the President's Commission suggested that in great measure the answer to such questions must be created rather than discovered by democratic processes, as well as by the forces of the market. "In a democracy, the appropriate values to be assigned to the consequences of policies must ultimately be determined by people expressing their values through social and political processes as well as in the marketplace."[39] The commission, however, also suggested that the concept of adequacy could in part be discovered by an appeal to that amount of care that would meet the standards of sound medical practice. "Adequacy does require that everyone receive care that meets standards of sound medical practice."[40] What one will mean by "sound medical practice" will itself be dependent on a particular culture and its societal choices. Criteria for sound medical practice are as much created as discovered.

Indeed, the arguments in chapters 2 and 5 lead to the conclusion that the concept of adequate care will not be discoverable outside of an appeal to a particular view of the good life and a particular understanding of the charge of medicine. In general, smaller social groups, insofar as they share a common view of the good life, may be able to appeal to such a vision in order to discover what should count as a decent minimum of health care within that understanding. In nations encompassing numerous communities, an understanding of what one will mean by adequate level of health care or a decent minimum will need to be created through open discussion and fair negotiation. In some communities such as the BaMbuti, there may be little commitment of resources to the endeavors of modern health care. For such communities, a decent level of such care will be no care at all. In nations such as the United Kingdom, the decent minimum of care may not include hemodialysis for individuals over the age of fifty-five or coronary bypass surgery for any but the most promising candidates for surgical treatment (or at least there are informal ways of discouraging such treatment). For many, such a minimal level of investment may not count as a decent level. But one must remember that one creates through negotiation an amount of health care that becomes de facto the decent amount for the community as a whole, though it always remains open to further critique, discussion, and alteration. In deciding what proportion of communal resources to invest in health care in general, and in specific forms of health care in particular, one may be compelled to fashion more or less stringent regulations for higher-level microallocational choices (e.g., determining whether or not fifty-six-year-old individuals with end-stage renal failure will receive hemodialysis through a national health care system). On the other hand, in deciding whether to provide hemodialysis or kidney transplantation for individuals over fifty-five through communal funds, one will be deciding what kinds of macroallocational choices will be acceptable.

In choosing the compass and character of the tier of health care provided for all out of communal resources, one will be deciding regarding the character of one's nation and society. In eschewing health care and in holding to their traditional way of life, the BaMbuti affirm their age-old values. They hold them to be more important than those protections against the losses in the natural lottery that could be provided by some form of communal health care insurance. So, too, the British, in investing less of their gross national product in health care than the Americans, the Germans, or the Scandinavians, make a choice among competing views of the good life. One will not be able to hide from this choice by pretending that the answer can be discovered. Though men and women do not have the resources of the gods and goddesses, like gods and goddesses they must participate in fashioning the web of values that will give character to their lives and to the life of their community.

If one measures a two-tiered system against the four desiderata for health care systems, such an approach substitutes a notion of minimal health care for the goal of equal health care. In a two-tiered system the goal of equal care for all with the very best of care for all will still be approachable only insofar as there are very ample communal resources and the will to invest them in health care, so as to make the minimum provided for all nearly approximate the character of health care purchasable by the affluent. In a two-tiered system the goal will only be approachable. A two-tiered system supports free choice in two ways. First, it defends individual providers and consumers against attempts to interfere in their free association and their use of private resources. Second, it includes a positive right of access to health care for individuals who have not been advantaged by the social lottery, not just a negative right of unobstructed access to the marketplace, insofar as a general insurance policy against losses at the natural and social lotteries is provided. The extent to which the insurance policy will allow choice of provider and services on the part of the insured will depend upon a society's vision of the good life and the extent of its communal resources. Such consumer choice within the minimal level of care will be achievable only insofar as there are ample communal resources and the will to invest them in health care. A two-tiered approach will not exclude charitable contributions to schemes to upgrade the care of those covered through a communal insurance program.

   Morally allowable opportunities for cost containment will exist primarily
in that tier of health care provided through communal resources. To place
restrictions on all payers, including individuals and private insurance carriers
with regard to the mode and extent to which they may reimburse for health
care services, is likely to constitute an unjustified interference in private
choices and in the use of private resources. To put this somewhat bluntly, an
all-payers prospective reimbursement system will not be morally justifiable
unless it is grounded in prior agreements by private payers.[41] It is difficult if
not impossible to imagine the circumstances in which all private payers
would have freely agreed to such a state of affairs. The same can be said with
regard to attempts such as that by the Canadian federal and provincial
governments to monopolize nearly all health care insurance, restricting the
opportunity for special levels of coverage and extra billing.[42] Though such
approaches may have contributed to controlling Canadian health care costs
(the percentage of the Canadian GNP invested in health care was 7.6 percent
in 1980, when the U.S. investment was 9.5 percent and that of the West
Germans was 9.4 percent), they did so by restricting the free market rights of
individuals and groups in Canada. In contrast, the West Germans, with less
success at cost containment, provided greater freedom, while effectively
insuring 99.8 percent of the population and paying for 92 percent of all
health care expenditures through third-party coverage.[43]
   A two-tiered system that would come to terms with the various justifiable
moral claims on it must thus be complex. However, there are rarely simple
answers in a complex world of conflicting rights and visions of the good life,
or in an approach that is a compromise among moral goals at tension. One
must acknowledge inequalities one does not have the moral authority to
overcome, while attempting to blunt the unfortunate outcomes of the social
and natural lotteries. It is peculiar that many who believe it is a good to sell
one's property and give the proceeds to the poor are not satisfied with being
charitable themselves unless they can use state force to constrain all others to
do likewise. One must pursue beneficence within the restraints of respect for
persons and be content with doing good to those in need even when one
cannot convince others to join in those endeavors. One must attempt, as far
as is possible, both to respect the freedom of individuals and to pursue their
good. Instead of a unified system, one will have a system with a mixed
justification: (1) a free market tier, justified in terms of the respect of free
choices and of private property, and (2) a tier supported by communal funds,
justified in terms of some vision of the good life and of beneficent action. The
difference between these two tiers will mean that in the future, as in the past,
some expensive lifesaving treatment may not be available to all because goals
other than health care may have been given greater priority. Moreover,

under nearly all circumstances, the rich will be able to circumvent shortages by seeking out providers who will supply the special care they seek. These reflections leave us with a justification for a system not far different from the one currently in place in the United States.

Is the allocation of organs special?

Up until now we have considered the allocation of the time and services of health care professionals and the resources of individuals, communities, and societies. Is the allocation of organs for transplantation in principle different from the allocation of time, services, or money? May societies with moral justification allocate organs to those in need or forbid individuals from selling their organs? In his criticism of Rawls's *Theory of Justice*, Robert Nozick tests his readers' intuitions about a society's right to distribute resources in general by asking whether a society may distribute organs.[44] One might imagine someone arguing that individuals in the original position would have agreed to the distribution of the second of a paired organ to those in need, if the surgical intervention carried only minimal risks, in order to protect themselves, should they be members of the least advantaged class with respect to functioning organs. Those who would question that removing a kidney was especially inhumane would likely receive the retort, which is more painful, having a kidney removed or being taxed? Which is more important for equal opportunity, minimal health or minimal economic resources?

Private property rights preclude a whole range of forced reallocations of resources, including organs. However, if one's organs are really one's own, may one not only keep them but sell them as well? The answer would appear to be in the affirmative. Though particular interpretations of the principle of beneficence and certain factual assumptions concerning the ways in which individuals can be exploited may support the notion that the sale of organs will lead to morally undesirable outcomes, the general freedoms of association and of the use of private resources should morally protect such practices, even if they are contrary to the general assumptions of Western mores. One might think here of the Roman Catholic view that one has a duty to God regarding oneself not to alter one's body except to preserve health as giving a basis for condemning such sales.[45] As was noted in chapter 7, this religious understanding of the prohibition finds a secular articulation in the writings of no one less than Kant, who argued that not only the sale but in fact the gift of part of one's body to another is morally forbidden.[46] However, such viewpoints require special theological premises, the existence of duties to oneself, or a duty of beneficence to override duties of mutual respect. None of these, as we have seen, has a sufficient standing in a general secular moral argument to override duties of mutual respect. Since selling oneself freely to another does not involve a violation of the principle of autonomy, such transactions should fall within the protected privacy of free individuals on the basis of the principle of autonomy. In addition, if one sells oneself at the right price and under the proper circumstances, one would suspect that one could maximize one's balance of benefits over harms. But the point in principle is that free individuals should be able to dispose of themselves freely.[47]

A sufficient supply of organs for transplantation can be acquired through a commitment on the part of numerous free men and women to make their organs available at death. If the actual expressed wishes of individuals were respected, independently of the wishes of relatives or others, the supply of organs would be significantly increased. As it is, the wishes of individuals are often not followed unless the next of kin concur, even if the dead donor had made an unconditional donation unrestricted by the wishes of relatives. Taking the actual free choices of individuals seriously would carry out the original intent of the Uniform Act for the Donation of Organs.

Respect for persons and their properties, including their bodies, provides an argument against proposals such as Arthur Caplan's to presume willingness to donate unless individuals have taken steps to indicate their unwillingness to participate.[48] Such a presumption might carry moral force in the case of abandoned organs, bodies unclaimed by relatives or friends. However, where friends and relatives do exist to claim a body, the presumption must be that they are the customary and intended inheritors of authority over the body and should be consulted. This does not mean that organs will not be available for transplantation. It means that such programs will need to depend on the actual free choices of actual free donors. Such dependence is inevitable for individuals and societies who take mutual respect seriously.

Conclusions: creating rights to health care and making obligations to care concrete

Our reflections leave us with familiar themes. We must distinguish between positive and negative rights to health care. There are negative rights to health care as rights to be unobstructed in free associations with others in the marketplace. One should be able without hindrance to trade one's private resources for the services of free men and women. Positive rights to health care, rights to the delivery of health care, arise only insofar as they are created by particular communities or nations. There is no basic human right to health care or a fundamental human obligation to provide heath care, though there may be very important reasons to create such a right or to see the obligation of being beneficent as including such a duty. There is nothing immoral, for example, about particular religious communities or the BaMbuti, the noble pygmies described by Colin Turnbull, not providing modern health care. On the other hand, ours, like most societies, has quite different commitments and concerns, such that the support of certain general programs of health care for all is seen as integral to the good life and to beneficent action.

The character of rights to health care delivery will depend on the moral vision of a particular community or the result of the negotiations among moral communities as occurs when a nation fashions its health care system. The meaning of health care rights can be construed as utilitarian, Rawlsian, or in terms of some other goals-based account of beneficence, depending on whether one appeals to the vision of a particular community as the foundation for those rights or to a particular process of negotiation. For example, if a society decides that the only rational and fair way to distribute commonly owned goods is to seek a pattern that maximizes the greatest balance of benefits over harms for the greatest number, the system will be clearly utilitarian in function and, depending on the history of its initiation, in intent as well. The same will obtain in a Rawlsian mode if a society decides that a fair distribution of commonly owned goods must be in a fashion that will advantage the least-well-off class (within constraints of assuring equality of opportunity and equal liberty).

Outside of a particular cohesive community, it may be difficult to determine an unambiguous rationale for a system of positive rights and obligations regarding health care: there may be both Rawlsian and utilitarian as well as other goal-oriented moral leitmotifs in the foundations of the system. This is as one would expect, insofar as a system of health care represents a compromise among various competing views of the good life and therefore of the way one ought to be beneficent. A particular health care system, as a *fair* compromise, will be *just*, in the sense of being the result of a *fair* procedure, one that respects the freedom of the participants in the compromise. However, it may still be regarded as inadequate from the point of view of particular understandings of beneficence. In that sense, from that viewpoint, it may be seen as morally incomplete, indeed wrong. A health care system for a peaceable, pluralist, secular society will have this character because the system will be offering health care across communities of moral commitment and therefore in ways that individual communities may regard as morally flawed but still integral to a fair compromise. In a peaceable, secular, pluralist society moral reflection with regard to rights and duties of health care delivery will thus lead to the familiar tension between respecting the freedom and achieving the good of others, between fair moral decisions and correct moral choices.

THE FOUNDATIONS OF BIOETHICS

Because of this complexity, it will at times be easier to describe the pattern sought through the compromise than the justification for the pattern, as in the case of an egalitarian system where different supporters may bring different justifications forward for the same system of health care. One will need to attend to both the justifications and the pattern, as well as to the history of the compromises, in order to give a meaning to the language of rights to health care (and obligations to provide health care) within any particular health care system. By attending to the justifications one can give an account of the moral grounding of the pattern of distributions in terms of visions of beneficent action. By attending to the pattern achieved one can give an account of the moral consequences of the pattern of distribution by determining how it bears upon those affected. By attending to the history one can determine whether the rights created through a compromise were fairly created, that is, with the free consent of those involved. There is no one unambiguous meaning of rights to the delivery of health care.

Rights and obligations regarding the provision of health care are then to be understood within the embrace of particular moral visions as well as within the history of particular sets of negotiations and compromises through which a people establishes a system of health care. The first is the level of the concrete moral life. It is because of their various visions of beneficence that individuals and their communities move to fashion systems of health care delivery. It is in this important sense that obligations to provide health care are prior to rights to the provision of health care. Rights are fashioned in terms of the content given to the duty to be beneficent to those in need. It is in terms of such visions of proper beneficent action that communities join together as nations to fashion large-scale webs of entitlements to health care and thus give content to beneficence through a system of rights to health care delivery. As always, however, particular communities may not wish fully to participate or may wish in various ways to have special health care systems with special rights and entitlements of their own (e.g., one might imagine Roman Catholics arguing that the provision of contraceptive, abortion, and sterilization procedures should not be provided through a national health insurance; on the other hand, one can easily imagine other communities wishing to provide such services through their communal insurance plans).

A web of concrete expectations is thus woven through the endorsement and negotiation of the men and women who constitute moral communities and who span moral communities through undertakings such as large-scale nations. In their weaving of patterns of commitment, they include certain goals and exclude others. Particular systems of health care are particular in choosing certain goals but not others, in ranking some goals higher and others lower. That patients in one system will receive care that they would not in another, that patients who would be saved in one system die for lack of care in another, is not necessarily a testimony to moral malfeasance. It may as well be the result of the different choices and visions of different free men and women. As we have seen, there are limits to our capacity as humans to discover correctly what we ought to do together. We humans must instead settle for deciding fairly what we will do together, when we cannot together discover what we ought to do. Even gods and goddesses must choose to create one world rather than another. So, too, must we.

Notes

1. Plato, *Republic* III, 407–8.
2. Plato, *Republic* III, 406a–b.
3. H. Tristram Engelhardt, Jr., "Shattuck Lecture—Allocating Scarce Medical Resources and the Availability of Organ Transplanatation," *New England Journal of Medicine* 311 (July 5, 1984): 66–77.
4. President's Commission for the Study of Ethical Problems in Medicine and Biomedical and Behavioral Research, *Securing Access to Health Care* (Washington, D.C.: U.S. Government Printing Office, 1983), vol. 1, pp. 43–6.
5. H. Newman, "Exclusion of Heart Transplantation Procedures from Medicare Coverage," *Federal Register* 45 (Aug. 6, 1980): 52296. See also H. Newman, "Medicare Program: Solicitation of Hospitals and Medical Centers to Participate in a Study of Heart Transplants," *Federal Register* 46 (Jan. 22, 1981): 7072–5.
6. President's Commission, *Securing Access to Health Care*, vol. 1, pp. 18–19.
7. I use the term *macroallocation* to identify allocations among general categories of expenditures; I use the term *microallocation* to indicate choices among particular individuals as to whether they will be recipients of resources and in what amount.
8. Nicholas Rescher, "The Allocation of Exotic Medical Lifesaving Therapy," *Ethics* 79 (April 1969): 173–86; and Robert M. Sade, "Medical Care as a Right: A Refutation," *New England Journal of Medicine* 285 (Dec. 2, 1971): 1288–92.
9. Leon Kass, "Regarding the End of Medicine and the Pursuit of Health," *Public Interest* 40 (Summer 1975): 11–24.
10. D. Wessel, "Transplants Increase, and so do Disputes over Who Pays Bills," *Wall Street Journal*, April 12, 1984, pp. 1, 12.
11. Charles Fried, "Rights and Health Care—Beyond Equity and Efficiency," *New England Journal of Medicine* 293 (July 31, 1975): 241–5.
12. For a thoughtful examination of the conflicts among the various goals set for health care in America, see Henry J. Aaron and William B. Schwartz, *The Painful Prescription: Rationing Hospital Care* (Washington, D.C.: Brookings Institution, 1984).
13. John K. Inglehart, "The British National Health Service under the Conservatives," *New England Journal of Medicine* 309 (Nov. 17, 1983): 1264–8.
14. Barry Newman, "Frugal Medical Service Keeps Britons Healthy and Patiently Waiting," *Wall Street Journal*, Feb. 9, 1983, pp. 1, 21.
15. John K. Inglehart, "The British National Health Service under the Conservatives—Part II," *New England Journal of Medicine* 310 (Jan. 5, 1984): 63–7.
16. Rudolf Klein, "The Politics of Ideology vs. the Reality of Politics: The Case of Britain's National Health Service in the 1980s," *Health and Society* 62 (1984): 82–109.

17. John Rawls, *A Theory of Justice* (Cambridge, Mass.: Harvard University Press, 1971), and Robert Nozick, *Anarchy, State, and Utopia* (New York: Basic Books, 1974).

18. See, for example, Norman Daniels, "Health Care Needs and Distributive Justice," *Philosophy and Public Affairs* 10 (1981): 146–79, and "Rights to Health Care and Distributive Justice: Programmatic Worries," *Journal of Medicine and Philosophy* 4 (1979): 174–91. Also Ronald Green, "Health Care Justice in Contract Theory Perspective," in R. Veatch and R. Branson (eds.), *Ethics and Health Policy* (Cambridge, Mass.: Ballinger, 1976), pp. 111–26. For a recent review of these issues, see John C. Moskop, "Rawlsian Justice and a Human Right to Health Care," pp. 329–38, and Lawrence Stern, "Opportunity and Health Care: Criticisms and Suggestions," pp. 339–61, both in *Journal of Medicine and Philosophy* 8 (Nov. 1983). A detailed review of issues in justice in health care is provided by Earl E. Shelp (ed.), *Justice and Health Care* (Dordrecht: Reidel, 1981).

19. Readers will recognize this island as one in the archipelago of philosophers' islands: fictive situations used to control for the usual variables of life. Here this island offers territory previously unowned and uninhabited, and therefore available for *original* possession. Using this example, one can ask how the process of distributing property in a just fashion should occur without addressing such special issues as making restitution for past injustices.

20. Rawls, *Theory of Justice*, p. 137.

21. Ibid., p. 302.

22. See, for example, Nozick's discussion of who should count as the worst-off class—representative depressives, alcoholics, or paraplegics? *Anarchy, State, and Utopia*, pp. 189–91.

23. Nozick, *Anarchy, State, and Utopia*, p. 160.

24. Ibid.

25. Flavius Petrus Sabbatius Justinianus, *The Institutes of Justinian*, trans. Thomas C. Sandars (Westport, Conn,: Greenwood Press, 1922; reprinted 1970), Book I.1, p. 5.

26. Fear of the blind forces of nature has been a theme throughout the history of man. With the development of preventive medicine, modern medical treatment, and health or sickness insurance schemes the fear of disease, pestilence, and plague has been blunted. To appreciate the full force of this fear within our culture one must look to the past when there was less of a sense of control over fate. This traditional fear of fate and the illnesses it brings is well expressed in the opening to the thirteenth-century collection of songs and poems Carl Orff set to music for the cantata *Carmina Burana: Cantiones Profanae* (Mainz: B. Schott's Soehne, 1953) [my translation]:

O Fortuna,	O Fortune
velut Luna	always changing
statu variabilis,	like the moon,
semper crescis	forever you wax
aut decrescis; . . .	and wane; . . .

This general appreciation of a lottery of fate in which one alternately wins and loses included a sense of the natural and social lotteries' bearing on health status. The second strophe begins:

Sors immanis	Lottery monstrous
et inanis,	and blind,
rota tu volubilis,	your turning wheel
status malus,	forever dissolves
vana salus	both misfortune
semper dissolubilis, . . .	and fruitless health, . . .

The third strophe begins:

Sors salutis	O Lottery of health
et virtutis	and of strength
michi nunc contraria, . . .	you are now against me, . . .

The poem captures what we have often forgotten, namely, the terror that seized our ancestors as plagues recurringly passed through cities and when life generally was much less secure. The majority of individuals in modern industrialized societies have little appreciation of these past realities and of the present life of millions in many developing countries who still live in such circumstances.

27. For an overview of the difficulties involved in delivering health care to those in need, see, for example, Isaac Ehrlich (ed.), *National Health Policy: What Role for Government?* (Stanford, Calif.: Hoover Institution Press, 1982); Steven Jonas (ed.), *Health Care Delivery in the United States*, 2d ed. (New York: Springer, 1981); John H. Knowles (ed.), *Doing Better and Feeling Worse: Health in the United States* (New York: Norton, 1977); Charles Lewis, Rashi Fein, and David Mechanic, *A Right to Health: The Problem of Access to Primary Medical Care* (New York: Wiley, 1976).

28. Some of the elements of the development of modern public health care are reviewed by George Rosen, *From Medical Police to Social Medicine* (New York: Science History Publications, 1974). For a case study that shows the developing contributions of state funds to hospital care toward the close of the nineteenth century, see Rosemary Stevens, " 'Sweet Charity': State Aid to Hospitals in Pennsylvania, 1870–1910," *Bulletin of the History of Medicine* 58 (Fall 1984): 287–314; and *Bulletin of the History of Medicine* 58 (Winter 1984): 474–95.

29. Robert Nozick, *Anarchy, State, and Utopia*, p. 160.

30. Robert G. Evans, "Health Care in Canada: Patterns of Funding and Regulation," *Journal of Health Politics, Policy and Law* 8 (Spring 1983): 1–43, at 30.

31. A utilitarian must also take account of the distress caused to individuals by the knowledge that the rich receive better health care than the poor.

32. Peter Singer, "Freedoms and Utilities in the Distribution of Health Care," in Robert M. Veatch and Roy Branson (eds.), *Ethics and Healthy Policy* (Cambridge, Mass.: Ballinger, 1976), pp. 175–93. Robert Evans makes this point in his defense of a comprehensive governmentally controlled health care system for Canada. He argues that since all in Canada are involved in the Canadian program, unlike Medicaid and Medicare in the United States, or even the United Kingdom where there is private insurance in addition to the National Health Service, "a reduction of public support for the Canadian insurance program affects every member of society, and thus generates much more intense political interest and scrutiny. When we are all in the same boat, the boat is maintained more carefully." "Health Care in Canada," p. 29.

33. As chapters 2 and 5 have shown, it will be difficult to discover those true medical needs that should be the object of medicine in the strict sense. Such a discovery of the boundaries of medicine would require the capacity to discover which needs

are more important and which should count as truly medical needs. In such a fashion one might hope to discover serious medical needs that should be the focus of an egalitarian health care system. However, such a hope is vain, not only because of the difficulty of ranking needs, but because of the difficulty of discovering a narrow range of the truly medical. Medicine has traditionally attended to the various worries, concerns, and vexations of individuals from infertility to unsightly complexions. Despite these difficulties, Norman Daniels attempts to argue for a fair equality of opportunity as the foundation for a basic right to health care—that health care necessary for the "maintenance of species-typical functional organizational function." He is, as he acknowledges, indebted to a Boorsian understanding of disease.

My approach abstracts a central *function* of health care, the maintenance of species-typical functional organization and function, and notes its central *effect* on opportunity. Specially, diseases, in different ways and to different degrees, impair the opportunity available to an individual relative to the *normal opportunity range* for his society. It is this effect on quality of life that makes health care more "special" than many other things which enhance life quality. I claim that *if* justice requires protecting fair equality of opportunity, then health-care institutions should be governed by an appropriately extended principle of fair equality of opportunity. Thus my analysis focuses on that general benefit of health care which is most relevant from the point of view of distributive justice.

Norman Daniels, "Fair Equality of Opportunity and Decent Minimums," *Philosophy and Public Affairs* 14 (Winter 1985): 106–10. As this volume has argued, justice does not require fair equality of opportunity. In addition, the appeal to species-typical functions will not perform the service that both Daniels and Boorse hope.

34. For a general overview of health care in the Soviet Union, see *Medical Care in the USSR: Report of the U.S. Delegation on Health Care Services and Planning* (Washington, D.C.: DHEW Publication no. [NIH] 72–60). For a general overview of the rising difficulties with that system see Constance Holden, "Health Care in the Soviet Union," *Science* 213 (Sept. 4, 1981): 1090–2, and David Satter, "Soviet Death Rates Rising, Report Says; Trend is Unique in the Developed World," *Wall Street Journal*, Oct. 18, 1982, p. 38. A more detailed analysis of some of the problems of the Soviet system can be found in Christopher Davis and Murray Feshbach, *Rising Infant Mortality in the U.S.S.R. in the 1970's* (Washington, D.C.: U.S. Department of Commerce, 1980). See also Murray Feshbach, "Between the Lines of the 1979 Soviet Census," *Problems of Communism* 31 (Jan. 1982): 27–37. Socialist health care systems in smaller, more homogeneous countries appear to function better than that of the Soviet Union. See Robert A. Greenberg, "Maternal and Child Health Services Policy in the German Democratic Republic," *Journal of Public Health Policy* (March 1984): 118–30.

35. From 5 to 15 percent of Polish health care is provided on a fee-for-service basis. Robert M. Veatch, "The Ethics of Critical Care in Cross-Cultural Perspective," in J. C. Moskop and L. Kopelman (eds.), *Ethics and Critical Care Medicine* (Dordrecht: Reidel, 1985), p. 204.

36. Pope Innocent III asked, "Who does not know that conjugal intercourse is never committed without itching of the flesh . . . whence the conceived seeds are befouled and corrupted." *Seven Penitential Psalms* 4 (*Patrologia latina* (Paris: J. P. Migne, 1844–1865) 217: 1058–9); cited in John T. Noonan, Jr., *Contraception* (Cambridge, Mass.: Harvard University Press, 1966), p. 150. Bernardin of Siena

joined in this position, adding that one committed a serious sin if one had intercourse "too frequently, with inordinate affection or with dissipation of one's strength." *Seraphic Sermons* 19.3; cited in Noonan, *Contraception*, p. 250.

37. There are many examples of the libidinous undertakings of the high Middle Ages, which coincided with the official Christian disapprobation of sexual pleasure, even in marriage. See, for example, songs from Orff's *Carmina Burana*, and "The Miller's Tale" by Chaucer. An engaging mockery of exceptionless purity is provided by Henry Fielding's parody of Samuel Richardson's *Pamela* (1740), *Joseph Andrews* (1742), in which Lady Booby asserts that she will not allow any fornicators or adulterers in her house and is met with the rejoinder that she will be reduced to employing hermaphrodites as footmen.

38. Nietzsche remarked in section 168 of *Beyond Good and Evil*, "Das Christentum gab dem Eros Gift zu trinken—er starb zwar nicht daran, aber entartete, zum Laster" (Christianity gave Eros poison to drink—he surely didn't die of it, but he degenerated, into a vice).

39. President's Commission, *Securing Access to Health Care*, vol. 1, p. 37.

40. Ibid.

41. The reader will undoubtedly conclude, and properly so, that I have in mind here an all-payers system similar to that instituted by New Jersey, which would attempt prospectively to determine reimbursements for health care in order to contain health care costs, as for instance through a set of related groups of diagnoses (DRGs). Though all health care in the U.S. is yet to be covered through such systems, insofar as any health care by unwilling private payers is involved, it would involve a restriction of the liberty of such payers to provide better care for themselves or their insured than would be provided to the insured of groups using such a prospective reimbursement system. One might wish to pay more than the rate provided through a prospective reimbursement system in order to allow for diagnostic and therapeutic procedures that, though they may be only marginally useful, may still offer some modest advantage. In addition, those paying more may simply receive prompter and more courteous care, an advantage not to be despised in a hospital. This may be seen as a general critique of the moral probity of price controls, the basis for which is found in chapter 4's treatment of private property and state authority.

My arguments here do not bear directly against the use of prospective reimbursement for such programs as Medicare, insofar as one interpreted Medicare as a voluntary system that does not exclude alternative systems. For an introduction to the prospective payment rule (DRGs) now in place for Medicare, see U.S. Department of Health and Human Services, Health Care Financing Administration, "Medicare Program; Prospective Payment for Medicare Inpatient Hospital Services. Interim Final Rule," *Federal Register* 48 (Sept. 1, 1983): 39752–890, and "Medical Program; Prospective Payment for Medicare Inpatient Hospital Services. Final Rule," *Federal Register* 49 (Jan. 3, 1984): 234–34. See also American Medical Association, Group on Health Service Policy, *DRGs and the Prospective Payment System: A Guide for Physicians* (Chicago: American Medical Association, 1983). For an introduction to the experience in New Jersey where the use of prospective reimbursement approaches being an all-payers system, see Andrew B. Dunham and James A. Morone, *DRG Evaluation Vol. 4-A: The Politics of Innovation—The Evolution of DRG Rate Regulation in New Jersey* (Princeton: Health Research and Educational Trust of New Jersey, 1983).

A case study of the ethical issues raised by such forms of reimbursement is provided by Jeffrey Wasserman, J. Joel May, and Daniel H. Schwartz, "The Doctor, the Patient, and the DRG," *Hastings Center Report* 13 (Oct. 1983): 23–4.

42. Robert G. Evans, "Health Care in Canada." This article provides an overview of the Canadian health care system and notes that in British Columbia and Quebec it is nearly infeasible for a physician to bill beyond the amount covered by the government health insurance. For a response to Evans's article, see Walter McClure, "Letter to the Editor," *Journal of Health Politics, Policy and Law* 8 (Winter 1983): 822–3.

43. J.-Matthias Graf Schulenburg, "Report from Germany: Current Conditions and Controversies in the Health Care System," *Journal of Health Politics, Policy and Law* 8 (Summer 1983): 320–65.

44. Robert Nozick, *Anarchy, State, and Utopia*, pp. 206–7.

45. Gerald Kelly, *Medico-Moral Problems* (St. Louis: Catholic Hospital Association, 1958), pp. 245–52.

46. Immanuel Kant, *Kants Werke*, Akademie Textausgabe (Berlin: Walter de Gruyter, 1968), vol. 6, p. 423.

47. The conclusions regarding the right of individuals to sell their organs depend on the general arguments devel░░░ in chapter 3, which support the right of individuals to do with th░░░ives and their consenting associates as they please. No one can demonstra░ justified authority to use consenting force against such peaceable undertakings. It should be clear that this argument supports the right to sell oneself into forms of indentured servitude such as through joining armed forces or to sell one's services as a prostitute. One is protected through the morality of mutual respect in making such choices, whether or not one considers selling one's organs, joining the military, or working as a prostitute to be ennobling endeavors.

48. Arthur Caplan, "Organ Transplants: The Costs of Success," *Hastings Center Report* 13 (1983): 23–32.

9

Reshaping Human Nature and the Pursuit of Virtue

We are alone and left to our own devices. The history of modern thought is marked by losses of ultimate orientation and purpose, which have forced us to turn to ourselves for meaning. The fact that we can no longer find a special place for ourselves in the universe sets the context for modern bioethics. We saw this in the introductory chapter. Secular bioethics is framed this side of a major moral and intellectual crisis. As Nietzsche recognized, modern science is a source of nihilism, and the Copernican revolution a metaphor for our loss of moral direction.[1] Nicolaus Copernicus, an employee of the Cathedral of Frauenburg in East Prussia, with his *De revolutionibus orbium coelestium* (1543) contributed to a vision that deprived us of our cosmic uniqueness and ushered in a secular view of reality. Even where his influence was not direct, the change in astronomical perspective became a metaphor for a radical alteration in the understanding of our condition. We are no longer the center of things. We now see ourselves as living on an obscure planet, orbiting a star, which is a member of one of innumerable galaxies. There is no longer anything special about where we are. There is also nothing special about what we are as humans. With the publication on October 24, 1859, of Charles Darwin and A. R. Wallace's *On the Origin of Species by Natural Selection, or the Preservation of Favoured Races in the Struggle for Life,* we moved toward seeing our nature itself as a result of chance. Rather than a descent of human nature from the gods, we have been offered a *Descent of Man, and Selection in Relation to Sex* (1871). Sexual selection, not divine providence, was seen as having fashioned the character of human nature.

375

We end this book where we began, with the difficulty of finding meaning in a world deprived of ultimate orientation. We began with the implications this has for moral issues in health care. We explored the extent to which moral standards could be erected when ultimate moral standards could not be discovered. Moreover, chapter 5 suggested that these difficulties do not bear solely on moral values, but on values in general, and in particular on the values associated with judgments of disease and health. We are concerned not only with what men and women ought to do, but with how or what they ought to be, since medicine and the biomedical sciences are becoming ever more a means for refashioning and reshaping human nature. Such judgments involve aesthetic values that indicate what is good human form and structure. Such judgments have also involved views about what is natural or unnatural, which in turn have traditionally been seen as having moral implications, insofar as unnatural acts have been taken to be immoral acts.

The appeal to human nature as a guide for moral action, though traditional, is taken from us as we acknowledge that we are shaped not by design but by the blind forces of mutation and natural selection. As chapter 5 has shown, this leads us to specifying diseases, in part at least, in terms of the values of particular individuals and cultures. As the values that structure the language of disease and health are as much created as discovered, we are again thrown back upon ourselves. The result is not only disorientation in the sense of a loss of transcendent moorings, but also a reorientation in terms of what one might call a transcendental mooring: persons as the center and source of meaning. Even if we do not have a special place in nature, and even if our very nature as humans is the arbitrary outcome of blind causal forces, we can understand the fact.

There is a distance between us as persons and us as humans. The distance is the gulf between a reflective and manipulative being and the object of its reflection and manipulation. From our perspectives as persons with particular views and hopes, we can decide whether this is the best of places in the cosmos. If we find it to be unsatisfactory, we can even plot ways of changing our location. We can decide whether this is the best of natures and seek ways to refashion it if we find it wanting. We as persons can make our bodies objects. We can discern ways in which we could have been better fashioned.

So far, our interventions have been humble ones. Through both passive and active immunization we have provided immunity to diseases without the morbidity of those diseases. We have developed prosthetic valves and joints. We have learned how to control the normal human mechanisms for rejecting foreign tissues so as to transplant organs. In developing contraceptives, we have come to understand hormonal mechanisms so that we can break the natural bond between recreational sex and reproduction. The very character of modern lifestyles in which women are fully engaged in the workplace and fully sexually active, while planning when they will have children, and how many, depends on the reliability of modern contraceptive technology. In this the traditional view of the Roman Catholic church is correct: artificial contraception is unnatural. It is a means for directing nature, if one means by nature the products of past evolutionary history. In the future our ability to constrain and manipulate human nature to follow the goals set by persons will increase. As we develop the capacities to engage in genetic engineering not only of somatic cells but of the human germ line, we will be able to shape and fashion our human nature in the image and likeness of goals chosen by persons. In the end, this may mean so radically changing our human nature that our descendants may be seen by subsequent taxonomists as a new species. If there is nothing sacred about human nature (and no merely secular argument could show it to be sacred), there is no reason why, with proper reasons and with proper caution, it should not be radically changed. In this critical assessment of our nature, we gain a clearer understanding of the remark of Protagoras, "Man is the measure of all things, of existing things that they exist, and of non-existing things that they exist not."[2] It is persons who are the measure of all things, because there is no one to measure but persons.

In praise of Dr. Feelgood and the pursuit of health

In his essay "Regarding the End of Medicine and the Pursuit of Health," Leon Kass shoulders a very important task.[3] He attempts to set limits to what is appropriately medical. If medicine is primarily focused on the cure of somatic diseases, and if norms for somatic health can be discovered, the compass of medicine will not depend on individual desires or cultural vagaries. One will be able to know truly what medicine ought to be doing. Through arguments such as these, Kass wants to exclude from medicine proper all interventions not aimed at remedying individual somatic difficulties. He wishes to exclude everything from cosmetic repairs of sagging anatomies to artificial insemination and in vitro fertilization.[4] As chapter 5 has shown, this attempt cannot succeed. Medicine is instead, as it has always been, focused on the myriad complaints patients bring regarding disabilities, pains, deformities, and the threat of premature death. Medicine, as a result, is directed to a range of diseases, disorders, and difficulties, from acne, sagging buttocks, neuroses, and clogged coronary arteries to cancer of the lung, unwanted pregnancies, sterility, and migraine headaches. One is unable to discover proper borders to the medical treatment of diseases, disorders, and difficulties in terms of a canonical notion of somatic form or structure. The limits must be found in moral arguments or in the ways in which we mark medicine from law and other endeavors on the basis of differences in concerns with pathoanatomical and pathopsychological causal explanations versus accounts of guilt, negligence, and liability. We find medicine marked off from other major social endeavors, insofar as it is, (1) because of special nonmoral values concerning human ability, freedom from pain, proper form, and scope of life, (2) because of the character of medical explanations, and (3) because of the character of the sick role versus the roles of criminal, sinner, and so on.[5]

A concern with wholeness, with health as other than the mere absence of disease, gives no deliverance from the ambiguity that results from a range of interests shaped by a range of values. Here Christopher Boorse is correct. Positive concepts of health turn on specific goals, or clusters of goals, which are often mutually exclusive.[6] Boorse has in mind the incompatible types of functional excellence that make one physique better for Olympic marathon racing and another for Olympic weightlifting. Sports medicine, insofar as it is directed not simply to repairing athletic injuries but also to achieving particular athletic capacities, becomes a pursuit of special understandings of health—of particular constellations of physical and psychological capacities, of particular senses of wholeness.

One might note here that there is nothing in principle wrong with attempting to determine how, by the use of drugs and hormones, one might best achieve certain goals in sports. It is rather that the use of such adjuvants would change the character of a sport that is supposed to be pursued without the medical enhancement of physical capacities, in addition to exposing the users to risks of side effects. But one might wish to employ medical intervention in order to be able to climb a very difficult slope of a very dangerous mountain. Such a successful climb might still be approvingly noted in the record books. The point is that one cannot discover the answer to such questions. One has to decide how one wishes to pursue particular excellences and goals and how one should balance possible risks and benefits.

A similar set of concerns underlies the arguments regarding different sexual orientations. If neither homosexuality nor heterosexuality is a disease, each will have its own virtues and vices. Each will realize a different human possibility, whose achievement medicine may at times aid through counseling and treatment. The use of transsexual surgery to achieve a particular sexual self-image, or artificial insemination for lesbians to achieve the goal of parenting in nontraditional settings, are examples of individuals employing medicine in the pursuit of different views of human excellence. One might imagine individuals pursuing through genetic engineering the goal of increasing sexual capacities and enjoyment in general, or for those in advanced years in particular. If octogenarians successfully achieved such a goal of enhanced sexual capacity and interest, one would substantially change one's views of the elderly and of the deportment one expects of great-grandparents.

Because medicine can not only control pains and anxieties, but at least in principle become the instrument for enhancing capacities and augmenting pleasures, the future of medicine is likely to be tied even more than in the past to the enterprise of making individuals perform well and feel good. Leon Kass condemns Dr. Feelgood, who "devotes his entire practice to administering amphetamine injections to people seeking elevations of mood."[7] However, it is difficult to mount a serious objection *in principle* to such activities. If such mood-elevating and controlling drugs had no serious side effects, but rather aided individuals in better realizing their professional goals, in being good spouses and lovers, and in acting with greater kindness and attention to others, what would be the grounds for objecting, other than a special view of the good life that held that happiness hard won through self-discipline was to be preferred to tranquillity acquired in part by medical intervention? This does not mean that one cannot criticize Dr. Feelgood. Particular current interventions by Dr. Feelgood can be seen as seriously wrongheaded in the same way that certain diseases can be recognized as diseases across cultures, or the past attempts of physicians to cure inflammatory diseases through bleeding can now be seen as harmful. Some side effects (e.g., forms of addiction) may undercut so many of the goals of persons that most individuals across cultures will be able to see them as harmful. In addition, the tranquillity or good feeling achieved may be superficial or stultifying. Many attempts to make life better, not just to cure disease, can be shown to cause more harm than good. When one is attempting to treat a disease rather than simply to augment human capacities, there is a background harm to overcome that may outbalance the iatrogenic harms associated with the treatment. The goal of simply making people feel better cannot trade on the substantial certain negative costs of failing to treat, as can interventions to cure arthritis or cancer. In short, when one tries to cure a serious disease with an established treatment, there is a greater chance of having a positive balance of benefits over harms. Such considerations do not provide an argument in principle against the goals of Dr. Feelgood. One finds instead objections to the dangers of particular modes of intervention and their possible side effects and failures. What one will need is prudence and care and the old maxim *festina lente* (make haste slowly).

The pursuit of wholeness, as the pursuit of healths in the plural,[8] underscores a recurring difficulty for finite men and women. Though they may have some of the aspirations and vision of the gods, their limited resources force them to choose among alternative goods. They do not have the capacity of an infinite being to realize all at one time.[9] It is not simply the limit on their purses, a limitation that plays such a major role in choices among modes of allocating resources for health care. It is a limit set by the fact that they must choose between a body or a mind developed primarily to achieve one set of goods rather than another. Given the limited capacities of both human bodies and minds, we need to choose which excellences to achieve. All finite beings must make such choices and live with such constraints. To be finite means one can do only some things, but not all things, at any particular time. Such constraints make us what we are. Different biological abilities give us different destinies. This is underscored by the fact that we are a dimorphic species. There are obvious ways in which there are differences between the wholeness or health of a woman and the wholeness or health of a man. A significant element of a woman's body is organized around the gestation of a fetus and the birth of a child. To achieve such goals requires physical capacities not required of men. But the differences are even more complex. Consider the different excellences of mental and physical health required of the sedentary philosopher, the hunter-gatherer, the healthy homosexual, the healthy heterosexual, and the healthy Trappist monk.

None of this need remain as we find it. Increasingly, we will not need so much to accept our destinies as to choose them, though we will always need to have a particular destiny. As in Aldous Huxley's *Brave New World*, we could set aside the primary sexual differences between men and women that depend on the gestation and the birth of children through the use of in vitro fertilization, in vitro gestation, and genetic engineering. One might even refashion human secondary sexual characteristics to achieve a unisex Brave New World, or one populated by the numerous sexes of Kurt Vonnegut's *Slaughterhouse-Five*.[10] Such possibilities for genetic engineering raise prudential issues, as does the case of Dr. Feelgood. One should be sure that the means for engineering will produce the desired goals without serious, undesired side effects. One must envisage with care the goals that one will seek and the values and circumstances they presuppose. Since human capacities are integrated as a whole, one will need to assess carefully the likely social and other changes that will result from the redesign of human nature. One will also need to make sure that particular individuals treated or produced through genetic engineering are not injured. However, restrictions with respect to this last point need not be any more severe than those currently required for experimental treatments or for parents reproducing despite the risk of having defective newborns.[11] One is concerned with the character of the harm, not the particulars of its production.

For those who fear that genetic reengineering may have unknown risks, one might protest that the failure to reengineer may possess similar unknown risks. There is evidence, for example, that human predispositions to belligerence have a genetic basis. About one-fourth of males in a state of nature (i.e., absent the controls of an organized state) die in fighting.[12] At one point this inclination to kill competing males may have contributed to the inclusive fitness of such belligerent individuals.[13] However, at present it may offer one of the most substantial risks for the total annihilation of mankind. In the end, the continued survival of humans may require engineering around such inclinations and such particular expressions of competitiveness.

Some have expressed the concern that genetic engineering might lead to uniformity among humans, to all being cloned in the same image and likeness. Such is unlikely if individuals and groups are allowed to choose freely in fashioning themselves. The polytheistic metaphor introduced in the second chapter should remind us that, absent coercive force, individuals may choose substantively different views of the good life. Given different views of the good life, different refashionings of human nature will appear more or less attractive. None of this is likely to happen in the short run. The first introductions of genetic engineering will most likely be modest attempts to alter somatic cells in order to aid suffering individuals. However, if one looks over the long run, in any serious sense of the long run, major changes will be unavoidable if we remain a free and technologically advancing species. Humans have been here for only a million years or so. If we are so fortunate as to have descendants who survive over millions of years to come (a short period in geological time), it is very likely that they will decide to refashion themselves so as better to live in the transformed environments of this earth and perhaps in the environments of other planets. What would hold them back from such genetic interventions, which over the long run would become both available and safe? In fact, there is no reason to presume that only one species would come from ours. There might be as many species as there were reasons for substantially refashioning human nature for this or new environments.

Here science fiction can be heuristic. In his 1931 novel, *Last and First Men*, Olaf Stapledon portrays the history of humans over a period of some two billion years from the present.[14] He pictures our descendants radically changing themselves during this period, so that they would no longer be members of our species, or perhaps even of our genus. However, they would be our descendants, no matter how nonhuman they would become. If one can envisage a conversation with extraterrestrials who have no common bond in history and biology, but a common bond in the capacity to analyze and reason, one will be able to imagine an even greater kinship with those descendant individuals, albeit they are no longer human. This science-fictional vision can give moral instruction on at least three points. First, it should remind us that there is nothing sacrosanct about human nature. Rather, second, we persons are free to refashion it, as long as we do so prudently, with consenting collaborators. Finally, the radical refashioning of human nature is likely to change the content of the virtues that mark human life. Even before we are able to engage in dramatic alterations in human nature, we will need to apply these points to the ways in which we manipulate our nature.

Virtues and vices

What are the virtues that should guide individuals engaged in the manipulation and the shaping of their very nature? What marks of character ought such individuals to have? Morally, what kinds of beings should they be? To answer these questions, we must first turn to the problem of virtue within a secular pluralist morality. Having examined the principles of autonomy and beneficence, what can we say about the character of a good physician or a good patient? Can these abstract analyses give us a sense of what virtues each should bear? What can one say of virtues within the compass of the secular philosophical morality this volume has offered? Aristotle held that virtue or excellence (*arete*) had to do with the mean, and that it was in fact a sort of mean.[15] But what is the context within which we are to understand such a mean? The Schoolmen held that virtue was what makes a person good and renders his actions good ("quae bonum facit habentem, et opus eius bonum reddit"). But if a concrete view of the good is attainable only within a particular understanding of the good life, what can be said generally about virtue? We will need to find the answer in a special interpretation of Kant's view that virtue is a strength of the moral will.[16]

The virtuous patient or health care giver in a secular pluralist society is one who has a developed habit of the will to respect the freedom of others and to attempt to achieve their good. The cardinal virtues will then be tolerance, liberality, and prudence. Tolerance is the cardinal virtue in the morality of mutual respect. Given the clash of conflicting views of the good life, each must have a developed disposition to let the other develop his or her own view of the good life, insofar as it is marked by similar tolerance. Intolerance becomes the cardinal vice. The morality of welfare and of social sympathies will for its part require liberality, the developed moral disposition of the will to give generously to the support of the good of others, even when that good seems strange and alien. Prudence will also be required so that one through sound judgment achieves a positive balance of benefits over harms. The vices that centrally undermine this morality are meanness and imprudence.

Each of these virtues will require others. The defense of the peaceable community may at times require gentleness, bravery, modesty, temperance, and endurance. The realization of the morality of welfare and of social sympathies will require temperance and friendliness. These, as well as other virtues, will be required to realize and to sustain the concrete fabric of a moral life. Within actual concrete moral communities, the virtues will have their full substance and fabric, as will the vices.[17] However, the singular task for a peaceable, secular morality spanning a pluralist society must be borne by those special marks of character and virtue that must be encouraged within the abstract context of secular pluralist morality. We will need to sustain tolerance and beneficence where there is no concrete bond to a particular vision of the good life. Here one must recall again Hegel's notion of bureaucrats as the universal class.[18] The good bureaucrat (including the individuals overseeing endeavors in human genetic engineering) in a secular pluralist society must at a minimum sustain tolerance and evenhandedness in caring for all who come for protection and welfare. All should receive their due, irrespective of their vision of the good life, their religious commitment, or their special ideological commitments. To be a good bureaucrat in that sense requires special dedication to that tier of the moral life that is articulated in secular pluralist morality and that has as its core the morality of mutual respect.

All citizens and all health care providers who do not closet themselves in special exclaves, as do the Amish, will need at times to shoulder these virtues of the good bureaucrat. Our tradition has given us little schooling in such austere virtues. Yet it is exactly such virtues that are required to sustain the mean between a dictatorial imposition of a particular view of the good life and a nihilist apathy that abandons all vision of the good. We must encourage a virtue that will sustain men and women in a perpetual commitment to tolerating the peaceful realization of many incompatible understandings of the good life and of good health care. The men and women who are exemplars in this moral context are those who are dedicated to avoiding all unconsented-to force against others and to achieving the abstract goal of prudently realizing the good of others. This dedication will not necessarily commit them to a further continuance of life in general or the life of persons in particular. They must even envisage the possibility that all might decide, for whatever reasons, to end their existence without progeny, and that even such a choice must be tolerated as well. To maintain such a range of toleration and to sustain liberality in such an abstract moral context will require constant moral resolve.

One may indeed decide that, though humans are capable of understanding the difference between right and wrong and of pursuing the right for brief periods of time, they do not have the capacity for an enduring commitment to the good. If such is the case, it will not be an argument against the moral point of view, but only for the judgment that human history is intrinsically bound to evil. There may, however, be remedies. The Judeo-Christian tradition has regarded human history as a conflict between the grace of God and the venality, cupidity, and inconstancy of human beings. A major element of this tradition saw the remedy not in human will itself, but in the grace of God. Somewhat tendentiously, one may interpret Christian dogma regarding baptism and grace as a form of supernatural genetic engineering. Grace was sought to make whole human nature, which was imperfect. We may now look forward to a time when we will be able in fact to engineer such grace, to fashion such constancy. Is there a moral bar to biotechnological grace? Some would undoubtedly argue that such pharmacologically achieved virtues or marks of character are not worthy of the same praise as those that have been achieved through years of struggle and moral self-mastery. Others might raise the concern that traditional practices of self-discipline and self-control might be challenged and weakened. Still others might argue that such easy pharmacological access to virtue would change the very fabric of society.

Such objections could not establish that such a goal would be intrinsically wrong, only that it might not be conducive to the realization of certain goods tied to moral struggle and travail. One could easily grant that pharmacologically produced marks of character and virtue do not merit praise as does that gained through personal struggle. But again, one would need to stress that such bioengineering of virtue would not in fact depart as radically from Western tradition as one might think, if one recalls the Christian concern with grace. Much of St. Paul's writings can be interpreted as arguing that individuals gain salvation not through their own merit, but by the grace of God. "There is a remnant according to the election of grace. And if by grace, then *is it* no more of works . . ." (Romans 11:5–6). This view took a major place in the reflections of the Christian church. It was central to Augustine's notion of the predestination of the saints[19] and was affirmed in the early church's condemnation of the Pelagians, who held that one could accept the grace of God without the prior divine prevenient grace to accept God's grace.[20] One might even note that Christian doctrine gives a metaphor for understanding the action that our successors might undertake for their children in engineering them for virtue. Aside from prudent concerns regarding foreseeable and unforeseeable deleterious side effects so as not to undermine but rather enhance self-conscious freedom, they would be acting as some Christian parents do in baptizing their children, so that the grace of God will inform and strengthen their character.

Whether the traditional practices of self-discipline would be challenged and eroded by engineering virtue would depend on the commitments of those individuals who wish to tough it out the old way. If the traditional ways of achieving and maintaining could not be sustained on their own, some cannot constrain others to abandon their pursuit of a new way of life for the old, just because those committed to the old cannot make it on their own. The price of freedom is that others may freely decide not to cooperate. This last point meets the last objection as well. As free men and women come to use new technologies, societies will change. Not all societies need change: one has always available the examples of the Amish and the Hasidim. Respect of the freedom of others will lead us, even in the future, to multiple visions of the good life and to a certain amount of uneliminable chaos. Beneficence will lead us to aiding others, where possible and permitted, to achieve their view of the good life. The genetic engineering of ourselves, as all serious undertakings, should be guided by tolerance, liberality, and prudence.

The vision of a secular pluralist morality

We return where we began, to a vision of the multiple interpretations of the good. Insofar as this volume succeeds, it establishes the possibility of a multiplicity of concrete moral views. One may recall that chapter 2 developed the metaphor of a polytheistic as opposed to a monotheistic world view so as to underscore the multiple ways in which men and women achieve the good and give concrete content to the moral life. There are innumerable ways in which men and women will wish to come to terms with their diseases, disorders, and disabilities, and to pursue a better control over their bodies so as to avoid vexations and to achieve particular visions of the wholesome life. Insofar as these are pursued within the morality of mutual respect, they will need to be tolerated, even if they are not endorsed and supported. This heterogeneous range of moral visions will need as its peaceable moral cement a commitment to a secular pluralist ethic.

This volume has offered a vision of that ethic. In doing so, it has supported propositions that many readers will find provocative, if not offensive. It has been argued that the views this volume offers are intellectually unavoidable even for the most committed Christian, Jew, Hindu, Buddhist, or Communist who does not wish to use force to resolve moral disputes. It has been an argument regarding the unavoidable moral limits of authority and the consequent moral requirements of toleration. Where rational arguments do not authorize force to dislodge others from their views of the good life, one will be left with an abstract morality of toleration and general commitment to beneficence, which will have many fewer moral prescriptions and proscriptions than the concrete moralities that have developed within the Judeo-Christian tradition.

The argument has not been that moral traditions, such as the Judeo-Christian, ought to be abandoned. Far from it. The propositions of a secular pluralist morality are, I have argued, unavoidable, not in the sense that they must supplant in the concrete moral life that individuals live with consenting others but rather in the sense that there is no rational warrant for the use of force in imposing any one particular view of the good life on others. One is forced to live one's life within two moral tiers. On the one hand, one will be committed to particular moral views about good health care, by virtue of being a member of an actual and concrete moral community. Here one should be a good Baptist, Hindu, Catholic, or Jew. However, as one's community does not include all others, one will need to reach to others within the constraints of a secular pluralist morality. If one's only contact with the secular pluralist morality occurs when one walks to the property line of one's peaceably established moral exclave, one's Communist commune or one's Amish community, one acknowledges secular moral constraints insofar as one does not carry the imposition of one's viewpoint beyond that line and insofar as one expects reciprocal tolerance of one's own way of life.

Secular pluralist morality is thus founded on limits: the limits of reason and of authority. It is unavoidable not because it is so well established but because other views are incapable of generally establishing the right to use force in controlling the lives of unconsenting others. Because of the limitations of our capacity in general rational terms to defend the discovery of a single correct concrete moral order or to establish authority for its imposition, and because of the ever-available intellectual standpoint of the peaceable community, we have a morality that allows many moralities to grow and flourish. The health care of finite men and women presupposes a moral vision of breadth and tolerance.

Notes

1. Nietzsche, in addressing "the nihilistic consequences of contemporary science," notes that "since Copernicus, man rolls from the center into the X." Friedrich Nietzsche, "Aus dem Nachlass der Achtzigerjahre," in *Werke in drei Baenden* (Munich: Carl Hanser, 1960), vol. 3, p. 882.

2. This fragment from Protagoras is preserved by Sextus Empiricus, *Outlines of Pyrrhonism*, trans. R. G. Bury (Cambridge, Mass.: Harvard University Press, 1976), I.216, p. 131. One should note that Protagoras was interpreted by Sextus Empiricus as arguing for a moral relativism. Making persons the center of the moral life is not the same as making a particular person or a particular group of persons the center of the moral life. The second, not the first, constitutes a true moral relativism.

3. Leon Kass, "Regarding the End of Medicine and the Pursuit of Health," *Public Interest* 40 (Summer 1975): 11–24.

4. Leon Kass, "Babies by Means of *In Vitro* Fertilization: Unethical Experiments on the Unborn?" *New England Journal of Medicine* 285 (Nov. 1971): 1174–9.

5. As we saw in section 4 of chapter 5, a problem (e.g., alcoholism) need not be seen as either a medical or a legal problem, but may be seen as a medical, legal, and religious problem.

6. Christopher Boorse, "Health as a Theoretical Concept," *Philosophy of Science* 44 (1977): 542–73.

7. Leon Kass, "Babies by Means of *In Vitro* Fertilization," p. 13.

8. Chester R. Burns, "Diseases Versus Healths: Some Legacies in the Philosophies of Modern Medical Science," in H. T. Engelhardt, Jr., and S. F. Spicker (eds.),

Evaluation and Explanation in the Biomedical Sciences (Dordrecht: Reidel, 1975), pp. 29–47.

9. Process theologians have argued that even God cannot do everything at one time. In deciding to create a world, God must decide among the worlds that could be created. Moreover, such a choice has an impact on the life and growth of God. Chief among the exponents of this view has been Charles Hartshorne, who has indicated ways in which his views bear on issues in bioethics; see Charles Hartshorne, "Scientific and Religious Aspects of Bioethics," in Earl E. Shelp (ed.), *Theology and Bioethics: Exploring Foundations and Frontiers* (Dordrecht: Reidel, 1985), pp. 27–44.

10. The Tralfamadorians, who communicate with Billy Pilgrim in *Slaughterhouse-Five*, have five sexes. They inform Billy that Earthlings come in seven sexes, though five of the seven sexes are sexually active only in the fourth dimension. Kurt Vonnegut, Jr., *Slaughterhouse-Five* (New York: Delacorte Press, 1969), pp. 98–9.

11. H. T. Engelhardt, Jr., "Persons and Humans: Refashioning Ourselves in a Better Image and Likeness," *Zygon* 19 (Sept. 1984): 281–95.

12. F. B. Livingstone, "The Effects of Warfare on the Biology of the Human Species," in M. Fried, M. Harris, and R. Murphy (eds.), *War: The Anthropology of Armed Conflict and Aggression* (Garden City, N.Y.: Natural History Press, 1967), pp. 3–15. For a classic study of a belligerent, primitive group, see Napoleon A. Chagnon, *Yanomamö: The Fierce People*, 2d ed. (New York: Holt, Rinehart and Winston, 1977).

13. Donald Symons, *The Evolution of Human Sexuality* (New York: Oxford University Press, 1979), pp. 144–58.

14. Olaf Stapledon, *Last and First Men* (1931; reprinted New York: Dover, 1968).

15. Aristotle, *Eudemian Ethics* II.3.1220b 35.

16. Immanuel Kant, *The Metaphysical Principles of Virtue: Part II of The Metaphysics of Morals*, Akademie Textausgabe, vol. 6, p. 17. For a comprehensive treatment of the virtues in medicine, see Earl E. Shelp (ed.), *Virtue and Medicine* (Dordrecht: Reidel, 1985).

18. G. W. F. Hegel, *The Philosophy of Right*, sec. 303.

19. Augustine of Hippo, *De corruptione et gratia*, pp. 34–8.

20. See, for example, the Council of Arles (A.D. 473), which condemned the Pelagian view that obedient human labor is not joined with the grace of God. ". . . qui dicit humanae oboedientiae laborem divinae gratiae non esse iungendum; . . ." "Concilium Arelatense," in Henricus Denzinger (ed.), *Enchiridion Symbolorum: Definitionum et Declarationum de Rebus Fidei et Morum*, 33rd ed. (Rome: Herder, 1965), p. 117. Similar views were expressed by the Second Council of Orange on July 3, 529. The question is the extent to which being aided by divine grace to do the good should be any more or less acceptable than being aided by bioengineering to do the good.

Index